Research Series on the Chinese Dream and China's Development Path

Project Director
Xie Shouguang, President, Social Sciences Academic Press

Series editors
Li Yang, Vice president, Chinese Academy of Social Sciences, Beijing, China
Li Peilin, Vice president, Chinese Academy of Social Sciences, Beijing, China

Academic Advisors
Cai Fang, Gao Peiyong, Li Lin, Li Qiang, Ma Huaide, Pan Jiahua, Pei Changhong,
Qi Ye, Wang Lei, Wang Ming, Zhang Yuyan, Zheng Yongnian, Zhou Hong

Drawing on a large body of empirical studies done over the last two decades, this Series provides its readers with in-depth analyses of the past and present and forecasts for the future course of China's development. It contains the latest research results made by members of the Chinese Academy of Social Sciences. This series is an invaluable companion to every researcher who is trying to gain a deeper understanding of the development model, path and experience unique to China. Thanks to the adoption of Socialism with Chinese characteristics, and the implementation of comprehensive reform and opening-up, China has made tremendous achievements in areas such as political reform, economic development, and social construction, and is making great strides towards the realization of the Chinese dream of national rejuvenation. In addition to presenting a detailed account of many of these achievements, the authors also discuss what lessons other countries can learn from China's experience.

More information about this series at http://www.springer.com/series/13571

Lan Xue · Guang Zeng

A Comprehensive Evaluation on Emergency Response in China

The Case of Pandemic Influenza (H1N1) 2009

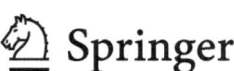

Lan Xue
Center for Crisis Management Research,
    School of Public Policy and Management
Tsinghua University
Beijing
China

Guang Zeng
Chinese Center for Disease Control
    and Prevention
Beijing
China

ISSN 2363-6866   ISSN 2363-6874   (electronic)
Research Series on the Chinese Dream and China's Development Path
ISBN 978-981-13-0643-3   ISBN 978-981-13-0644-0   (eBook)
https://doi.org/10.1007/978-981-13-0644-0

Jointly published with Social Sciences Academic Press, Beijing, China

The printed edition is not for sale in the Mainland of China. Customers from the Mainland of China
please order the print book from Social Sciences Academic Press.

Library of Congress Control Number: 2018941972

Printed on acid-free paper

This Springer imprint is published by the registered company Springer Nature Singapore Pte Ltd.
part of Springer Nature
The registered company address is: 152 Beach Road, #21-01/04 Gateway East, Singapore 189721,
Singapore

Series Preface

Since China's reform and opening began in 1978, the country has come a long way on the path of Socialism with Chinese Characteristics, under the leadership of the Communist Party of China. Over 30 years of reform, efforts and sustained spectacular economic growth have turned China into the world's second largest economy, and brought many profound changes in the Chinese society. These historically significant developments have been garnering increasing attention from scholars, governments, and the general public alike around the world since the 1990s, when the newest wave of China studies began to gather steam. Some of the hottest topics have included the so-called "China miracle", "Chinese phenomenon", "Chinese experience", "Chinese path", and the "Chinese model". Homegrown researchers have soon followed suit. Already hugely productive, this vibrant field is putting out a large number of books each year, with Social Sciences Academic Press alone having published hundreds of titles on a wide range of subjects.

Because most of these books have been written and published in Chinese, readership has been limited outside China—even among many who study China—for whom English is still the lingua franca. This language barrier has been an impediment to efforts by academia, business communities, and policymakers in other countries to form a thorough understanding of contemporary China, of what is distinct about China's past and present may mean not only for her future but also for the future of the world. The need to remove such an impediment is both real and urgent, and the *Research Series on the Chinese Dream and China's Development Path* is my answer to the call.

This series features some of the most notable achievements from the last 20 years by scholars in China in a variety of research topics related to reform and opening. They include both theoretical explorations and empirical studies, and cover economy, society, politics, law, culture, and ecology, the six areas in which reform and opening policies have had the deepest impact and farthest-reaching consequences for the country. Authors for the series have also tried to articulate their visions of the "Chinese Dream" and how the country can realize it in these fields and beyond.

All of the editors and authors of the *Research Series on the Chinese Dream and China's Development Path* are both longtime students of reform and opening and recognized authorities in their respective academic fields. Their credentials and expertise lend credibility to these books, each of which having been subject to a rigorous peer-review process for inclusion in the series. As part of the Reform and Development Program under the State Administration of Press, Publication, Radio, Film, and Television of the People's Republic of China, the series is published by Springer, a Germany-based academic publisher of international repute, and distributed overseas. I am confident that it will help fill a lacuna in studies of China in the era of reform and opening.

Xie Shouguang

Acknowledgements

The 2009 Influenza A (H1N1) pandemic was a test of China's public health system and of its national emergency management. In 2010, commissioned as a third party of independent evaluation by the joint prevention and control mechanism against Influenza A (H1N1) and the Emergency Management Office of the State Council, the task force which the Tsinghua University (School of Public Policy and Management) assembled in collaboration with the China CDC, the Institute of Medical Information of the Chinese Academy of Medical Sciences, the Center for Health Management and Policy of Shandong University, and the Academy of Military Medical Sciences accepted this evaluation project.

We would like to express our heartfelt thanks to the member agencies of the joint prevention and control mechanism against Influenza A (H1N1) and to related departments and agencies of Beijing, Fujian, Guangdong, Henan, and Sichuan among other provinces and cities, for their active cooperation and great support—searching data for us, providing us with a large amount of documents, and participating in our workshops or interviews. Also, we would extend special thanks to the members of the advisory panel who gave us professional guidance and help from the very beginning. Still, we would like to thank Horizon Research Consultancy Group and 12320 Health Hotline for their hard work done for our surveys. Finally, we should also express sincere thanks to all task force members and other researchers who took part in the discussion, research, preparation, and revision of this report.

December 2011

The Task Force of the Comprehensive Expert
Evaluation Report on Influenza
A (H1N1) Prevention and Control
in the Chinese Mainland

Contents

Summary

Comprehensive Expert Evaluation Report on Influenza A (H1N1) Prevention and Control in the Chinese Mainland

Commissioned by the Ministry of Health (MOH)—the former lead agency for the national mechanism of joint prevention and control of Influenza A (H1N1), the School of Public Policy and Management (SPPM) of Tsinghua University organized a multidisciplinary expert evaluation team ("evaluation team") which launched in May 2010 an evaluation of prevention and control regimes in the Chinese mainland. This effort was soon afterward designated as a special research project by the Emergency Management Office of the State Council. It was also the country's first systematic expert evaluation of the whole emergency management process of a major public health emergency.

The evaluation, underscored by the principles of independence, objectivity, rationality, and comprehensiveness, focused on, among other things, emergency management processes, prevention and control strategies, operational features of the joint mechanism, primary prevention and control efforts, their cost-effectiveness, and social impact. During an evaluation over the course of a year and half, the evaluation team carried out considerable investigations into the task forces, ministries, and commissions responsible for the mechanism, as well as into the governments, centers for disease control and prevention, port quarantine authorities, hospitals, enterprises, neighborhoods, and schools in Beijing, Fujian, Henan, Guangdong, and Sichuan, while also having commissioned professionals surveys into 3,262 unaffected people, 893 patients with Influenza A (H1N1), and 646 people having close contact with such patients. These surveys resulted in a large amount of firsthand data and a 150,000-character evaluation report. Below is a summary of the primary conclusions and policy suggestions resulting from the evaluation.

Effects of Influenza A (H1N1) Prevention and Control

Facing tremendous pressure from the outbreak of a highly uncertain new strain of influenza within the context of the global financial crisis, the Chinese government insisted on placing people and public health first and foremost. It took vigorous and effective measures, achieved set goals relating to disease prevention and control, effectively safeguarded public health and economic and social stability, and markedly improved the government's credibility, international image, and capabilities in the response to public health emergencies.

Epidemic Controlled and Public Health Safeguarded Effectively

Upon the outbreak of the epidemic, China introduced a series of measures which paid equal attention to prevention and treatment—not only in biomedical terms but also from public health and social perspectives. These measures effectively curbed the spread and reduced the intensity of the epidemic. During the first 3 months that the global epidemic developed rapidly, the epidemic in China remained at a considerably low level, which allowed the country time to prepare for the research and development, production, and storage of drugs and vaccines for combating a possibly more devastating epidemic. At the same time, the country's proactive use of advantageous medical resources and adoption of a strategy in which centralized treatment was provided for serious patients proved to be very effective. In addition, China is one of the first countries to have developed an Influenza A (H1N1) vaccine and to have vaccinated target groups relatively early for immunity protection.

Epidemic Prevention and Control Safeguarded Economic and Social Stability in a Cost-Effective Manner

The country's Influenza A (H1N1) prevention and control effort, well planned and organized in the midst of the global financial crisis, made it possible to ensure economic and social development as well as stability, and prevent severe damage on society. According to the cost–benefit analysis conducted by the evaluation team, from April 25, 2009 through to December 31, 2009, for every one RMB spent on Influenza A (H1N1) prevention and control, there was a yield of about 7.99–11.55 RMB, suggesting that the country's prevention and control effort was cost-effective. This also demonstrated that the price that the Chinese government paid for its early adoption—in light of the national situation—of a well-structured prevention and control strategy, to avoid possible losses from lack of preparedness or response, was worth the investment. The investment could in a sense be seen as "insurance" against worst outcomes. The survey findings showed that nearly 70% of the people interviewed thought the epidemic has not caused inconvenience to their work and life. Moreover, the rigorous Influenza A (H1N1) prevention and control ensured that preparations were well under way for such important events as the 60th anniversary of the founding of the People's Republic of China, the 11th National Games of China, and Expo 2010.

People-Centered Epidemic Response Strategy Widely Recognized, and Government Credibility and Global Image Significantly Increased

The Chinese government was widely acclaimed for its positive, responsible, open and transparent strategy, its prevention and control practices which put people first and exhibited a high esteem for the health and safety of the public, and the evident progress it made in emergency management and public communication. The evaluation team found that public satisfaction with central and local governments regarding their work on the epidemic reached 92 and 85%, respectively. After the epidemic, the public had greater trust in the government's capabilities in terms of managing emergencies, with the degree of their trust in central and local governments rising to 96 and 94%, respectively. While thought highly of at home, the country's international image was also improved. Margaret Chan Fung Fu-chun, Director-General of the World Health Organization, noted that following the outbreak of the epidemic the Chinese government had played a strong role of leadership with active and effective measures of prevention and control. International mainstream media organizations generally reported favorably on China, considering China's move against Influenza A (H1N1) to have been open and proactive. *The New England Journal of Medicine*, one of the most authoritative of its kind, remarked that China's effort on Influenza A (H1N1) prevention and control and research was very fruitful. At the same time, China actively participated in international cooperation and assistance regarding epidemic prevention and control, creating an image of a responsible big country.

Significantly Increased Capabilities for Coping with Public Health Emergencies

The Influenza A (H1N1) prevention and control regimes produced far-reaching effects on the country's capacity building regarding infectious diseases and public health emergency. It had become a real-life drill for professionals of various sorts, and as a result the country's capabilities of influenza monitoring, field epidemic management, and medical treatment were improved. After the epidemic broke out, with a prompt investment of nearly 400RMB million, China strengthened its disease monitoring system in a short time and expanded its influenza monitoring network to include 411 laboratories and 556 sentinel hospitals, with remarkably enhanced capabilities for the identification, diagnosis, and treatment of new infectious diseases as well as coping mechanisms. The Chinese National Influenza Center, of the Chinese Center for Disease Control and Prevention, was designated as the world's fifth World Health Organization Collaborating Center (WHOCC), and China was the first developing nation to have a WHOCC. The Influenza A (H1N1) prevention and control effort also led to improved medical capabilities at local levels, including rebuilt negative pressure rooms and purchased medical apparatuses—which will play a crucial role in future prevention and control of major infectious diseases. In addition, the country exhibited strong emergency research capabilities in terms of vaccine development, clinical research, and other factors, making it one of the first countries to develop an Influenza A (H1N1) vaccine. Its fast influenza testing technology has attained globally leading level.

Basic Experience in Influenza Prevention and Control

During the country's fight against Influenza A (H1N1), governments at various levels as well as the private sector worked hard in dealing with the crisis, and accumulated a large amount of experience which would be useful for public health emergencies that may occur in the future.

Strengthening Emergency System, Laying a Solid Foundation for Influenza A (H1N1) Prevention and Control

In the wake of the SARS epidemic that broke out in 2003, remarkable progress was made in the country's emergency management effort structured around preparedness plans, systems, mechanisms, and legislation. Public health investment was ramped up at central and local levels, giving a boost to the development of disease prevention and control institutions and hospitals. The establishment of public health emergency response mechanisms, the improvement of public health emergency legislation and preparedness system building, the strengthening of health emergency monitoring and warning capabilities, and the broadening of international and regional communication and cooperation have laid a good foundation for the country's success in Influenza A (H1N1) prevention and control.

Taking Advantage of Institutional Strengths and Fostering a Climate in Which the Government Took the Lead with the Widest Possible Public Participation

The Chinese government stood out worldwide, especially among developing nations, when it comes to how much attention it was giving and how fast it responded to the Influenza A (H1N1) epidemic. The central government established a cross-departmental prevention and control mechanism and strengthened communication and coordination among the government departments involved. Local governments also established corresponding systems and mechanisms as appropriate. At the same time, the active participation of all the stakeholders helped create a society-wide prevention and control mechanism comprising communities, schools, enterprises, and villages, forming a climate in which the government took the lead with participation of the whole society.

Striving to Safeguard the Health and Safety of the General Public and the Interests of Special Groups with great responsibilities

Our governments at all levels acted prudently and responsibly with a view of lowering the risks and potential harm that the epidemic might cause to public health. After fully considering the interests and needs of special groups, they then formulated the priority strategy of curing and vaccinating the high-risk population, coordinated and improved the measures in support of the isolation policy, and made proper efforts to ensure that some ethnic and religious activities were normally carried out. The surveys found that 96.7% of respondents thought that the government's disease prevention and control measures fully embodied an attitude of significant responsibility and humanitarianism.

Employing Science and Technology to Make Disease Prevention and Control More Efficient and Effective

The country made full use of science and technology to make prevention and control measures as efficient and effective as possible. Strengthened epidemic monitoring and warning and the swift launch of emergency research programs provided the scientific basis on which epidemic prevention and control plans were made and improved in good time. Under the national joint mechanism, a special expert committee was set up, and governments at various levels also paid great attention to the roles of experts. These experts were instrumental in scientific decision-making about Influenza A (H1N1) prevention and control. According to surveys by the evaluation team, over 84% of the medical workers interviewed believed that the employed medical treatment measures were scientific.

Insisting Upon Openness and Transparency, Effectively Conducting Risk Communication and Health Education

The country stuck to the principle of "timeliness and accuracy, openness and transparency, positive guidance, and moderateness in amount" when it comes to information disclosure, and for the first time applied systematically the ideas and methods of risk communication to communicate over the epidemic and vaccination and step up health education. By so doing, it strengthened epidemic monitoring and fostered public participation in epidemic prevention and control while maintaining the stability of society as a whole.

Enhancing International and Regional Collaboration

The Influenza A (H1N1) prevention and control agencies in China actively participated in international collaboration and acted upon the *International Health Regulations 2005* (IHR 2005). China worked closely with the WHO, communicated the epidemic situation to the WHO and involved countries, and provided Mexico with support and assistance at the earliest possible time following the epidemic outbreak there. At the same time, China received timely technical guidance from the WHO as well as significant support from countries such as the United States, Canada, and Mexico.

Problems with and Specific Policy Suggestions about China's Influenza A (H1N1) Prevention and Control

During the course of the epidemic prevention and control, some problems concerning public health emergency management also surfaced. The evaluation team suggests such solutions as further revising the *Infectious Disease Prevention and Treatment Law*, the *Emergency Response Law* among other laws as well as relevant emergency plans, continuously improving emergency command systems and mechanisms, strengthening risk evaluation and communication, clarifying rights and obligations of enterprises and related organizations in responding to public health emergencies, and improving the regulations on the system of coordination and communication among governments, enterprises and the rest of society. At the same time, considering the growing uncertainty and globalization of public health emergencies, China should continue to strengthen capacity building for coping with them, and implement a "go global" strategy in the public health field, including enhancing international and regional collaboration and actively working with other countries and regions to build an epidemic monitoring, prevention, and control network. Below are some specific policy suggestions.

Create a Permanent, Cross-Departmental National Public Health Emergency Command Agency, Distinguish Between and Improve Upon Warning Standards and Response Standards, Improve Concrete and Viable Peacetime–Wartime Switch Procedures and Operational Rules

During the course of the epidemic prevention and control, the mechanism that highlights shared responsibility, joint action, coordination and communication played a crucial role, and it marked a significant innovation the country had introduced into the emergency management system and advancing with times. Due to a lack of explicit legislative support, however, this mechanism has its limitations at lower levels, including facing the issue of having inadequate authority, lack of clarity in accountabilities, and a dearth of coordination in decision-making. At the same time, how to play the full role of the existing permanent emergency response system (including the emergency management offices at various levels) and how to deal with their relations with the agencies under the joint prevention and control mechanism at local levels are also problems warranting prompt attention.

In addition, the country's *Emergency Response Law, Public Health Emergency Response Regulation, National Overall Preparedness Plan for Public Emergency*, and *National Preparedness Plan for Public Health Emergencies* among others, though comprising provisions relating to such aspects as emergency warning and response, are still lacking in explicit provisions in certain areas. For instance, they do not provide clearly for the transition from warning phase to response phase, between peacetime and wartime status, as well as related operational rules, which make it difficult to identify the right time for the shift to and from emergency response, response procedures, and specific rules for multi-departmental participation, thus affecting the efficiency of emergency response.

The evaluation team's suggestion: Create a permanent, cross-departmental national command center for public health emergencies, integrate the innovative joint prevention and control mechanism with the existing emergency management systems, and incorporate the joint prevention and control mechanism into the center's decision-making and coordination process. This center has its office at the Ministry of Health (MOH) which also works as its convener, directing and coordinating emergency management effort while accepting guidance from the

Emergency Management Office of the State Council. The center's response level and form of organization depend on different degrees of public health emergencies.

At the same time, efforts should be made to improve preparedness plans and to optimize processes and strengthen and improve operability requirements. It is necessary to further clarify the specific standards and management systems relating to warning and response levels in the *Emergency Response Law*, the *National Preparedness Plan for Public Health Emergencies*, and other emergency preparedness plans, and pay attention to the difference and correlation between these warning and response levels. It is necessary to ensure smooth transition from emergency warning to response, to further clarify the authority that related government departments have in states of emergency, to improve policymaking and adjustment procedures, and to revise the articles of the *Infectious Disease Prevention and Control Law* relating to infectious disease confirmation and adjustment.

Abide by the Principle of Responsibility by Level and Jurisdiction, Further Clarify the Scope of Authority and Operational Rules Concerning Emergency Management for Governments at Central, Local or Other Levels, Delegate, as Necessary, the Power to Release Information on an Epidemic and Other Events, and Further Strengthen Timeliness, Pertinence and Flexibility of Epidemic Response

During the course of the epidemic prevention and control, the WHO provided China with suggestions in proper time based on global epidemic developments, and China made clear the principle of "taking threats to public health seriously, responding actively, and coping with the epidemic in a scientific manner according to law through joint prevention and control efforts," organized experts to conduct surveys in time according to epidemic developments, and established measures for timely adjustment in prevention and control strategies. But perhaps because actual conditions varied widely from region to region given the vast territory of the country, in understanding and implementing related policy measures, some local governments and departments failed to give full consideration to actual situations and consequently were lacking in flexibility, timeliness, and pertinence in their prevention and control action. Therefore, the country's general epidemic prevention and control policies have yet to be refined in terms of their pertinence and operability with local governments and departments. Surveys by the evaluation team showed that 70% of the public thought prevention and control measures adjusted in time, while the remaining 30% disagreed, suggesting that there was still room for further improvement in this regard.

In terms of epidemic response, due in part to local administrative pressure, various degrees of overreaction existed at the grassroots level. Some medical institutions, for example, complained that the local government requested "zero death" which was not scientifically justifiable, causing unnecessary pressure to be placed on local medical workers.

The evaluation team's suggestion: Give more consideration to actual epidemic situations in regions and differences in their response capabilities when giving directions at the central level, allowing room for local decision-making. Furthermore, strengthen and improve local capabilities of making well-informed and scientifically based decisions without being compromised by misleading factors. Improve expert participation mechanisms at various levels in a way that ensures decisions are made based on actual circumstances and can be implemented by local governments and at grassroots institutions. With strict epidemic monitoring and detection, local governments may, as permitted by relevant laws and regulations, release information and evaluation results about an epidemic that has occurred (or a suspected epidemic) or other public health emergencies, and determine their warning and response levels based on actual circumstances. Create a risk evaluation and overall analysis mechanism with participation of multidisciplinary experts, who perform risk evaluations as needed by epidemic developments in the process of prevention and control and revise prevention and control strategies and measures based on an overall analysis of evaluation results, so as to ensure that the prevention and control effort is appropriate and effective on the whole.

Amend as Soon as Possible the Infectious Disease Prevention and Treatment Law and its Detailed Rules for Implementation, Fully Revise National Influenza Pandemic Preparedness and Emergency Response Plans, Provide Against Emerging Infectious Diseases, and Improve Universal Measures and Procedures Against Such Diseases

During the course of the epidemic prevention and control, evidence shows some policy measures not adequately grounded in law. For instance, the process of downgrading the epidemic from Category A to Category B infectious disease was not adequately substantiated, causing deviation in the implementation at local levels of policy. At the same time, there also existed the problem of not having adequate regulations as to authority that local governments had in emergency management, such as the lack of charity in procedures for emergency requisition and compensation. There was a lack of continuity and consistency between some prevention and control policies developed by government authorities, with unconformity and even conflicts in documents reported.

Problems still existed with emergency preparedness system. In response to the WHO's call for global preparedness, the MOH used what was primarily intended for a highly pathogenic H5N1 pandemic, as a guideline for the prevention and control of an Influenza A (H1N1) pandemic. This was clearly not completely appropriate.

The evaluation team's suggestion: Amend and improve the Infectious Disease Prevention and Treatment Law and its detailed rules for implementation to the extent that it can be flexibly applicable to Influenza A (H1N1) and epidemics of other types; further revise existing influenza pandemic preparedness plans at health authorities, and gradually create a comprehensive, networked, and coordinated pandemic emergency response system at the national level. Moreover, given the uncertainty and complexity of emerging infectious diseases for which the existing single-disease preparedness plans are not suitable, it is suggested that the country formulate emergency response plans dedicated to emerging infectious diseases, regulate universal measures, procedures, and powers and responsibilities of participating agencies in prevention and control, and establish as quickly as possible mechanisms that allow flexible adjustment in strategies against unknown diseases.

Governments at Various Levels Should, Taking Into Consideration New Healthcare Reform, Create Feasible Emergency Funding, Stockpile and Compensation Mechanisms

The process of Influenza A (H1N1) prevention and control revealed problems such as inadequate resource reserves and flawed policies on local government procurement payment and prevention and control compensation. In addition, there was a lack of policies on compensation for medical services delivered against pandemic diseases. Of the 26 designated hospitals surveyed by the evaluation team, only 55% received government subsidies, and nearly 84% paid medical expenses on behalf of Influenza A (H1N1) patients. The 26 hospitals paid a total of 14,235,500RMB in medical expenses, representing approximately 550,000RMB per hospital. As of the present time, some provinces still have not yet addressed the issue of payments that designated hospitals made on behalf of patients, and some locations have yet to pay vaccine manufacturers for the purchase of Influenza A (H1N1) vaccine.

In addition, medical stockpile mechanisms dedicated to pandemic diseases have yet to be improved, alongside systems relating to repositories at central and local levels. In case of emergency, related ministries and commissions lacked complete information on national and local repositories. More works need to be done in terms of the standards, forms, and types of emergency supplies.

The evaluation team's suggestion: Take the opportunity presented by implementation of new healthcare reforms to further increase the coverage of basic medical insurance, to improve commercial medical insurance schemes, and to increase the benefits of medical insurance against major infectious diseases.

Establish as soon as possible at provincial and municipal levels public health emergency funding and compensation mechanisms, including advance payment, so as to ensure that action for public health emergencies is not affected by shortage of funds and that participants can be reasonably compensated for their investment toward coping with public health emergencies. Establish stable and effective mechanisms for multichannel compensation to medical institutions at grassroots levels. Establish funding and compensation tracking and supervision mechanisms. In addition, review the financial spending on the Influenza A (H1N1) epidemic by local governments at various levels, as well as the financial compensation to related hospitals, vaccine manufacturers among other participants, so as to deal well with all aspects of work in the aftermath of the epidemic and consequently increase government credibility.

Further Strengthen Capacity Building of Grassroots Medical Institutions to Ensure the Availability of Public Health and Medical Services Along Fault Lines in Emergency Management Such as the Education Settings, Large Construction Sites, and Important Transportation Hubs

In recent years, the country has ramped up basic public health services, but still places inadequate attention on the major fault lines in emergency management represented by schools, large construction sites, and important transportation hubs. There is a lack of emergency supplies and resources within certain key departments, fields and sectors, and grassroots disease prevention and control workers, in particular, are inadequate both in number and capabilities. At the Ministry of Education (MOE) as well as education departments at lower levels, for example, there is a dire shortage of health workers and funds, making it hard for them to undertake the tremendous tasks of health guidance, monitoring, and physical examinations of students. General hospital capabilities in relation to detecting, identifying, and treating clinical cases of infectious diseases still need to be improved. The evaluation team found in surveys that during the Influenza A (H1N1) prevention and control, nearly 90% of the disease control and prevention institutions met with manpower shortages, while 45% complained of financial shortages. In less-developed regions, medical resources are limited, and there are severe shortages of medical equipment and facilities, antivirus drugs, and protective appliances, with intensive care unit (ICU) facilities and equipment being hard-pressed to meet medical needs in dealing with major infectious diseases. Moreover, expenditure is inadequate on research concerning life sciences, medical frontiers, public health prevention and control, emergency management, and other respects.

The evaluation team's suggestion: Further strengthen capacity building as required by the new healthcare reform at grassroots healthcare institutions, accelerate investment into health monitoring and disease prevention, and control in vulnerable settings such as schools, large construction sites, and important transportation hubs—especially in relation to outreach and education directed at schools of various types, and improve the public health management mechanisms in schools. Enhance support to less-developed regions in such aspects as medical infrastructure and training. Increase expenditure on research in frontier fields while strengthening basic medical research.

Boost IT Development as Required by the Healthcare Reform, Strengthen Disease and Epidemic Monitoring and Warning Systems Based on Risk Management, and Improve Information Reporting Mechanisms

Though the country's influenza monitoring capacity has been improved over the years, an imbalance exists between monitoring networks at the provincial level. A full-coverage, high quality, epidemiological, and laboratory-based surveillance system—especially a worldwide public health information and monitoring system, is not yet built. There is still an inadequacy in comprehensive, in-depth analysis of existing monitoring data, and international and domestic public opinion monitoring network concerning epidemic developments needs to be further strengthened.

The contents and standards for information collection and submission overlap and vary between different departments, causing difficulties to local work and increasing administrative costs. The country has established information systems relating to epidemic surveillance, including a direct epidemic reporting system, but no information interconnection and sharing mechanism have been created between CDC and medical institutions at various levels. Within medical institutions at the county level, in particular, the data collection and submission system are so weak that the decision-making process is poorly coordinated and there is no access to an information sharing system, which weakens their capacity in making well-informed decisions about emergencies.

The evaluation team's suggestion: Enhance IT applications as required by the healthcare reform in the country's emergency command and decision-making systems, accelerate IT application at healthcare institutions based on resource integration, and boost information interconnection at various levels and between regions, departments, specialized institutions, and monitoring network nodes.

Expert Panel

Chief Project Experts:
Xue Lan, dean and professor of School of Public Policy and Management, Tsinghua University
Zeng Guang, chief epidemiologist and research fellow of Chinese Center for Disease Control and Prevention

Advisory Team Members: (In surname stroke order)
Ma Huaide, vice president of China University of Political Science and Law
Wang Chen, vice president of Beijing Hospital under the Ministry of Health, and deputy director of the Beijing Respiratory Disease Research Institute
Wang Ke'an, former president of the ThinkTank Research Center for Health Development and the Chinese Academy of Preventive Medicine
Wang Ruotao, research fellow at the Chinese Center for Disease Control and Prevention
Wang Longde, academician of Chinese Academy of Engineering, and president of the Chinese Preventive Medicine Association
Yin Yungong, director of the Institute of Journalism and Communication Studies, Chinese Academy of Social Sciences
Feng Zijian, director of Public Health Emergency, Chinese Center for Disease Control and Prevention
Bai Chong'en, director of Department of Economics and associate dean, School of Economics and Management, Tsinghua University
Shan Chunchang, counselor of the State Council and leader of State Council Expert Panel of Emergency Management
Liu Peilong, former director-general of the Department of International Cooperation, Ministry of Health
Li Xiguang, director of Tsinghua International Center for Communication
Chen Siyi, former editorial board member and deputy editor-in-chief of Xinhua News Agency's *Outlook Weekly* magazine
Chen Zhaoying, director of the National Center for Science and Technology Evaluation, Ministry of Science and Technology

Chen Huanchun, academician of Chinese Academy of Engineering, and vice president of Huazhong Agricultural University

Qiu Renzong, research fellow at the Institute of Philosophy, Chinese Academy of Social Sciences

Zhang Kan, former director of the Institute of Psychology, Chinese Academy of Sciences

Hou Yunde, academician of Chinese Academy of Engineering, and research fellow at the National Institute for Viral Disease Control and Prevention, Chinese Center for Disease Control and Prevention

Zhao Kai, academician of Chinese Academy of Engineering, and director of the National Vaccine & Serum Institute

Yuan Ming, associate dean of the School of International Studies, Peking University, and director of the Institute of International Relations

The late Huang Jianshi, dean of the School of Public Health, Peking Union Medical College

Evaluation Team Members:

From Tsinghua University

Xue Lan, dean and professor of School of Public Policy and Management

Peng Zongchao, professor at the School of Public Policy and Management, and director of the Center for Crisis Management Research

Wei Wuming, postdoctoral researcher at the School of Public Policy and Management

Zhong Kaibin, part-time research fellow for the Center for Crisis Management Research, and associate professor at the Chinese Academy of Governance

Shen Hua, postdoctoral researcher at the School of Public Policy and Management

Wang Zhiqiang, postdoctoral researcher at the School of Public Policy and Management

Hu Yinglian, part-time research fellow for the Center for Crisis Management Research, and lecturer at the Chinese Academy of Governance

Ma Ben, part-time research fellow for the Center for Crisis Management Research, and associate professor at the School of Political Science and Public Administration, Shandong University

He Jing, part-time research fellow for the Center for Crisis Management Research, and associate professor at China Youth University of Political Studies

Zhou Ling, part-time research fellow for the Center for Crisis Management Research, and lecturer at the School of Social Development and Public Policy, Beijing Normal University

Tang Tian, Ph.D. student at the School of Public Policy and Management,

Fan Shiwei, Ph.D. student at the School of Public Policy and Management

Xue Wenjun, Ph.D. student at the School of Public Policy and Management

Li Fang, research assistant at the School of Public Policy and Management

From Chinese Center for Disease Control and Prevention

Zeng Guang, chief epidemiologist and research fellow

Ma Huilai, guiding teacher and chief physician for the Chinese Field Epidemiology Training Program

Shen Tao, guiding teacher and assistant researcher for the Chinese Field Epidemiology Training Program

Liu Huihui, guiding teacher and assistant researcher for the Chinese Field Epidemiology Training Program

Chen Jing, physician in charge, and a trainee (from the Tianjin Center for Disease Control and Prevention) of the 8th session of the Chinese Field Epidemiology Training Program

Tang Xuefeng, physician in charge, and a trainee (from the Sichuan Center for Disease Control and Prevention) of the 8th session of the Chinese Field Epidemiology Training Program

Xing Xuesen, physician in charge, and a trainee (from the Hubei Center for Disease Control and Prevention) of the 8th session of the Chinese Field Epidemiology Training Program

Zhang Zewu, physician in charge, and a trainee (from the Dongguan Center for Disease Control and Prevention) of the 8th session of the Chinese Field Epidemiology Training Program

From Shandong University

Wang Jian, professor at the Center for Health Management and Policy

Bian Ying, professor at the Center for Health Management and Policy

Li Hui, lecturer at the Center for Health Management and Policy

Li Shunping, lecturer at the Center for Health Management and Policy

Kong Peng, lecturer at the Center for Health Management and Policy

Sun Xiaojie, lecturer at the Center for Health Management and Policy

Bian Xuefeng, lecturer at the Center for Health Management and Policy

From Chinese Academy of Medical Sciences

Dai Tao, director and research fellow of the Institute of Medical Information

Wang Fang, associate professor at the Institute of Medical Information

Wei Xiao, assistant researcher at the Institute of Medical Information

Liu Xiaoxi, assistant researcher at the Institute of Medical Information

Wang Min, assistant researcher at the Institute of Medical Information

Sun Xiaobei, research associate at the Institute of Medical Information

From Academy of Military Medical Sciences

Cao Wuchun, director and research fellow of the Institute of Microbiology and Epidemiology

Liu Lijuan, associate professor and leader of the Foreign Infectious Disease Team, formerly at the Institute of Microbiology and Epidemiology and now at the Institute of Health Quarantine, Chinese Academy of Inspection and Quarantine

From Chinese Center for Disease Control and Prevention

Kong Qiang, chief epidemiologist and research fellow

Ma Huilai, senior lecturer and chief physician of the Chinese Field Epidemiology Training Program

Shen Tao, guidance teacher and assistant researcher for the Chinese Field Epidemiology Training Program

Hu Guang, guiding teacher and assistant researcher for the Chinese Field Epidemiology Training Program

Jiang Hua, physician in charge and trainee from the Tianjin Center for Disease Control and Prevention of the 4th session of the Chinese Field Epidemiology Training Program

Luan Xuefeng, physician in charge and trainee from the Sichuan Center for Disease Control and Prevention of the 4th session of the Chinese Field Epidemiology Training Program

Kang Xiaoping, physician in charge and trainee from the Hubei Center for Disease Control and Prevention of the 5th session of the Chinese Field Epidemiology Training Program

Zhang Zewei, physician in charge and trainee from the Dongguan Center for Disease Control and Prevention of the 6th session of the Field Chinese Field Epidemiology Training Program

From Shandong University

Wang Jian, professor at the Center for Health Management and Policy

Bao Yong, professor at the Center for Health Management and Policy

Hu Reman, at the Center for Health Management and Policy

Lv Shaohua, lecturer at the Center for Health Management and Policy

Kong Peng, lecturer at the Center for Health Management and Policy

Sun Xiaojie, lecturer at the Center for Health Management and Policy

Ren Zeliang, lecturer at the Center for Health Management and Policy

From Chinese Academy of Medical Sciences

Dai Tao, director and research fellow of the Institute of Medical Information

Wang Fang, associate professor at the Institute of Medical Information

Wei Ran, lecturer at the Institute of Medical Information

Qi Shuxia, assistant researcher at the Institute of Medical Information

Wang Min, assistant researcher at the Institute of Medical Information

Qiu Wuhua, research associate at the Institute of Medical Information

From Academy of Military Medical Sciences

Cao Wuchun, director and research fellow of the Institute of Microbiology and Epidemiology

Liu Quan, associate professor and leader of the Force Publication, Disease Control at the Institute of Microbiology and a backbone arrow at the Institute of Health Quarantine, Disease Academy of military and Quarantine

Chapter 1
Introduction

1.1 Background of Influenza A (H1N1) Prevention and Control in China

In March 2009, the "Human Swine Flu," which first appeared in Mexico and then rapidly spread across the globe, captured the attention of the world. On April 24th of that year, the World Health Organization (WHO) issued a global notification on the "Swine Influenza A subtype H1N1" in the United States and Mexico. On April 26th, 2009, the WHO Director-General declared this event a "Public Health Emergency of International Concern." On April 27th, the WHO raised the pandemic alert from Phase 3 to Phase 4, and two days later, to Phase 5. On April 30th, the WHO, the United Nations Food and Agriculture Organization, and the World Organization for Animal Health issued a joint statement, agreeing to refer to the pandemic as Influenza A (H1N1) and to end the usage of the term "Human Swine Flu." The pandemic influenza was thus officially renamed "Type A (H1N1)" [referred to as Influenza A (H1N1)].

On June 11th, the WHO raised its pandemic alert to its highest level of Phase 6, indicating the beginning of a global pandemic and another global health war for the 21st century! Could established global influenza prevention and control mechanisms contain the spread effectively? Could the national public health emergency systems muster orderly responses? Could countries and regions coping with on-going global financial crisis withstand this kind of attack? Thankfully, related state institutions and organizations provided quick responses and implemented a wide range of prevention and control policies and measures. With the guidance and coordination of the WHO, states worked closely together and managed to prevent the spread of Influenza A (H1N1), and in the process acquired knowledge and experience that would be useful in mitigating similar challenges in the future.

After the SARS crisis in 2003, the outbreak of Influenza A (H1N1) was yet another test of China's abilities in constructing emergency management systems.

© Social Sciences Academic Press and Springer Nature Singapore Pte Ltd. 2019
L. Xue and G. Zeng, *A Comprehensive Evaluation on Emergency Response in China*, Research Series on the Chinese Dream and China's Development Path, https://doi.org/10.1007/978-981-13-0644-0_1

At the National Conference for the Prevention and Control of SARS held on July 28th, 2003, President Hu Jintao and Premier Wen Jiabao emphasized the importance of securing a public health emergency system, requiring relevant authorities to "earnestly build up our emergency response mechanisms and capabilities as well as strive to secure an efficient, responsive, full-fledged and fully-functional emergency response system under centralized leadership so as to improve our capabilities in tackling various emergencies and risks." In the years that followed, China made strenuous efforts in formulating and revising public emergency preparedness plans, and worked hard in building and improving systems, mechanisms, and legislation, all of which were geared toward emergency management (This whole effort was referred to as the "One Plan, Three Systems"). The country's remarkably improved modern emergency management system played a crucial role in the most recent pandemic prevention and control efforts.

The Influenza A (H1N1) prevention and control efforts also benefitted greatly from China's unremitting efforts in bolstering their public health emergency system. In his 2004 *Report on the Work of the Government*, Premier Wen Jiabao highlighted the importance of strengthening the public health system, stating for the first time that we must attempt to establish a fully functioning system for disease prevention and control and medical treatment that covers both urban and rural areas, with the goal of strengthening our countermeasure capabilities in handling epidemics and other public health emergencies. As a result of increased government investment over the years, significant progress has been made in the construction of public health systems. Disease prevention and control systems have been established across the nation through the construction of multi-tiered centers for disease control. The construction of public health emergency response systems has also grown through the development of hospitals (or wards) for infectious diseases and emergency medical centers. At the same time, reforms for disease prevention and control organizations along with health supervision and law enforcement at the provincial, city, and county levels have also been progressing smoothly with the formation of a disease prevention and control system and public health emergency response system, both with Chinese characteristics. These two systems in turn have provided a strong foundation for the prevention and control of Influenza A (H1N1).

1.2   The Necessity and Importance of Influenza A (H1N1) Prevention and Control Evaluations

Beginning in early 2010, the Joint Influenza A (H1N1) Prevention and Control Mechanism set about preparing a comprehensive evaluation of all the processes in countering Influenza A (H1N1) in mainland China. The goals of this evaluation were to summarize the experience and lessons China had drawn from its Influenza A (H1N1) prevention and control efforts since April 2009, and to further improve the country's public health emergency management system. On August 10th, 2010,

WHO Director-General Margaret Chan Fung Fu-chun declared the pandemic finished, signaling more favorable conditions for a full evaluation of countries' prevention and control efforts. In the spring of 2010, the State Council's Influenza A (H1N1) Joint Prevention and Control Mechanism and the State Council's Emergency Management Office came together and officially commissioned Tsinghua University's School of Public Policy and Management (SPPM) to organize an Influenza A (H1N1) Prevention and Control Work Evaluation team. This team consisted of multidisciplinary experts, and its mission was to provide an independent, comprehensive evaluation of prevention and control efforts in mainland China since 2009. This was the country's first open, systematic, and objective evaluation of countermeasures and processes in mitigating a public health emergency, which held great historical significance.

Firstly, Influenza A (H1N1) was yet another major challenge posed to China's public health system in the 21st Century. This evaluation can aid us in the creation of a timely review of the experiences and lessons learned, the improvement of the country's public health emergency management system, and the guarantee of timelier decision-making for a variety of future public health emergencies; and thus when the next one occurs, countermeasures will be better suited and the damage to life and property will diminish. The evaluation also has a positive, demonstrative effect that can be used in the mitigation of other public crisis, enabling the government and society to better respond to, and recover from a crisis. Additionally, given the importance of coordinated mechanisms in determining the effectiveness of emergency response, an evaluation of the Joint Influenza A (H1N1) Prevention and Control Mechanism will contribute significantly to setting future standards and to the development of objective and scientific evaluation indicators.

Secondly, a comprehensive evaluation of the national efforts on Influenza A (H1N1) prevention and control was necessary in order to build a responsible, transparent government. One of the defining features of a modern, trustworthy government is its courage to take the moral, political, legal and administrative responsibilities in the face of mistakes or losses. An evaluation of a government's response to a public emergency is a part of the accountability process, and it provides a factual basis for future improvement. At the same time, building a transparent government requires the evaluation of government performance.

Moreover, an evaluation on the response to major public emergencies is a concrete manifestation of learning from advanced countermeasures and experiences from foreign countries in similar situations. Many developed countries, regions, and international organizations are taken great effort in post-emergency evaluations. For instance, the U.S. Government, after the 9/11 terrorist attacks in 2001, established an independent commission, whose evaluation of the response to the attacks was presented as *The 9/11 Commission Report*. After the WHO removed its recommendation for tourists to consider postponing travel to Hong Kong on May 28th, 2003, the Chief Executive of the Special Administrative Region declared the establishment of the SARS Expert Committee, which carried out an evaluation of Hong Kong's emergency management during the outbreak. They released their report globally in both Chinese and English. On September 8th, 2005, in the wake of the underground bombings that took place on the morning of July 7th, 2005, the London Parliament established the 7 July Review Committee, which also served as a Recovery and Reconstruction Committee. Its purpose was to investigate and evaluate the underground bombings and to begin reconstructive work; this committee published its first evaluation report on their website in July 2006. On September 15th, 2006, U.S. President George W. Bush ordered the federal government to complete an investigation and evaluation regarding the preparation for, response to and recovery from Hurricane Katrina, in order to see what lessons could be drawn from the disaster. Congress also commissioned experienced experts and cabinet members to perform a meticulous evaluation on the disaster, and this resulted in a report released by the House of Representatives. All of the countries mentioned above revised their emergency preparedness and mechanisms based on the evaluation findings to be better equipped for similar events in the future. It's clear that these evaluations were an important driving force for improving government emergency management systems, and they provide concrete references that can benefit China in the construction of our own emergency evaluations.

After the peak of the Influenza A (H1N1) pandemic, everyone—from the WHO to countries across the globe, from government departments to the academic community—all began reflecting upon the pandemic. In April 2010, the WHO established an independent panel of leading experts in the field for the following purposes: to review the global pandemic responses and the functioning of the International Health Regulations, and to evaluate the decision in raising the pandemic alert to the highest warning level. The European Union (EU) evaluated the responses of its member states from April 24th to August 31st, 2009, and independently reviewed their vaccination policies. The Australian government also assessed its response to the pandemic.[1]

1.3   The Framework, Characteristics and Principles of This Influenza A (H1N1) Prevention and Control Evaluation

1.3.1   Evaluation Framework

This evaluation is based on the characteristics of the pandemic at both home and abroad and its purpose is to discuss how China's public health emergency management system worked in the face of Influenza A (H1N1) through its coping strategies, joint prevention and control mechanisms, prevention and control cost effectiveness, and social impact. The overall effectiveness of the government's Influenza A (H1N1) prevention and control mechanisms are evaluated through the

---

[1]Hamilton (2009).

use of field surveys, statistical analysis, and a range of other methods, and with the summation of experiences and discussion of practical issues, this evaluation will help improve emergency management capabilities of China's public health system. The evaluation focuses on the following areas.

1.3.1.1   Prevention and Control Strategies

An evaluation was conducted on the overall prevention and control strategy, the preparedness plan, and policies and measures adopted in the different phases of the pandemic. The policies were then assessed to see if they were human-centered, relevant, timely, effective, and whether they suited the country's conditions.

1.3.1.2   The Joint Prevention and Control Mechanism

The actual operation effectiveness and efficiency was assessed on how the various components of the coordination mechanism worked in disease surveillance and response, with particular emphasis on decision-making, communication and coordination mechanism between and within departments, expert advice, and public participation.

1.3.1.3   Prevention and Control Measures and Emergency Response Capabilities

An evaluation was conducted on pre-pandemic preparedness and the following capabilities: disease monitoring, prevention, and control; the flexibility of medical treatment policies and the treatment itself; vaccine development and support capabilities; provision of financial and physical resources for major public health emergencies; news dissemination and risk communication, international cooperation; and when appropriate, the assessments on the emergency response research measures and capabilities.

1.3.1.4   Actual Response Effectiveness

This part of the evaluation focused on the three following areas:

A. Assessment on Public Health Effectiveness
    This provided an overview of the pandemic and evaluated the overall efficacy of maintaining public safety and the prevention and control policies and measures in containing the spread of Influenza A (H1N1).

B. Cost and Benefit Assessment
    Cost-benefit analysis was utilized to evaluate the overall cost or benefit of
    national investment in Influenza A (H1N1) prevention and control, and to
    analyze the advantages and disadvantages of relevant policies and measures.
C. Social Impact Assessment
    This assessment mainly evaluated the following areas: the satisfaction of the
    general public, international community (WHO included), and other stake-
    holders (patients, close contacts, medical staff, and disease control staff) with
    the government's response; the impact on the image of the government (in-
    cluding the impact of the prevention and control policies on the reputation,
    image, and trustworthiness of the government); the impact of pandemic pre-
    vention and control on economic growth and social stability; the potential
    impact on future influenza prevention and control, responses to major public
    health crises, and social progress.

1.3.2   The Characteristics of This Influenza A (H1N1) Prevention and Control Evaluation

The characteristics of this evaluation are based upon China's conditions and its
current mechanisms in the public health sector. The major characteristics are listed
below.

1.3.2.1   First Ever Comprehensive Evaluation of the National Response to a Public Health Emergency

Although it has become common practice amongst countries to perform emergency
response evaluations, this was the first time in which China had a public health
emergency evaluated systematically and comprehensively. The Chinese government reviewed the 2003 SARS epidemic in its aftermath but didn't provide a
systematic evaluation of the country's response to the crisis from the perspective of
coping with a public health emergency. In the wake of the Influenza A (H1N1)
epidemic, both the State Council and the Ministry of Health (MOH) continued to
give their full attention to the outbreak, and the MOH and the State Council's
Emergency Management Office requested the SPPM to take the initiative and
conduct a comprehensive evaluation of the national crisis response. This evaluation
is the first systematic and comprehensive evaluation in the country's history of
public health emergency management, and the first full evaluation of a major
emergency since the country began strengthening emergency system building in
2003. It will provide an invaluable model for future development.

1.3.2.2 Adoption of a Third-Party Evaluation Mechanism

In the past, public emergency reviews were conducted within the central or local governments by internal working groups. But for various reasons, it's difficult for such reviews to be objective and unbiased. However, this evaluation of the Influenza A (H1N1) epidemic was conducted by a third party with the participation of authoritative experts from various fields, all of whom took part in or gave guidance during the evaluation process. This was done in the hopes of gaining a better understanding of the entire response process and to ensure the evaluation was as independent and objective as much as possible.

1.3.2.3 Comprehensive Evaluation Concerning the Process and Effectiveness of Coping with the Public Health Emergency

This evaluation focused both on the effectiveness of the Influenza A (H1N1) prevention and control efforts and its entire process. The efficacy portion not only highlighted traditional health effects, but it also paid particular attention to economic benefits and social impact. The process review portion placed emphasis on related central policies, alongside the process of their top-down implementation. Therefore, this evaluation is comprehensive in scope as it combines "points, lines, and areas."

1.3.3 Evaluation Principles

Combining general international requirements and China's specific conditions, especially in regards to emergency response, this evaluation was formed by gathering first-hand information and organizing authentic, on-scene data, all with the hopes of establishing a real picture of the entire crisis. We abided by the following principles.

1.3.3.1 Independence

An evaluation is a process of discovering and organizing information; it is an unbiased information channel that provides more than just conventional data. Therefore, independence is the first and foremost principle for an evaluation. Through institutional design, evaluator selection, and the application of the scientific approach, we endeavored for independence in this evaluation, so that it was not influenced by any related decision-makers, attitudes of executive agencies, interest groups, public or media opinion, and economic benefits.

1.3.3.2   Objectivity

One of the goals of independence is to ensure objectivity. Although any evaluation is to a certain degree subjective, this evaluation team tried to make its evaluation as objective and authentic as possible by employing available knowledge, information, technology, and methods. We were able to avoid using the assessors' own subjective assumptions and instead conduct logical and deductive reasoning through the use of objective data collection and organization.

1.3.3.3   Normativity

To protect independence and objectivity, definite and detailed evaluation regulations were established regarding the following: the subject, procedures, evaluation principles, the use of evaluation funds, evaluation accountability, and the use and disclosure of evaluation outcomes.

1.3.3.4   Scientifically Justifiable

On one hand, this evaluation examined the efficiency and effectiveness of the joint prevention and control mechanism from the angles of both the public health system and the national disease prevention and control system, thus ensuring that the evaluation process was systematic. On the other hand as Influenza A (H1N1) is a new virus, this evaluation sought to critically evaluate the relevant decision-making processes and decisions under uncertain conditions, taking into account the objective knowledge and information available at the time, rather than conducting a post-event evaluation.

1.3.3.5   Holistically Comprehensive

From team composition, evaluation process initiation, to evaluation plan review, efficient participation of multidisciplinary experts was always a top priority. The evaluation team was not only comprised of experts in public health, emergency management, public policy and performance evaluation, but also experts in international relations, sociology, ethics, medicine, healthcare, and many more.

The advisory panel was also comprised of multidisciplinary experts, including those in biomedicine. Biomedical specialists came from fields such as inspection and quarantine, agriculture, public health, clinical medicine, medical biology, and traditional Chinese medicine; and other members mainly hailed from public administration, economics, law, diplomacy, and media. Other professionals were also engaged temporarily as needed during the evaluation, and participated in multidisciplinary discussions about the evaluation plan and outcomes.

1.4 The Methods, Processes and Limitations of This Influenza A (H1N1) Prevention and Control Evaluation

1.4.1 Evaluation Methods

According to the overall principles, subject matter, and characteristics of the evaluation, the specific evaluation work was divided into two main parts, i.e. investigation and post-evaluation. Field research and surveys were first conducted on related government departments and on local governmental efforts, and then a comprehensive analysis and evaluation was carried out by various specialists. During this investigative process, the evaluation team also studied international collaboration and actively sought opinions on China's crisis response from international organizations like the WHO as well as from noted international experts. Specifically, the following methods were employed during the evaluation.

1.4.1.1 Comparative Analysis

There was a robust combination of vertical and horizontal comparative analysis which included a historical comparison between Influenza A (H1N1) and SARS prevention and control, a horizontal comparison in practices and lessons learned in tackling Influenza A (H1N1) from different departments, regions and entities, and international research that delved into experiences and lessons learned from other countries battling the same virus.

1.4.1.2 Questionnaires

Questionnaires were given out regarding risk perception, behavior choice, and level of satisfaction among different groups and departments concerning the epidemic response measures. Interview and telephone surveys were also conducted. A legitimate and comprehensive indicator system was developed to ensure survey and evaluation quality. These evaluation methods were chosen based on this indicator system, and calculations, analysis, and explanations were all done using specific indicators.

1.4.1.3 Symposiums

Department officials and relevant experts participated in these symposiums where they discussed opinions and reviewed the results and issues associated with epidemic prevention and control.

1.4.1.4   In-depth Interviews with Officials and Specialists as Well as Local Case Investigations

In-depth interviews were held as needed for evaluation purposes with some key decision-makers and specialists. Individual local cases were surveyed on site to determine regional similarities and differences in epidemic prevention and control.

1.4.2   Evaluation Process

Starting in March 2010, according to general requirements of the mandators, the evaluation team proposed their overall plan, key points, and major research issues for the evaluation. Shortly afterwards, the evaluation team held a symposium for members of the joint prevention and control efforts, where they invited various experts to discuss the evaluation plan and provide their feedback. Building on that, the evaluation team revised and finalized the overall evaluation, work plans, and the labor division.

After sifting through a large amount of domestic and foreign data, documents, and news reports, the evaluation team visited and conducted field research in some chosen areas- including Fujian, Guangdong, Sichuan, Henan, and Beijing. They held symposiums and interviews in those locations with the following: local government officials, workers from local disease prevention and control institutions, commercial enterprises, communities, and school administrators and students who had partook in Influenza A (H1N1) prevention and control. Questionnaires were sent out and the evaluation team also visited related health care institutions. At the same time, in order to obtain more information on the implementation of relevant policies and the local experience with the prevention and control process, the evaluation team conducted on-site surveys and in-depth interviews with the following entities: various departments in these regions involved in Influenza A (H1N1) prevention and control, concentrating on health authorities, disease prevention and control institutions, hospitals, port inspection and quarantine agencies, schools affected by the epidemic that were isolated and under medical observation, and journalists.

In addition, the evaluation team accumulated a large amount of first-hand data through in-depth interviews with central level work groups under the joint prevention and control mechanisms along with related government departments and officials.

Meanwhile, in order to learn more about the public's understanding of Influenza A (H1N1) and their opinion on the national epidemic response, the evaluation team commissioned the Horizon Research Consultancy Group who then conducted a national household survey and 3262 valid samples were obtained. The evaluation team also entrusted the 12320 Health Hotline to conduct telephone surveys in Beijing, Fujian and Henan of 893 patients in different stages of Influenza A (H1N1) development and 646 people with close contact with Influenza A (H1N1) patients.

During the evaluation process, the evaluation team also engaged—when necessary—specialists and scholars in health care, disease control, public policy, media, international relations, and ethics fields for multiple consultation meetings and internal discussion sessions, through which problems arising from the evaluation were discussed and solved in timely manner. This ensured that the entire evaluation proceeded smoothly and without incident. After the evaluation report was initially formulated, several experts were invited to review it and provide their feedback.

1.4.3 Evaluation Limitations and Explanations

Due to time, resource, and experience constraints, certain limitations arose in terms of evaluation perspective, scope and methodology.

Firstly, in regards to the difficulty of the evaluation, we were conscious of the following realities: China is a populous, developing country with a large migrating population, urban and rural development is of a dualistic pattern, a considerable developmental gap exists between the east and west regions of the country, characteristics of public health emergencies vary widely between different areas (at the provincial, municipal, and county levels), and there is an imbalance both in the distribution of public health resources and in the scope of health emergency management. Owing to the uncertainty of public health emergencies, the complexity of the public health system, the incompleteness of information gathering mechanisms, complex regional characteristics, and the dynamic nature of the administrative system in China, many difficulties are still present in achieving a comprehensive analysis on the effectiveness of national measures against Influenza A (H1N1). That being said, since there similar post public health emergency evaluations are lacking in comparative references, this evaluation also served as an exploration by which to provide lessons and a foundation for similar evaluations in the future.

Secondly, in terms of evaluation perspective, the strategies, mechanisms, processes, effectiveness and impact of Influenza A (H1N1) prevention and control efforts were all viewed through the lens of public health emergency management and policies. This evaluation has no assessment regarding specific scientific issues found in healthcare (e.g. vaccine safety, efficacy of traditional Chinese medicine, etc.).

Thirdly, at the core of it, this evaluation focused mainly on the assessment of prevention and control at the national level. There were two considerations pertaining to this. On the one hand, the Influenza A (H1N1) prevention and control efforts were considered nationwide countermeasures to a public health emergency, all under the joint national prevention and control mechanisms, with the core strategies and plans established at a national level. On the other hand, the nature of the countermeasures varied because different regions faced different epidemic issues. While an all-inclusive summation of such experiences would be beneficial, such an evaluation would be impossible given the issues involved and time and resources constraints. It is of course true that prevention and control strategies along with emergency responses constructed at a national level must be implemented through local governments. Therefore, for our subject matter, we endeavored to research and present as much as possible the characteristics of, and problems with, the local governments we had surveyed. Nevertheless, such a reflection was far from enough in representing all of the local, multifaceted efforts that did occur.

Fourthly, in regards to research targets, as it was impossible to research and present all countermeasures that took place in every location, after conducting preliminary surveys in Fujian, we selected sample regions from the coastal, central and western parts of the country. Among the coastal regions we selected Guangdong, which, in addition to its being a coastal province, it also borders the special administrative regions of Hong Kong and Macau—which is one of the factors we considered. From the central regions we selected Henan, mainly because of its role as a major national transportation hub. Because China's first case of Influenza A (H1N1) occurred in Sichuan, we selected Sichuan to represent the west. At the same time, Beijing was added to our research targets because of its special role as the capital in epidemic response system. It should be noted that we selected and researched these regions to showcase the diversity of the prevention and control of Influenza A (H1N1), and not to provide a statistical representation or analysis of this subject.

Fifthly, we provide here an explanation for our cost-benefit analysis of the nation's Influenza A (H1N1) prevention and control efforts. It has long been an international challenge to conduct a cost-benefit analysis of response efforts to a public health emergency, as it involves not only estimating policy intervention costs but also its effects. Given the myriad of issues concerning data sources and analysis methods for intervention costs and effects, the evaluation team also struggled with the decision to conduct a cost-benefit analysis regarding this epidemic. After multiple internal discussions, we felt that as Chinese society continues to advance and develop, the public will have increasingly higher requirements for government performance, so performing a cost-benefit analysis of the state's response to a public health emergency will help related departments in improving their efficiency. This analysis will also help the public better understand and support emergency management efforts. It is precisely because of the difficulties in data collection and the immaturity of research methods, that we must try all means possible to pave the way for better collection and research methodology in the future. In light of this, we decided to conduct this analysis and make the information publicly available with the hopes of encouraging more counterparts in relevant fields to conduct similar analysis so we may improve the caliber of our national policy cost-benefit assessments. On the other hand, although the evaluation team made great efforts in their data collection and analysis, a large portion of the data obtained can only be approximated due to lacking relevant data and to the limitations of analysis methods employed. Moreover, some analysis methods were also based on many relevant assumptions, some of which purported ideal scenarios. Prudence is therefore when interpreting the final cost-benefit analysis outcomes. However, it is not the statistics that hold weight for our analysis, but instead the knowledge we gain regarding the magnitude and relevant factors of the costs and benefits from the Influenza A (H1N1) prevention and control.

1.5   Report Style and Structure

Because systematic evaluations of public emergencies are still something of a rarity in China, there are very few examples available to follow. It is quite a common practice abroad to perform an investigation or evaluation in the wake of a major emergency. Such reports track the developments of the event with comments and analyses inserted throughout, as in the case of the 9/11 investigative report or the 7 July 2005 London bombings investigative report. Others focus on main issues involved in the event, with more emphasis placed on analyzing the issues than on recording the event itself. We believe a combination of the two styles better suits this evaluation report. Above all else, we must provide a complete account of the entire epidemic, so that an entire record might exist and the public will be able to get a quick glimpse of the sequence of events. But, given the evaluation report's purpose and its focus on several subjects, we must dive deeper to analyze specific relevant issues. We thus strived for a suitable balance between narration and analysis.

Given the above considerations, this evaluation report is structured as follows: Following Chap. 1 Introduction, Chaps. 2 and 3 form the first narrative and analysis part of the evaluation report. Chapter 2 provides an overview of the global spread of Influenza A (H1N1) as well as of response strategies and measures in various countries, and Chap. 3 introduces in detail China's response to the epidemic and its coping strategies. These two chapters provide a more macro view of international and domestic responses to the Influenza A (H1N1) pandemic, alongside an intro-duction to and an analysis of the change in domestic coping strategies—providing a basis for the subject-specific analysis that follows. From Chaps. 4 to 7—which form the second main narrative and analysis portion of the report, the focus is on describing and analyzing, in succession, the systems and mechanisms, emergency response measures, costs and benefits, and social comments regarding Influenza A (H1N1) prevention and control. Chapter 8, the third main analysis portion of the report, sums up the preceding chapters as well as primary outcomes, experiences and lessons learned from the country's Influenza A (H1N1) prevention and control efforts, it discusses issues that require further deliberation, and it proposes some important policy recommendations on how to better our responses to public health emergencies (Fig. 1.1).

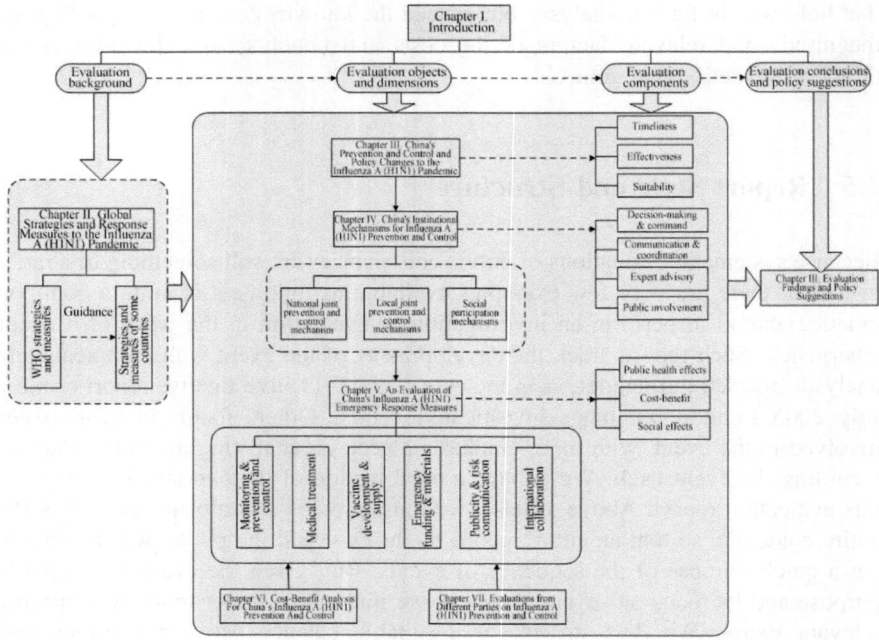

Fig. 1.1 China's influenza A (H1N1) Prevention and control evaluation framework

Reference

Hamilton, A. (2009). Swine flu—An assessment of the Australian response. *Rural and Remote Health*. http://www.rrh.org.au/articles/subviewnew.asp?ArticleID=1251.

Chapter 2
Global Strategies and Response Measures to the Influenza A (H1N1) Pandemic

2.1 The Global Pandemic Influenza A (H1N1)

As an infectious respiratory disease, influenza is prone to cause pandemics for its fast mutation, easy dissemination, susceptibility to humans, and its elusive nature in terms of treatment. Three influenza pandemics occurred in the 20th century which caused huge losses worldwide. According to historical estimations, in 1918 the Spanish Influenza (H1N1) may have resulted in roughly 20–40 million deaths worldwide.[1] It was so deadly that some scholars view it as one of the deadliest events in human history. The Asian Influenza (H2N2) in 1958 claimed about two million lives and the Hong Kong Influenza (H3N2) in 1968 caused an estimated one million deaths.

This pandemic originated from a new Influenza A virus that was discovered in North America in March–April of 2009. The spread of this virus sparked the first influenza pandemic of the century, which swept the globe in less than half a year. By June 11th, 2009, 28,744 confirmed cases, including 144 deaths, had been reported in 74 countries and regions in North America, South America, Europe, Oceania, Asia and Africa, and on that very day the WHO raised the alert level to Phase 6 and declared it a global Influenza A pandemic.

Two peak phases occurred during the pandemic on a global and regional level, one in the spring of 2009 and the other in the autumn and winter period of the same year. Beginning in April 2010, the global death rate from the pandemic decelerated along with its scope, as shown in Figs. 2.1 and 2.2.

By August 1st, 2010, more than 214 countries and regions throughout the world reported confirmed cases of Influenza A, with a total of 18,449 deaths. The WHO believed that actual number of cases and deaths exceeded those reported.

On August 10th, 2010, the WHO declared the end of the Influenza A Pandemic, and announced the beginning of the global post-pandemic period. According to

---

[1]WHO (2009a).

© Social Sciences Academic Press and Springer Nature Singapore Pte Ltd. 2019
L. Xue and G. Zeng, *A Comprehensive Evaluation on Emergency Response in China*, Research Series on the Chinese Dream and China's Development Path, https://doi.org/10.1007/978-981-13-0644-0_2

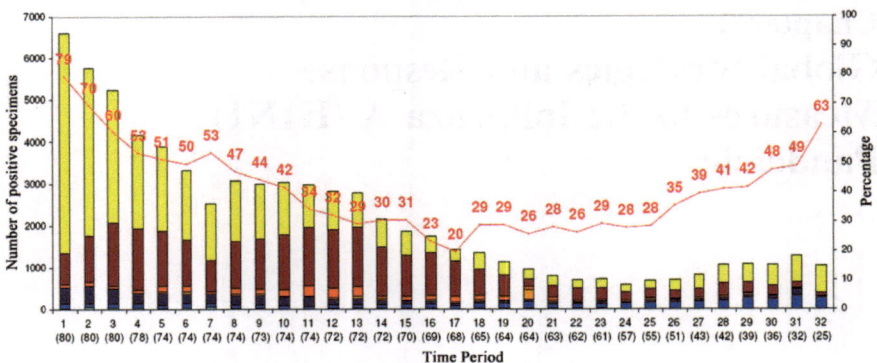

Fig. 2.1 Global Spread of Influenza Viruses from April 19th, 2009 through August 14th, 2010 (WHO. Weekly virological update on 26 August 2010. http://www.who.int/csr/disease/swineflu/laboratory27_08_2010/en/index.html)

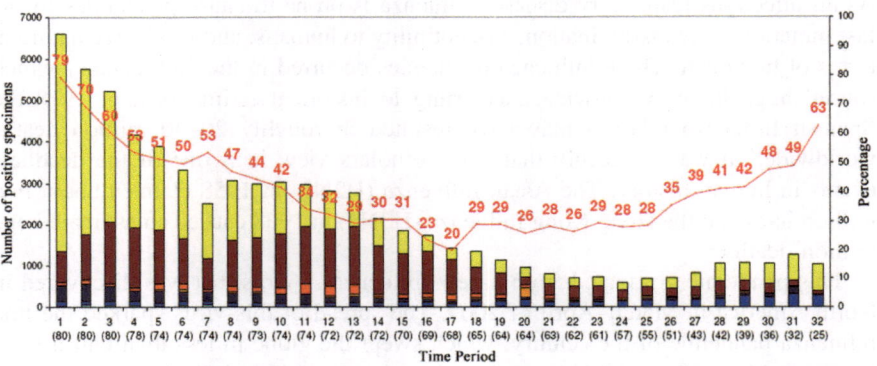

Fig. 2.2 Global Spread of Influenza Viruses from January 3rd, 2010 through August 14th, 2010 (WHO. Weekly virological update on 26 August 2010. http://www.who.int/csr/disease/swineflu/laboratory27_08_2010/en/index.html)

analysis by the WHO, after the global peak in the winter of 2009, there were no signs of any further widespread dissemination of the virus, thus proving the end of the Influenza pandemic. Nevertheless, the organization warned that entering the post-pandemic period didn't mean the Influenza A virus would disappear completely, as epidemic outbreaks were still likely to occur in some regions. Additionally possibilities of virus variation were evident and so countries were advised to be on alert during this time.

2.2 WHO's Global Pandemic Strategies and Response Measures

In response to the threat of a global influenza pandemic, the WHO as per the International Health Regulations 2005 (IHR 2005), put a large amount of work into global prevention and control efforts, and also adjusted prevention and control strategy priorities to fall in line with this global influenza outbreak. Countries worldwide have been proactive in their responses to the WHO's strategies and recommendations.

2.2.1 Capacity Building and Preparedness

2.2.1.1 Publishing the *Pandemic Influenza Preparedness and Response*

In order to tackle possible influenza pandemics and minimize losses, in 1999 the WHO published its official guidance, the *Influenza Pandemic Plan: the Role of the WHO and Guidelines for National and Regional Planning*, which was then later revised in 2005 and 2009, respectively.[2] In the 2005 revised WHO *Global Influenza Preparedness Plan*, an influenza pandemic was divided into six different phases: Phases 1–2 are interpandemic, i.e., no new influenza viruses have been detected in humans but an influenza virus subtype is circulating among animals and could potentially pose a threat to humans; Phases 3–5 consist of the pandemic alert phases where a new influenza virus has been detected in humans but its spread among humans remains limited; Phase 6 is the warning phase, declaring that the new influenza virus has spread widely across human populations.

In its 2009 revision of the *Pandemic influenza preparedness and response*, the WHO retained the use of a six-phase approach, but made some changes to the criteria. Phases 1–3 are characterized by the transmission of an influenza virus among animals and few humans, and correlate with preparedness, including capacity building and response planning activities. Phase 4 is characterized by sustained human-to-human transmission of an influenza virus, while in Phases 5–6 the virus becomes widespread and prevalent among humans. Phases 4–6 clearly signal the need for response, prevention, and control measures. During the post-peak period, pandemic activity drops, but there are still possibilities of recurrent outbreaks, before levels finally return to those seen in seasonal influenza[3] periods.

These plans from the WHO were made mainly based on the threat levels from the highly pathogenic avian influenza (H5N1), which are much different from the

---

[2]WHO. Pandemic influenza preparedness and response. http://www.who.int/influenza/resources/documents/pandemic_guidance_04_2009/en/.

[3]WHO. Current WHO phase of pandemic alter for pandemic (H1N1) 2009. http://www.who.int/csr/disease/swineflu/phase/en/index.html.

threats posed by Influenza A (H1N1) in 2009, and which are not likely to be the same as future influenza threat levels. These documents have nevertheless played a crucial role in pandemic response efforts and have provided some basic guidance that can be utilized in the outbreak of any infectious disease. The *Pandemic influenza preparedness and response* also summarized the lessons learned from coping with SARS and the highly pathogenic avian influenza, which will be a great asset in responding to future outbreaks of infectious diseases.

2.2.1.2   Assessing Global Laboratory Diagnostic Capabilities for Influenza A (H1N1)

On May 2nd, 2009, the WHO published its first ever list of countries and laboratories with the capacity to perform PCR (polymerase chain reaction) testing used to diagnose the Influenza A (H1N1) virus in humans, which was updated and re-published on May 4th, 2009. The WHO's criteria for diagnostic capabilities are: "Scoring 100% in the last two or more WHO external quality assurance programme panels (EQAP) received by the laboratory; or scoring 100% in the last panel and having a history of consistent results for earlier panels." On the list published were 98 institutions in 73 countries which were able to perform PCR to diagnose the Influenza A (H1N1) virus in humans.

2.2.2   Pandemic Alert and Risk Assessment

2.2.2.1   Revising Alert Levels

In response to the outbreak and spread of Influenza A, in the initial stages of the pandemic, the WHO began working on various alert and preparedness plans. On April 25th, 2009, the WHO held an emergency meeting, swiftly determining the severity of the pandemic situation and announced that it constituted a public health emergency of international concern.[4] On the evening of April 27th, 2009, the WHO raised the influenza pandemic alert level from Phase 3 to Phase 4,[5] and again to Phase 5 on the evening of April 29th.[6] Then in May during the World Health Assembly, it called on the international community to stay alert. On June 11th, the

---

[4]Statement by WHO Director-General Margaret Chan. Swine influenza. 25 April 2009, http://www.who.int/mediacentre/news/statements/2009/h1n1_20090427/en/index.html.

[5]Statement by WHO Director-General Margaret Chan. Swine influenza. 27 April 2009, http://www.who.int/mediacentre/news/statements/2009/h1n1_20090427/en/index.html.

[6]Statement by WHO Director-General Margaret Chan. Swine influenza. 29 April 2009, http://www.who.int/mediacentre/news/statements/2009/h1n1_20090427/en/index.html.

level was raised to Phase 6, the highest level the WHO has declared in the past 41 years—signalling the onset of a global influenza pandemic. On August 10th, 2010, based on its global assessment, the WHO removed the Phase 6 alert level and announced that the world was moving into the post-pandemic period.[7]

While adjusting pandemic alert levels, the WHO proposed that countries stay flexible in tailoring their specific response measures to their local epidemic situations, and warned that Influenza A (H1N1), as highly infectious as it is, would continue to do harm in the infected countries and could potentially spread to more countries. As the virus continued to spread in the southern hemisphere, which was at that time entering winter, the risk of its combination and mutation with other local epidemic influenza viruses increased, and so the international community was still required to closely monitor the situation.

2.2.2.2 Assessing the Risk of the Influenza A (H1N1) Pandemic

In the early days of the pandemic, the WHO's Influenza Pandemic Assessment Team published its assessment results on May 11th, 2009, in which a comparison was made with the 1957 and 1918 pandemics.[8] The assessment came to the following conclusions: this was a new subtype of the Influenza A virus; the Influenza A (H1N1) virus was likely to become more contagious than seasonable influenza viruses; differences in clinical symptoms were related to the patient's overall health situation; young people were more susceptible to the virus; the mortality rate was expected to be far lower than the 1918 pandemic; and there were still many uncertainties surrounding the pandemic.

After the pandemic tapered off, on April 12th, 2010 the International Health Regulations Review Committee held its first meeting in Geneva to assess the global response and the functioning of the IHR in relation to the pandemic, as well as to summarize related experiences and lessons learned. The assessment work is still under way and completion is expected in May 2011.[9]

2.2.3 Response Measures

In addition to its preparation and alert efforts, the WHO also strengthened pandemic monitoring and introduced a series of strategies and measures relating to pandemic response, treatment, vaccine development, inoculation, and distribution.

---

[7]Director-General's opening statement at virtual press conference. H1N1 in post-pandemic period. 10 August 2010. http://www.who.int/mediacentre/news/statements/2010/h1n1_vpc_20100810/en/index.html.

[8]WHO (2009b).

[9]WHO. International Health Regulations (IHR) Review Committee. External review of pandemic response. http://www.who.int/ihr/review_committee/en/index.html.

2.2.3.1 Integrating Global Pandemic Information

Beginning on April 24th, 2009, when it first published information on the outbreak of human swine influenza in the U.S. and Mexico, the WHO continually released pandemic and epidemiological information to the globe with the intention of facilitating international communication and sharing.

From April 24th through July 6th, 2009, during the early days of the pandemic, every day or every other day, the WHO published new laboratory-confirmed cases and deaths in affected countries, and at the same time it closely tracked the global transmission of Influenza A (H1N1).

2.2.3.2 Adjusting Pandemic Monitoring Methods

As the pandemic developed, WHO experts considered that as far as pandemic risk monitoring and response strategies were concerned, continued laboratory virus testing to all patients was no longer necessary, as it could overburden laboratories and thus influence their capacity in caring for critically ill patients and other unusual circumstances.[10] On July 16th, 2009, the WHO announced that countries affected by the epidemic were no longer required to report new confirmed cases, and recommended that attention be placed on monitoring influenza viruses and unusual epidemic events. But countries where Influenza A was not present still needed to report cases as they were discovered.

After April 2010, although the increasing rates of the fatality were on the decline and the pandemic activity remained relatively low, the WHO continued the monitoring of the pandemic and remained in close contact with public health experts in countries across the globe in order to determine whether the virus activity had returned to levels and patterns normally seen for seasonal influenza. Global pandemic activity had remained low over the past few months, and there was little evidence of higher pandemic influenza activity than what was normally caused by the seasonal influenza. The transmission of the Influenza A virus still persisted in the Southern Hemisphere, but it was still impossible to determine if countries there had transitioned to levels and patterns expected for seasonal influenza. Therefore, the WHO continued conducting epidemiological monitoring of the global pandemic situation and reported on relevant information.[11]

---

[10]Zhang (2009).

[11]WHO. Monitoring patterns and levels of worldwide activity. http://www.who.int/csr/disease/swineflu/notes/briefing_20100721/en/index.html.

2.2.3.3   Issuing Technical Guidance on Influenza Prevention and Control

On April 25th, 2009, the WHO released its first *Viral Gene Sequences to Assist Update Diagnostics for Influenza A (H1N1)*. By August 2010, the WHO had published more than 60 guidance documents on public health topics related to the influenza pandemic, including clinical care, medical treatment and management, laboratory and etiological detection, alert and response, surveillance, epidemiology, vaccines, travel, and personal protection.[12]

In the early days of the Influenza A Pandemic, the WHO's guidance documents were primarily about pandemic preparedness and responses as well as laboratory and hospital management. On May 6th, 2009, the WHO published a guidance document on biorisk management for laboratories handling specimens of Influenza A that were suspected or confirmed to have caused the pandemic, including recommendations of checklists for laboratory managers and staff members as well as minimum operating conditions for special related laboratory operations.[13] In addition, the WHO also published the *Case management of Influenza A (H1N1) in air transport*,[14] the *Clean hands protect against infection*,[15] and the *Clinical management of human infection with pandemic (H1N1) 2009*,[16] all of which provided valuable technical guidance in the early stages of the pandemic for containing its transmission and treating those infected.

With the spread of the virus along with a growing understanding of it, the WHO revised previously published guidance documents such as the *Clinical Management of Human Infection with Pandemic (H1N1)*, and the *Laboratory Diagnosis of Influenza A (H1N1)*. Published on May 21st, 2009, the *Clinical Management of Human Infection with Pandemic (H1N1)*, was formulated based upon updated virus information as well as data relating to seasonal influenza and the highly pathogenic avian influenza because at that time there was little case data available on H1N1. As experts and researchers began to learn more about the virus and evidence mounted for possible treatments, in October 2009, through a panel of experts in public

---

[12]WHO. Guidance documents on pandemic (H1N1) 2009. http://www.who.int/csr/disease/swineflu/guidance/en/index.html.

[13]WHO. Laboratory biorisk management for laboratories handling pandemic influenza A (H1N1) 2009 virus http://www.who.int/entity/csr/resources/publications/swineflu/Laboratorybioriskmanagement.pdf.

[14]WHO. Case management of Influenza A (H1N1) in air transport. http://www.who.int/csr/resources/publications/swineflu/air_transport/en/index.html.

[15]WHO. Clean hands protect against infection. http://www.who.int/csr/resources/publications/swineflu/AH1N1_clean_hands/en/index.html.

[16]WHO. Clinical management of human infection with pandemic (H1N1) 2009. http://www.who.int/csr/resources/publications/swineflu/clinical_management/zh/index.html.

health, laboratory, pathological and clinical fields, the WHO published their revised guidance in November 2009,[17] providing updated technical support for the diagnosis and treatment of patients with Influenza A (H1N1).

2.2.3.4 Coordinating Vaccine Research and Development

After the outbreak of Influenza A (H1N1), the WHO consulted related pharmaceutical manufacturers about developing vaccines, encouraging worldwide support of Influenza A (H1N1) vaccination production. The organization also collaborated with drug authorities in related countries ensuring that newly developed Influenza A vaccines met as many safety standards as possible. Meanwhile, the organization helped China in efficiently obtaining live strains of the Influenza A (H1N1) virus, which accelerated the country's research and development of relevant vaccines and drugs.

While ensuring an adequate amount of seasonal influenza vaccines were available, the WHO also initiated research and development for Influenza A (H1N1) vaccinations in the early stages of the pandemic.[18] Given that global limited production capacity for antiviral drugs and influenza vaccines could never meet the healthcare needs of 6.8 billion people, the WHO recommended governments to have clear and targeted prevention and control measures to avoid waste of resources.[19]

2.2.3.5 Planning for Vaccination Distribution

On July 2nd, 2009, a meeting of the world's health ministers was held in Mexico to assess the influenza pandemic and discuss countermeasures and inoculation distribution. At the meeting, WHO Director-General Margaret Chan called for international collaboration and solidarity, while stressing that special attention must be paid to high-risk groups like pregnant women and patients with chronic diseases. The WHO also called on vaccine manufacturers to provide them a certain amount of free vaccines so as to help developing countries better cope with their epidemics.[20]

In response to the ongoing global pandemic, the WHO stressed the importance for countries to carry out inoculations and to set forth three goals for their vaccination strategies, i.e. ensuring the normal operation of national healthcare systems,

---

[17]WHO. Clinical management of human infection with pandemic (H1N1) 2009: revised guidance. http://www.who.int/csr/resources/publications/swineflu/clinical_management/en/index.html.

[18]WHO Says Old Vaccines Production and New Vaccines Development Equally Important. Ecns. cn, May 16, 2009. http://world.people.com.cn/GB/9311296.html.

[19]Liu and Yang (2009).

[20]World Health Ministers' Meeting Discusses Measures against Influenza A (H1N1). Xinhuanet.com, July 4, 2009. http://medicine.people.com.cn/GB/9593164.html.

lowering morbidity and mortality, and minimizing possibilities of community-level outbreaks. To ensure continued normal operations of healthcare systems, the WHO recommended medical workers first be vaccinated, then pregnant women, patients aged six months and older with such chronic illnesses like asthma and obesity, healthy people aged 15–49, healthy children, healthy people aged 50–64, and people aged 65 and older—in that exact order.[21] The WHO also urged pharmaceutical manufacturers to produce vaccines at full capacity, to ensure fair distribution among developed and developing countries. Countries such as China, Italy, France, the United States, Germany, the United Kingdom, Norway, Sweden, Finland, Australia, and Japan took steps to vaccinate domestic residents, based on their own epidemic situations, healthcare resources, and ability to acquire vaccines. Some of the countries placed orders for more vaccines in order to cope with potential outbreaks.[22,23]

Response strategies varied widely across countries (see a detailed description in the next section) because each was faced with outbreaks and developments with different characteristics, in addition to political, economic, and cultural dissimilarities, especially in their public health systems which varied in both management and operation. While developed countries already had fairly effective response measures in place thanks to their advanced economic and social development as well as robust healthcare systems, some developing countries with poor economic foundations and weak public healthcare had a much harder time dealing with public emergencies. Therefore, they had an even harder time in dealing with Influenza A (H1N1). After the pandemic broke out, countries showed varied responses to the WHO's recommended response strategies and measures; in particular developing countries that had greater reliance on these strategies and measures as well as technical assistance from the WHO, were much more proactive. There is no doubt that the WHO played a crucial role in helping countries worldwide—especially developing ones—in coping with the pandemic, whether it is pandemic monitoring, clinical diagnosis and treatment of the virus, or vaccine development and distribution. However, because this pandemic originated in North American countries, taking into account the political, economic and cultural differences between countries as well as their different response capabilities, the WHO was also faced with new challenges like how to provide tailored guidance to developed and developing countries. The purpose of this guidance was to increase the effectiveness of related strategies and measures, mitigate and contain the spread of the pandemic, and minimize the negative effects of the virus on society and populations. Such targeted guidance was not particularly prevalent in their guidance regarding

---

[21]Influenza A (H1N1) Is More Pathogenic Than Common Flu, WHO Deems Vaccination Necessary. People.cn, July 15, 2009. http://medicine.people.com.cn/GB/9654341.html.

[22]Sweden Begins Vaccinating Its People against Influenza A (H1N1) in Autumn. Xinhuanet.com, July 15, 2009. http://medicine.people.com.cn/GB/9658730.html.

[23]Developed Countries Rush to Buy Influenza A (H1N1) Vaccines, Leaving Poor Countries Worried about Epidemic Control. People.cn, July 28, 2009. http://medicine.people.com.cn/GB/9732375.html.

response strategies and measures as the requirements placed on developed countries were quite low, resulting in an overall devaluation of said proposed strategies and measures. Therefore, when confronting similar public health emergencies in the future, the WHO should present more pertinent strategies and tailored measures which could play greater roles in pandemic preparation and response.

2.3 National and Regional Response Strategies and Measures

The outbreak in late April 2009 of Influenza A (H1N1) in several North American countries quickly attracted attention in related countries. Responding promptly to the crisis, government agencies and related departments in multiple countries immediately initiated public health emergency mechanisms and put into action a wide range of prevention and control strategies and measures.

2.3.1 National and Regional Influenza Response Systems and Mechanisms

2.3.1.1 National Response Mechanisms for Influenza A (H1N1)

Considering the serious economic, social, and public health consequences that could happen due to the outbreak, coping with the pandemic would demand participation, coordinated preparation, and enhanced collaboration from governments and different departments. Some countries specifically established unified leadership bodies and related mechanisms to deal with the pandemic, while others did so through existing government bodies or departments.

For example, countries like the United Kingdom, India, Japan, and Mexico set up a special coordination and management mechanism, and established an emergency decision-making, command and coordination body which was directed by the heads of government with the guidance and participation of relevant agencies. The British government specifically established a ministerial committee consisting of related government departments to strengthen inter-departmental communication and coordination and ensure the formulation and execution of preparation and response policies. The Indian Ministry of Health and Family Welfare established the Inter-Ministerial Task Force and Joint Monitoring Group for AI/pandemic to direct and coordinate the national response to the pandemic.[24] France's public health emergency mechanism was run by the "Inter-ministerial Risk Group" with

---

[24]Dr. Shashi Khare. Pandemic influenza A H1N1: Preparedness & response in India. CDC New Delhi. http://209.61.208.233/LinkFiles/RCE_DAY02_H1N1_INDIA-Dr_Shashi_Khare.pps.

the responsibility of decision making, situational tracking, and publicity, and the Minister of the Interior acted as the lead and was responsible for approving and initiating such decisions. Japan established the New Influenza Response Headquarters directed by the Prime Minister, and transformed the Risk Management Center's Information Liaison Office under the Prime Minister's Official Residence into the Official Residence's Liaison Office for directing and coordinating national pandemic response efforts. Mexico, whom in the past responded to public health emergencies mainly through direct government interventions and temporary emergency groups, established the National Committee for Health Security (CNHS) for analyzing, monitoring, and assessing the security issues of national health policies and for proposing relevant policies.

The United States, Australia and some other countries didn't specifically establish a governing body in response to the pandemic. After its incorporation in 2003 into the United States Department of Homeland Security (DHS), the Federal Emergency Management Agency's (FEMA's) responsibilities were expanded from natural disaster response to counter terrorism and pandemic diseases. The FEMA Director, appointed by the President, reports directly to the Secretary of Homeland Security and may, in response to a crisis, be summoned by the President to attend ministerial-level meetings and take part in the decision-making process. After the influenza pandemic outbreak in 2009, the United States launched its standard emergency response procedures, which included close collaboration and coordination among the federal, state and local governments along with the private sector. The U.S. Congress was charged mainly with funding public health efforts at the federal, state, and local levels,[25] while it was the responsibility of the federal government to update response plans, strengthen the development and revision of community-based plans, and enhance response capabilities. The DHS oversaw the distribution of antiviral medications and the dissemination of pandemic information to the public.[26] The U.S. Department of Health and Human Services (HHS), the executive body of pandemic preparation and response, was in charge of deploying, directing, and overseeing various response efforts, and they also completed the following: issued guidance on the influenza pandemic,[27] provided technical, financial, and medical support to states, and based on pandemic analysis announced a national state of emergency. As the national public health institute under the HHS, the Center for Disease Control and Prevention (CDC) played a crucial role in virus monitoring, prevention, and control. Similarly, Australia established a mechanism in which an inter-agency committee under the leadership of the prime minister and the cabinet was in charge of determining the federal government's preparation and

---

[25]Weissman (2009).

[26]Department of Homeland Security. Testimony of Alex Garza, MD, MPH, Office of Health Affairs, before the Senate Homeland Security and Governmental Affairs Committee on "H1N1 Flu: Getting the Vaccine to Where it is Most Needed". November 17, 2009. http://www.dhs.gov/ynews/testimony/testimony_1258473176155.shtm.

[27]Craig Vanderwagen (2009).

response strategies as well as pandemic countermeasures,[28] with state governments making and implementing relevant policies under the guidance of the federal government.

Whether or not a governing body was established for management of the pandemic, countries worldwide attached great importance to collaboration among government institutes and departments. For example, interim pandemic assessment reports by U.S. departments all mentioned that the timely response to, and rapid progress made in coping with the influenza pandemic, were due in large part to the clear divisions of labor and close collaboration among federal government institutes, departments, and state, and local governments.[29,30] The Indian government also stressed that pandemic responsibilities did not fall solely on the health department, and that it was necessary for multiple departments to collaborate with one another; the following departments of India were involved in pandemic preparation and response: the Ministry of Finance which provided cash, budgets, risk management, and insurance; the Ministry of Commerce and Industry which provided medical equipment; the Ministry of Road Transport and Highways which was charged with handling relevant transportation and communication issues; the Ministry of Defense and related military departments which was charged with public services, laws and regulations, security, and human rights; the Ministry of Information and Broadcasting which guaranteed the transparency of strategic communication, the dissemination of information, etc.; the Ministry of Environment and Forests and the Ministry of Health and Family Welfare which ensured biosafety, sanitation, wildlife conservation, etc.

2.3.1.2 Examples of National Pandemic Response Strategies (Plans)

To effectively curb the transmission of the pandemic and its negative effects on society, many countries formulated a national strategy or plan against possible influenza outbreaks from 2003–2005, outlining the duties and division of labor among government departments as well as their preparation and response strategies. Their policies on Influenza A (H1N1) were generally built on these strategies.

In 2005, pursuant to the *Pandemic Preparedness Guidance* published by the WHO, the United States developed the *HHS Pandemic Influenza Plan* and the *National Strategy for Pandemic Influenza*, according to which preparation and response strategies and measures would be chosen based upon phases that measured the pandemic's development. Included in the documents are detailed provisions about the duties along with preparation and response strategies of related government departments and mechanisms, i.e.: inter-departmental collaboration,

---

[28]Council of Australian Governments/Working Group on Australian Influenza Pandemic Prevention and Preparedness. National Action Plan for Human Influenza Pandemic. 2010.
[29]Sebellus (2009a).
[30]Sebellus (2009b).

public risk communication, vaccine production and distribution, and the stockpiling of antiviral medications.

In accordance with the WHO *Pandemic Preparedness Guidance*, the United Kingdom published their *Influenza Pandemic Contingency Plan* in 2005, and their *National Framework for Responding to an Influenza Pandemic* in 2007, which stipulated that strategies and measures for both preparation and response would be selected based upon pandemic phases.

In 2005, Australia formulated the *Australian Heath Management plan for Pandemic Influenza* and later revised it in 2008, and it remains as the country's national-level health plan for an influenza pandemic.[31]

India formulated the *Influenza Pandemic Preparedness and Response Plan* in 2005, which was used as a foundation for prevention and control policies against Influenza A (H1N1).

In 2006, the Mexican government issued the *National Preparedness and Response Plan for Pandemic Influenza*,[32] on which the country's prevention and control policies against influenza A were built.

On May 11th, 2009, the Japanese government swiftly issued the *Action Plan for Measures against Influenza A (H1N1)* to curb its domestic transmission. This plan contained response measures formulated according to four phases of distinct pandemic phases, i.e. occurrence overseas, early occurrence at home, infection expansion—spread—recovery, and stabilization.

2.3.1.3 National Funding for Influenza Pandemic Prevention and Control

For countries across the globe, central governments primarily provided the funds for prevention and control efforts against Influenza A (H1N1), and these funds were made available to related departments in the different pandemic phases. During the initial period and at the peak of the pandemic, these funds were mainly used for stockpiling antiviral drugs; purchasing relevant equipment, facilities, protective supplies and other materials; establishing points of distribution for antiviral drugs; providing patients with free antiviral drugs; and carrying out pandemic monitoring. During post-peak periods, funds were mainly utilized to purchase unified Influenza A vaccines from manufacturers, which were then distributed to the public with no charge.[33] Some developed countries also specifically established foreign assistance funds that provided developing countries both monetary and material assistance in combatting the pandemic.

---

[31] Australian Health Management Plan for Pandemic Influenza. http://www.health.gov.au/internet/panflu/publishing.nsf/Content/ahmppi-2009.

[32] Plan Nacional de Preparación y Respuesta ante una Pandemia de Influenza. http://www.dgepi.salud.gob.mx/pandemia/FLU-aviar-PNPRAPI.htm.

[33] DH. Pandemic H1N1 (2009) Influenza: Chief Medical Officer's Fortnightly Bulletin for Journalists. 21 January 2010.

The United States Congress invested heavily in pandemic prevention and control. In 2006, the Congress provided an appropriation of more than seven billion U.S. dollars (USD) for implementing the pandemic preparedness strategy. On April 28th, 2009, the U.S. President received another appropriation of 1.5 billion USD from Congress which was specifically designated for combatting the swine flu. In July of that year, Congress provided 1.85 billion USD to be used as funds for emergency resource deployment and an additional 5.8 billion USD for emergency preparation and response against the influenza pandemic.[34] In September, the Congress went on to make 1444 million USD available to states and hospitals for carrying out vaccination programs.[35] Meanwhile, the United States Agency for International Development (USAID) provided Mexico with five million USD in emergency aid funds, 900,000 sets of personal protective equipment for virus monitoring personnel, and Tamiflu for 400,000 courses of treatment. Additionally, the HHS provided 147 countries with 769 laboratory diagnostic kits, and donated to the Pan American Health Organization (PAHO) medications for 420,000 courses of treatment in aid of Latin American and Caribbean countries.

In Australia, funds for prevention and control against Influenza A (H1N1) originated mainly from the federal government, which was used specifically for monitoring pandemic development, stockpiling and distributing antiviral drugs, training medical personnel, providing free vaccinations for citizens, and assisting developing countries with prevention and control efforts. The federal government spent 43 million USD on antiviral drugs, 1.4 million USD on the purchasing of automatic detection equipment for the National Influenza Center and other public health laboratories, 4 million USD on training general practitioners across the country, and 3 million USD on a donation to the WHO which was used in aiding developing countries, especially those neighboring Australia, with pandemic monitoring, detection, preparation and response.

In the United Kingdom, funds for responding to Influenza A (H1N1) came mainly from the British government; by January 20th, 2010, the Department of Health had dispensed to the nation 1.26 million doses of Pandemrix, an influenza vaccine developed by GlaxoSmithKline, and 370,000 doses of a Baxter-developed vaccines.[36]

The Indian government established a one billion rupee disaster response fund in accordance with the *Disaster Management Act*, which was administered by the Ministry of Home Affairs, and this disaster fund accepted donations from individuals and organizations. In addition, a national disaster fund was specifically established to finance disaster relief and recovery efforts. State governments also

---

[34]William Corr (2009).

[35]See Footnote 29.

[36]DH. Pandemic H1N1 (2009) Influenza: Chief Medical Officer's Fortnightly Bulletin for Journalists. 21 January 2010.

established disaster response funds and relief funds in accordance with the law at the state and regional levels.[37]

Mexico invested a total of 350 million USD in Influenza A (H1N1) preparation and response, including the purchasing of drugs and vaccines, and the adoption of other prevention and control efforts.[38]

2.3.2 *National Prevention and Control Policies and Measures*

2.3.2.1 Outbreak of the Influenza Pandemic

Pandemic Outbreak Alert

After the outbreak of the Influenza A (H1N1) Pandemic, some countries, in accordance with WHO pandemic alert phases as well as their domestic situations, initiated and adjusted their pandemic alert levels. The United States, for example, declared a public health emergency on April 26th, 2009, and made several updates afterwards[39] until the stage of emergency was lifted on June 23rd, 2010.[40] Declaring a state of emergency helped the HHS prepare for and respond to the influenza pandemic, and prompted the Food and Drug Administration (FDA) to issue Emergency Use Authorizations (EUAs) for the use of antiviral drugs and therapeutic tools—i.e. they approved the use of Relenza and Tamiflu as stockpiled antiviral drugs for prevention and control of the virus, RT-PCR for virus detection, and N95 masks, which protected pandemic-affected communities. On April 29th, 2009, in light of the WHO's pandemic alert phases and its national pandemic situation, Singapore raised their alert level in its five-level disease warning system from Green to Yellow, and again to Orange the next day.

Inspection and Quarantine

To prevent the influenza virus from spreading into and circulating within their territories, many countries adopted strict inspection and quarantine measures in the early days of the pandemic. The United States screened travelers from Mexico and other countries, conducting both temperature and medical inspections. Cargo—especially

---

[37]Xiaoming (2009).

[38]Mexico Announces Pandemic Influenza Alert Removed. http://www.chinadaily.com.cn/micro-reading/mfeed/hotwords/20100811734.html.

[39]See Footnote 34.

[40]HHS declares public health emergency for swine flu. April 26, 2009. http://www.hhs.gov/news/press/2009pres/04/20090426a.html.

baggage and raw meat products from epidemic affected areas—were strictly quarantined; many airlines required their service staff to observe and question passengers suspected of illness, and when necessary, have them examined. American border officials between the United States and Mexico also were required to examine the physical condition of travelers crossing the border and be prepared to take necessary measures. Additionally, citizens were asked to stop all unnecessary travel into epidemic areas.

Australia also implemented strict border control, requiring all flights from the Americas to report the health status of passengers on board before landing; any individual with influenza-like symptoms had to be assessed by Australian quarantine authorities in order to determine if further treatment was required; eight major airports across the country were equipped with body temperature measuring instruments, and every incoming passenger was required to complete a health declaration card.

India adopted pandemic monitoring measures at airports, sea ports, and inland ports across the country; all incoming passengers to the twenty two international airports were screened, especially those from epidemic areas or with influenza symptoms, who were then quarantined and treated for at least three days. Medical personnel were trained in advance, and were required to wear masks, gloves, and protective clothing at work. Influenza A (H1N1) inspection standards and operational rules were formulated and implemented national widely at that time.

Japan's Ministry of Health, Labor and Welfare required all flights from Mexico, United States, and Canada arriving at the Narita, Kansai and Chūbu Centrair International Airports be inspected while aboard the plane. Local airports not included on the list of airports for quarantine measures, for example in Niigata, Akita and Hiroshima, also decided to follow suit and expanded the scope of quarantine to include flights from South Korea, Hong Kong, and some other countries and regions. Japanese border inspection and quarantine authorities screened people from Mexico, the United States and had cargo strictly quarantined, especially baggage and raw meat products from epidemic areas.

Preparedness

While applying strict control measures against the importation of the virus, in the early days of the pandemic countries also began strengthening preparation capacity building. For example, in the United States, during the initial stage of the outbreak, the HHS dispensed medication from the Strategic National Stockpile enough to treat three million people, the Department of Defense (DOD) separately readied enough medication for seven million soldiers, and the CDC allocated antiviral drugs, protective equipment, and testing kits. At the same time, the HHS provided training for medical personnel with the goal of enhancing their abilities in treating and handling the pandemic. The German government required each state to stockpile enough antiviral drugs to use for 20% of their populations. South Korea increased budget spending so that by the end of October the country's had enough drugs stored for 10% of its population. In an effort to mitigate the spread of the virus, the Indian government designated specific hospitals to treat Influenza A (H1N1) cases.

Health Education

To increase public awareness of the pandemic, countries developed large scale health education and communication projects. The U.S. CDC provided health recommendations to society, communities, clinical workers and other professionals, and launched an online live-broadcast health education program, "Know What to Do about the Flu," to help strengthen the public's abilities in protecting themselves against the virus. The United Kingdom updated pandemic situations and work priorities on a regular basis via an official government website, and provided technical support relating to virus prevention and treatment. India published a "public notice' through national media channels with the aim of disseminating knowledge and increasing public awareness of Influenza A (H1N1) prevention and control. The government also set up a toll-free service hotline to answer questions about the influenza pandemic. In Japan, an information, education and communication campaign was launched targeting high-risk groups of people arriving at and departing from the country's international airports, and the Ministry of Health, Labour and Welfare opened an information window to answer questions from the public.

2.3.2.2 The Spread of the Influenza Pandemic

Focusing on Clinical Treatment

As the pandemic developed and more cases emerged, it was found that the majority of cases were coming from local communities instead of from abroad. At this point in time, the continued use of containment strategies had been ineffective, and medical personnel were having to dedicate more time and energy to the increasing number of patients.

According to the National Response Framework, the HHS in the United States needed to stockpile enough antiviral drugs for one-fourth of the country's population during the pandemic, and to prepare at least six million treatment courses during the pandemic's initial phase. In the spring of 2009, the HHS allocated eleven million treatment courses that could be used for rapid response against the pandemic. The CDC and the FDA also worked together to address potential options for treatment of severely hospitalized patients.[41] In October, the HHS shipped an additional 300,000 bottles of the antiviral oseltamivir in oral suspension formula to

---

[41] Anna Schuchat (2009a).

states in order to mitigate a predicted national shortage. The FDA worked closely with the CDC, the Office of the Assistant Secretary for Preparedness and Response (ASPR), manufacturers, and others to increase production and availability of personal protective equipment such as gloves, masks, and respirators. At the same time, the 2009 Influenza (H1N1) Consumer Protection Team, established by the FDA, put in place an aggressive strategy to combat fraudulent influenza products.[42]

The British Secretary of State for Health declared on July 2nd, 2009, that the United Kingdom's response efforts were transitioning from a "containment phase" to a "treatment phase." In order to cure patients more efficiently, the British government created a national stockpile by the purchasing of more antiviral drugs, and drug distribution centers were also established across the country, with the National Health Service (NHS) playing a leading role in treatment provisions. To relieve pressure on medical institutions, on July 23rd, 2009, the British government launched the National Pandemic Flu Service (NPFS).[43] The NPFS was a self-help healthcare system which, through a dedicated website and call centers, provided people worried about flu-like symptoms with professional assessment services, including the suggestions on whether they should receive treatment or contact a general practitioner, etc. A person, if assessed as indeed having Influenza A (H1N1) symptoms, would be given an authorization number by the system, which he or she could use to pick up antiviral drugs from one of local distributions centers. The launch of this system effectively mitigated the pressure on primary healthcare institutions and allowed general practitioners to dedicate their attention to critically ill patients.

In order to quickly detect and treat critically ill patients, and also to ensure an adequate number of hospital beds as the number of cases increased, the Japanese government readjusted its guidelines on pandemic response efforts, and discarded the practice of classifying regions according to rate of transmission in that area. According to the revised guidelines, regular hospitals received patients infected with Influenza A (H1N1); all mildly ill patients were instructed to medicate and rest at home, rather than being hospitalized. For patients with asthma or other illnesses whom had contracted Influenza A (H1N1) and whose conditions were likely to worsen, a PCR (polymerase chain reaction) test or other Influenza A virus test was performed, and effective antiviral drugs were administered as early as possible. When necessary, decisions would be made to get them hospitalized. Japan gradually used the confirmed cases reported from a certain number of hospitals as estimations and predictions for that area's infected population.

Australia used antiviral drugs from their national medical stockpile to treat moderately and critically ill patients, especially those with severe breathing difficulties or those whose conditions were rapidly worsening. All medical personnel, who contracted Influenza A (H1N1) and developed moderate symptoms of

---

[42]Jesse Goodman (2009).

[43]DH. Launch of the National Pandemic Flu Service. http://webarchive.nationalarchives.gov.uk/+/www.dh.gov.uk/en/Publichealth/Flu/Swineflu/DH_102909.

infection, or were more prone to develop serious symptoms, were eligible for antiviral treatment. Patients with fairly mild symptoms were encouraged to self-medicate.

India issued clinical management guidelines, where the Indian Committee on Infectious Diseases published guidance on the screening and clinical treatment of laboratory-diagnosed cases of Influenza A (H1N1); the Ministry of Health and Family Welfare issued guidelines on family isolation, clinical examinations, and hospitalization by categories of Influenza A (H1N1) cases—where Categories A/B patients were asked to be isolated and reduce contact with their family and others and Category C patients required immediate hospitalization. All suspected cases were tested at the National Institute of Communicable Diseases (NICD) in New Delhi, or at the National Institute of Virology in Pune, and then examined further at relevant laboratories. India currently has forty four laboratories dedicated to the early management of controlling confirmed cases.[44]

Policies for Community-based Non-drug Pandemic Mitigation

Given the dynamic nature of the pandemic, involving each and every citizen in its mitigation became a very important part of global response efforts.

To contain the pandemic, Mexico mobilized a large force of police officers and soldiers to execute the following: distribute masks among citizens for free, shut down public places, cancel or delay large-scale events, halt teaching activities in all schools—including universities, primary and secondary schools, and kindergartens —in Mexico City and in the State of Mexico. On April 29th, 2009, the Mexican government declared a suspension of all nonessential public affairs and economic activities from May 1st through May 5th. Moreover, the Mexican government also adopted a wide range of measures to strengthen pandemic information communication and sharing, i.e.: reporting pandemic developments via media channels, setting up 800 hotlines, launching influenza prevention websites, giving out leaflets on pandemic information that called for personal hygiene and increased public awareness of the virus.[45]

In the United States, the HSS launched a one-stop influenza information website (www.flu.gov), which gathered information from regular media briefings conducted by the HHS and other federal agencies,[46] and provided the public with scientific and effective information services. In collaboration with federal, state, and local partners, the HHS also developed a wide range of community-based intervention guidelines which were being evaluated simultaneously. The CDC and the DHS provided specific recommendations targeted to a wide variety of groups, including the general public, people with certain underlying health conditions, infants, children, parents,

---

[44]John and Moorthy (2010).
[45]Del Rio and Hernandez-Avila (2009).
[46]See Footnote 41.

pregnant women, seniors, health care workers, workers in relevant industries, laboratory workers, and homeless people. With these recommendations, people were equipped to take appropriate action in reducing the transmission of the virus, especially in early autumn before vaccines were widely disseminated. The CDC also provided, and updated on a regular basis, scientific guidance on influenza prevention and control to schools, daycares, universities, large and small businesses, and federal agencies. These comprehensive guidelines provided not only advice on how individuals and institutions could protect themselves against the virus and mitigate its spread, but also recommendations for healthcare providers about the appropriate use of anti-viral drugs, especially in treating patients who were at the highest risk of suffering complications from the influenza.[47,48]

In Japan, after the alert level transitioned from an "overseas pandemic" phase to the heightened "early onset of a domestic pandemic" phase, the local governments of Osaka and Hyōgo Prefectures required the following for areas where infections had occurred: gatherings and collective recreational activities be suspended, entertainment venues be temporarily closed, social service workers be required to wear masks, teaching activities of varying levels at more than one thousand educational institutions be suspended for one week, citizens avoid trips and gatherings, and business activity be reduced for the time being.

In Australia, patients with mild symptoms were allowed to stay at home as a means of isolation.

Revising Pandemic Monitoring

With the rapid spread of the pandemic, the United States didn't take stock in counting cases, but instead focused on the evolution process of the virus.[49] The United States' advanced and unique monitoring system for bacteria and viruses uses dynamic and standardized methods to collect data related to virus occurrence, virus developments, and basic medical trends, and employs national demographic data to compute virus incidence and describe its epidemiological characteristics. This system brings together and facilitates cooperation within the CDC, state health authorities, academic partners, hospitals and infection control centers. Moreover, it contains special research platforms, i.e., socio-economic evaluations of disease risk factors, effects of the disease and vaccinations, data on resources for vaccine research and development, and data on approved vaccines.

In Australia, laboratory testing focused on critically ill patients, high-risk groups with severe diseases, and personnel in relevant institutions. Monitoring was also conducted to see if any resistance or mutations of the virus had occurred.

---

[47]See Footnote 29.
[48]See Footnote 41.
[49]United States Becomes Eye of Pandemic Influenza Storm, Puts out But Not Protect against Fire. Ecns.cn, May 19, 2009. http://news.xinhuanet.com/world/2009-05/19/content_11398140.htm.

Vaccine Development and Inoculation

Understanding that vaccinations were the best means for combatting the virus, countries focused a large amount of resources on vaccination development and inoculation methods.

In its influenza pandemic preparedness and response plan, the HHS in the United States set two objectives for vaccine preparation[50]: to stockpile twenty million vaccinations for key personnel, and to increase manufacturing capacity to cover the population in the United States, in other words, produce 300 million doses within six months of the pandemic outbreak. Immediately following the outbreak, the National Institute of Allergy and Infectious Diseases (NIAID) subordinate to the U.S. National Institutes of Health (NIH) began its research on the virus and vaccination development. In July 2009, the NIAID initiated a series of clinical trials on the effectiveness of newly developed vaccines. In September, the FDA approved manufacturing for four vaccination types, which were then made available for distribution among the states. The federal government then identified priority groups for vaccination and formulated an inoculation policy.[51] Starting on October 5th, a national Influenza A (H1N1) voluntary inoculation program begun targeting high-priority groups including pregnant women; people between the ages of 6 months through 24 years of age; people aged 65 years or older with chronic health disorders like asthma, diabetes and heart disease; and healthcare and emergency services personnel.[52] During the two months that followed, vaccine manufacturers provided 10–20 million vaccination doses each week, an amount which reached roughly 250 million by the end of 2009.[53,54] According to statistics, the federal government ordered a total of 229 million doses of the vaccine with the plans of vaccinating 158 million people, and in the end 90 million people were actually inoculated.

On October 21st, 2009, the United Kingdom launched its national Influenza A (H1N1) inoculation program. The first phase of the plan provided the vaccine to the high risk population of fourteen million people, including critically ill patients, pregnant women, and healthcare personnel working in hospitals. Soon afterwards, general practitioners across the country began encouraging people with health disorders or immunity problems, and pregnant women to get vaccinated. On December 8th, 2009, the British government went on to include children ages six months to five years old in the vaccination program.

---

[50]See Footnote 30.

[51]See Footnote 41.

[52]See Footnote 30.

[53]President Obama Declares a National Influenza A (H1N1) Emergency. Ecns.cn, October 25, 2009. http://medicine.people.com.cn/GB/10252536.html.

[54]EU Approves First Influenza A (H1N1) Vaccines. CRI Online, September 30, 2009. http://news.sina.com.cn/w/2009-09-30/024718754642.shtml.

In August 2009, Australia approved a national vaccination program and began providing free vaccinations to healthcare workers, pregnant women, and individuals with chronic health disorders who were susceptible to the virus. On September 30th, the Australian government announced that all adults and children aged ten years and older could also receive free vaccinations.

In May 2009, the Mexican government announced an appropriation of 6.2 million USD for the establishment of a dedicated committee composed of 12 authoritative medical experts, and this committee's mission was to mobilize and coordinate research efforts for carrying out etiological, epidemiological, diagnostic reagent and vaccine research relating to Influenza A (H1N1). It was also responsible for providing policy recommendations on pandemic prevention and control and medical treatment options to the government.[55]

In July 2009 Japan began distributing permits authorizing the utilization of Influenza A (H1N1) vaccines, and they also launched a national vaccination program. The first groups to receive it included healthcare personnel, police officers, as well as high-risk groups like pregnant women, patients with chronic diseases, and seniors.

2.3.2.3 Post-peak Period

As Influenza A (H1N1) cases gradually declined, some countries readjusted their pandemic response levels as well as their measures for virus prevention, control, and treatment. Countries set about making summaries and conducting evaluations while continuing their pandemic monitoring and information sharing.

Readjusting Alert Levels and Measures for Virus Prevention and Control

In 2010, most regions across the globe saw a decline in Influenza A (H1N1) activity, and though in some regions the virus still sustained its intensity (level), the overall virus transmission dropped. Additionally, it was discovered in most cases that the Influenza A virus only caused mild infections, and that its virulence had not increased since it was first reported in April 2009. Effective vaccinations had been in circulation since November 2009. It was for these reasons that the Singaporean Ministry of Health decided on February 12th, 2010, to downgrade its alert level from Yellow to Green.

Beginning in February 2010, the United Kingdom deactivated the National Pandemic Flu Service (NPFS), an act done in line with ensuring the operational response was appropriate to the threat level posed by the virus and also because general practitioners and primary care trusts could now manage the clinical

---

[55]Mexico Sets up Special Committee for Influenza A (H1N1) Research. Xinhuanet.com, May 12, 2009. http://news.xinhuanet.com/world/2009-05/12/content_11357428.htm.

caseload by themselves.[56] Anyone concerned about flu-like symptoms were advised to contact their doctor for assessment, who could then issue an antiviral authorization voucher if needed. The NPFS would be reactivated should the pandemic virus regained its virulence. Starting on April 1st, 2010, free antiviral medication from the national stockpile was no longer available to patients with Influenza A (H1N1). Normal treatments and prescription charges were reinstated for those suffering from influenza.[57]

In June 2010, the United States declared the end of the public health emergency.

Expanding Vaccination Coverage

As confirmed cases declined and the spread of the virus continued to slow, the U.S. federal, state, and local health authorities began to readjust their response strategies. In addition to continued efforts in strengthening public health education and inter-agency collaboration, other measures included bolstering the vaccination campaign,[58] strengthening virus monitoring, and continuing focus on virus mutations.

Commencing Summarized Pandemic Evaluations

As the pandemic developed in the United States, especially after the wide distribution of vaccinations to the public, some U.S. agencies and institutions evaluated the results of a range of their prevention and control measures. The purpose of these evaluations were to identify problems that existed in the national pandemic response measures, and correct them to better the response in the future. For example, the Institute of Medicine (IOM) Forum on Microbial Threats analyzed the domestic and global impact of the Influenza A (H1N1) pandemic, while the Department of Defense (DOD) and the Global Emerging Infections Surveillance (GEIS) reviewed influenza response programs, including management and planning, monitoring, laboratory research, response capacity, capacity building, collaboration and coordination, guidance, contact lists, contingency plans, and so on. The evaluation report, *Sustaining Global Surveillance and Response to Emerging Zoonotic Diseases*, analyzed global influenza A (H1N1) detection, reporting, and response systems, and expounded upon shortcomings and challenges surrounding the pandemic. On March 5th, 2010, the University of Pittsburgh Medical Center's

---

[56]Written Ministerial Statement announcing National Pandemic Flu Service to stand down. http://collections.europarchive.org/tna/20100509080731/,   http://dh.gov.uk/en/Publichealth/Flu/Swineflu/DH_111890.

[57]Pandemic H1N1: stand down of the antiviral distribution arrangements. http://www.dh.gov.uk/en/Publicationsandstatistics/Lettersandcirculars/Dearcolleagueletters/DH_114769.

[58]The United States Advertises Public Vaccination against Influenza A Virus. Evening News, December 8, 2009. http://news.sina.com.cn/h/2009-12-08/124319215143.shtml.

(UPMC's) Center for Biosecurity held a conference to summarize important lessons learned from pandemic responses and raised policy suggestions in mitigating future infectious disease emergencies. On May 4–5th, 2010, the CDC, the National Association of County and City Health Officials (NACCHO), and other stakeholders met to review the federal, state and local policies that had an impact on local health departments' pandemic detection, response, and recovery efforts.

2.4 An Overall Analysis of Global Prevention and Control for the Influenza Pandemic

While modernized health care systems, antiviral drugs and vaccines represented the advantages of global response efforts this time around, factors like globalization and urbanization allowed the fastest transmission of any pandemic ever witnessed. After outbreaks occurred in multiple countries, governments worldwide immediately adopted a wide variety of proactive containment measures. While there were many successful responses, shortcomings were also exposed which incited doubt and controversy surrounding the pandemic.

2.4.1 General Characteristics of Global Prevention and Control

2.4.1.1 Governments Played Proactive, Even Leading Roles in Response Efforts

In regards to prevention and control measures, governments in most of the affected countries did not look lightly upon the pandemic, and they played leading roles in policy making, resource collection and allocation, as well as organization and coordination. Firstly, governments identified and allocated prevention and control organizations and accountability mechanisms at the national level. As mentioned before, some countries such as the United Kingdom and India specifically established bodies for comprehensive coordination in response to the influenza pandemic, while others like the United States—where established emergency response agencies were already in existence—launched their emergency response efforts upon the outbreak of the pandemic. The U.S. government then oversaw an organized response from varying agencies. Secondly, countries developed national-level pandemic strategies or response plans as general outlines for prevention and control efforts. Thirdly, funds for response efforts in most cases originated from the central government, where the capital was then allocated to appropriate departments based upon their responsibilities. Lastly, central governments were in charge of across-the-board organization and coordination in all aspects of the response efforts, especially in the provision of services, drug supplies, and vaccinations, while at the same time playing a crucial role in communication and coordination with other social service organizations, businesses, and the general public.

2.4.1.2   WHO Facilitated Global Coordination and Guidance

In the course of global responses to the sudden outbreak of the influenza pandemic, the WHO made good use of its expertise and networking strengths. With a global approach, the organization disseminated information, pushed coordination, and strengthened guidelines. It played an important role in coordinating and guiding countries' efforts to raise awareness, develop technical guidance, release pandemic information, develop vaccines, etc.

2.4.1.3   Most Countries Emphasized Domestic Collaboration in Pandemic Response Efforts

Most countries possessed an influenza prevention and control system comprised of a variety of collaborative relationships, i.e.: partnerships between central, provincial (state), and local governments, the private sector, and individuals, as well as international partnerships established through bilateral or multilateral collaboration. Each party within this system had its function and standard operating procedures, with the division of labor already institutionalized; and in implementing specific prevention and control measures, these parties were expected to fulfill their expectations and duties as stakeholders. Each stakeholder understood their role to play during the preparation, prevention, and control of the pandemic, and no major changes occurred in that respect during the pandemic. At the same time, capacity building and positioning was constantly being improved according to the different functions of each party. In addition to inter-departmental coordination and collaboration, countries like the United States also called upon the public for participation and global collaboration, which expanded collaboration as it brought in community and societal involvement.

2.4.1.4   Most Countries Focused on Policy Adjustments in Prevention and Control

During different phases of the pandemic, countries emphasized the integration of comprehensive measures and key response issues, and efforts were adjusted according to the development of the pandemic. In the early phases, prevention and control strategies were "strict," as they focused largely on containment with inspection and quarantine measures. Cases diagnosed early were treated in a timely manner to better the odds of developing a successful vaccination. At the spreading period of the pandemic, the focus shifted to clinical treatment of patients, alongside strengthening virus monitoring. During the post-peak period, while some countries quickly revised alert levels which reduced social impact, others had no readjustment mechanisms for policy changes in place which resulted in inefficient prevention and control.

2.4.1.5 Most Countries Emphasized International and Bilateral Collaboration

During this time, most countries recognized the importance of international collaboration. Firstly, faced with the grim situation of a pandemic gripping the globe, affected countries followed the WHO's pandemic strategies and recommendations. Combining the domestic situation with WHO's proactive policies and recommendations, most countries adopted relevant response measures. However, there were many countries that didn't adopt all of the WHO's policies and recommendation, nor did they follow all of the policy readjustments. Instead in light of their domestic situation, governments formulated their own response strategies and measures. Secondly, relatively close collaboration between countries did occur. The United States, for instance, deployed 16 personnel to Mexico including experts in influenza epidemiology, laboratory, health communications, emergency operations, information technology and veterinary sciences, who worked under PAHO, the WHO and a trilateral team of Mexican, Canadian and American experts.[59] The personnel provided both technical support on the epidemiology of the virus as well as laboratory support for confirmed cases. Japan donated 100 million Japanese Yen worth of emergency materials to Mexico—the country hit the hardest by the pandemic—including 190,000 masks, 3000 pairs of goggles, 3000 surgical gowns, 3000 pairs of surgical gloves, and 1370 bottles of disinfectant agents.

2.4.1.6 Some Countries Focused on Risk Communication

Strengthening risk communication has increasingly become an important part of public health emergency management. The United States' routine monitoring system provided a good foundation for risk communication. Its fast multidisciplinary information sharing, multi-level public communication (national and local), and online information management and dissemination, were crucial in coordinating programs and carrying out public health emergency management and response efforts among federal agencies and departments. The HHS continued to develop and strengthen communication as it was an important part of the public health response efforts,[60] this included broad distribution of public service announcements, news reports, and other traditional media, use of social media such

---

[59]Anna Schuchat (2009b).
[60]See Footnote 30.

as podcasts and blogs, and frequent phone conferences. The HHS issued a series of risk communication guidance documents like *Communicating in a Crisis: Risk Communication Guidelines for Public Officials*. Working with the DHS, the HHS also developed a *National Situation Report*, which was published on the DHS' website. That being said, most other countries didn't possess such robust epidemic monitoring and information collection systems, and so governments' timely explanations and communication took the forefront in response efforts. For example, India's Ministry of Health and Family Welfare appointed officials to announce latest developments to the public, disseminate public health information such as disease-related risks, personal protection measures and disease prevention guidelines via media and leaflets, and launch round-the-clock hotlines to provide citizens with pandemic guidance and facilitate the reporting of influenza cases.

2.4.2   Controversy over WHO Response and National Prevention and Control Strategies and Measures

2.4.2.1   Controversies surrounding the appropriateness of the countries' prevention and control strategies

Due to the many uncertainties surrounding the occurrence and development of the Influenza A (H1N1) pandemic, the level of "appropriateness" of response strategies —i.e. were they considered "lax" or "strict," "ineffective" or "overreacting"— became a major controversial point surrounding the pandemic prevention and control policy.

On the one hand, based on their own pandemic situations, their preparation evaluation, and cost-benefit analyses, developed countries such as the United States, Canada, the United Kingdom, and France, adopted policies that focused more on treatment than on control. The United States, for example, in the early days of the pandemic considered Influenza A (H1N1) no bigger a threat than the seasonal influenza, so the government failed to take strict response measures, like quarantine and medical observation, which resulted in a spike in domestic infections. On October 23rd, 2009 the United States declared a national health emergency, sparking questions about the government's response efforts. While some critics questioned whether there indeed existed such an emergency, others argued that a state of emergency should have been declared from the very beginning. An article published in the *New York Times* in early January 2010, gave full recognition to the country's response strategy, insisting that apart from luck, the federal government's appropriate, rapid, and conservative response successfully contained the virus and minimized potential harmful effects it could've had on the economy.

On the other hand, some countries began with strict measures and relaxed them later on, causing difficulties in latent response efforts. For example, countries like Mexico declared a state of high alert immediately upon the outbreak, leading to a certain extent, a public panic. But after the WHO elevated the pandemic alert phase, the Mexican government rushed to lower its domestic alert level in order to ease public anxiety. Thus the public became careless, causing the increased transmission rate.

Moreover, media in Japan, France and other countries exaggerated pandemic situations that embellished "the widespread transmission" of the virus in home countries through imported cases. People became panic-stricken and it became increasingly difficult to implement proper response measures. Japan and other countries failed in resource management as they placed too much emphasis on border control and quarantine, and not enough on domestic control and detection, thus making it difficult to contain the spread of the pandemic. These actions also led to widespread criticism of government response efforts.

2.4.2.2 Controversy over the WHO's Response

Though the WHO's role in the global pandemic response efforts was widely recognized, the organization also suffered criticism as there were varied opinions about the timeliness of alert level changes and their investments in personnel and equipment. Reuters reported on April 12th, 2010, that the WHO admitted to having problems in their response efforts, including its failure to communicate the uncertainty of the new virus before it swept the globe. Some critics held that from the perspective of pandemic development, the Influenza A (H1N1) pandemic was not as dreadful as it was initially anticipated, and it was the WHO that created a global panic in its response—which caused an excess in vaccination stockpiling among some countries. Some even suspected that the IHR Emergency Committee might have had an "affair" with some drug manufacturers and was suspected of helping them seek profit by deliberately exaggerating pandemic situations so that the WHO would raise its pandemic alert to the highest level.[61] In response, on April 12th, 2010, the WHO commissioned a panel of external experts to conduct an overall evaluation of the global response to the influenza pandemic in the hope of providing lessons for the future, and simultaneously to assess the global implementation of the IHR 2005. The WHO's policy evaluation comprised three main parts, i.e. capacity and preparedness, pandemic alert and risk assessment, and response. On June 10th, 2010, the WHO officially responded to and clarified such issues as to the Influenza A (H1N1) virus met the criteria for a pandemic, the severity of the pandemic, and related conflicts of interest.[62]

---

[61]Central People's Government of the People's Republic of China. WHO Experts Warn Global H1N1 Pandemic Still Not Over Yet. http://www.gov.cn/jrzg/2010-04/15/content_1581776.htm.

[62]WHO. The international response to the influenza pandemic: WHO responds to the critics. http://www.who.int/csr/disease/swineflu/notes/briefing_20100610/en/index.html.

2.4.2.3 Controversy over Vaccine and Antiviral Drug Policies and Technology

There are no international standards for vaccine allocation in mitigating the global burden of disease. While the United States began vaccinating its citizens in early October 2009 after the FDA approved on September 15th the marketing of Influenza A (H1N1) vaccines produced by CSL, MedImmune, Novartis Vaccines and Diagnostics, and Sanofi Pasteur, Mexico, which had been suffering a severer pandemic situation, was unable to launch a vaccination program until January 2010. Building a powerful global vaccine production infrastructure for influenza pandemics where countries and regions in need could acquire adequate vaccines at affordable prices became one of the hot international topics at this time.

The WHO stated that although antiviral drugs used at that time to combat influenza enjoyed complete patent protection, the organization proposed that these drugs be acquirable in the cases of public health crises. The use of antiviral drugs was hit heavily upon in the WHO's guidance documents, but, given cost issues, the use of such drugs and vaccines had little operability in most middle and low-income countries.

Moreover, some international media held that the outbreak in the United States brought to the forefront the many flaws in their healthcare system, most notably the use of old-fashioned vaccine technology and excessive reliance on vaccine manufacturers abroad. A highly controversial event also occurred during vaccination distribution: The New York City Department of Health and Mental Hygiene decided to give the small amount of vaccine available in the early phases of the pandemic to big corporations on Wall Street such as Goldman Sachs and Citibank, an act which experts believe only exacerbated public relation issues. Vaccine production and distribution became a controversial focal point during prevention and control of the pandemic as it involved multi-faceted issues such as vaccine patents, mass psychology, and social justice.

References

Anne Schuchat, M. D. (2009a). *H1N1 preparedness: An overview of vaccine production and distribution*, November 18, 2009. http://www.hhs.gov/asl/testify/2009/11/t20091118b.html.

Anne Schuchat, M. D. (2009b). *U.S. global health response to a novel 2009-H1N1*, May 6, 2009. http://www.hhs.gov/asl/testify/2009/05/t20090506b.html.

Craig Vanderwagen, W. (2009). *HHS' effort to provide science-based pandemic influenza guidance for the U.S. workforce*, June 16, 2009. http://www.hhs.gov/asl/testify/2009/06/t20090616b.html.

Del Rio, C., & Hernandez-Avila, M. (2009). Lessons from previous influenza pandemics and from the Mexican response to the current influenza pandemic. *Arch Med Res, 40,* 677–680.

Jesse Goodman, M. D. (2009). *H1N1 preparedness: An overview of vaccine production and distribution*, November 18, 2009. http://www.hhs.gov/asl/testify/2009/11/t20091118a.html.

John, T. J., & Moorthy, M. (2010). 2009 pandemic influenza in India. *Indian Pediatrics, 47*(2010), 25–31.

Liu, G., & Yang, L. (2009) *WHO Director-General Margaret Chan says international community cannot afford to take influenza A (H1N1) pandemic lightly.* Xinhuanet.com, May 19, 2009. http://news.xinhuanet.com/world/2009-05/19/content_11397804_1.htm.

Sebellus, K. (2009a). *Preparing for the 2009–2010 influenza season*, September 15, 2009. http://www.hhs.gov/asl/testify/2009/09/t20090915a.html.

Sebellus, K. (2009b). *2009 H1N1 influenza: Monitoring the nation's response*, October 21, 2009. http://www.hhs.gov/asl/testify/2009/10/t20091021a.html.

Weissman, D. N. (2009). *Protecting the protectors: An assessment of front-line federal workers in response to the 2009-H1N1 influenza outbreak*, May 14, 2009. http://www.hhs.gov/asl/testify/2009/05/t20090514a.html.

WHO. (2009a). *Global surveillance during an influenza pandemic.* Version1, updated draft April 2009. http://www.who.int/csr/resources/publications/swineflu/surveillance/en/index.html.

WHO (2009b). *Assessing the severity of an influenza pandemic*, May 11, 2009. http://www.who.int/csr/disease/swineflu/assess/disease_swineflu_assess_20090511/en/index.html.

Willam Corr, J. D. (2009). *2009-H1N1 influenza: HHS preparedness and response efforts*, July 29, 2009. http://www.hhs.gov/asl/testify/2009/07/t20090729b.html.

Xiaoming, R. (2009). Characteristics of the India's public health emergency management system: From a perspective of influenza A (N1H1) preparedness and response. *Global Science, Technology and Economy Outlook*, Issue 7.

Zhang, Z. (2009) *Influenza A pandemic moves into a new phase, WHO changes way of epidemic reporting.* Xinhuanet.com, July 17, 2009. http://news.xinhuanet.com/newscenter/2009-07/17/content_11723758.htm.

Chapter 3
China's Prevention and Control and Policy Changes to the Influenza A (H1N1) Pandemic

3.1 Influenza A (H1N1) Epidemic in China: An Overview

The first case of Influenza A (H1N1) in China was found in Hong Kong, on May 1st, 2009, where the patient had flown from Mexico to Hong Kong via Shanghai. On May 11th, Sichuan Province reported the first imported Influenza A (H1N1) case in mainland China, and the first domestic case was reported on May 29th. In June, the epidemic spread from eastern provinces where there are more airports and land ports to the inland provinces (Fig. 3.1). By mid-August, most cases were imported and virus activity level was low. Beginning in late August, the epidemic spread rapidly and widely, with increasing outbreaks especially in primary and secondary schools. Cases peaked at the end of November, after which the epidemic tapered off. From mid-January 2010, the Influenza A (H1N1) virus had a lower share in influenza cases than Influenza B viruses. Beginning in April, Influenza A (H1N1) activity remained low, and there were fewer influenza outbreaks than in the same period of previous years. On August 10th, the WHO announced the Influenza A (H1N1) pandemic had moved into the post-pandemic period, which meant that global influenza activity—including Influenza A (H1N1)—had returned to normal seasonal levels.

3.1.1 Time Distribution for Confirmed Cases of Influenza A (H1N1)

By 24:00 p.m., August 29th, 2010, the national Influenza A (H1N1) information management system showed that a total of 128,080 confirmed cases had been reported across the country (excluding Hong Kong, Macao, and Taiwan; the same below), including 8349 severely ill cases (2785 critically ill) and 805 fatalities. Admittedly, however, due to a variety of factors such as the limitations of the

© Social Sciences Academic Press and Springer Nature Singapore Pte Ltd. 2019
L. Xue and G. Zeng, *A Comprehensive Evaluation on Emergency Response in China*, Research Series on the Chinese Dream and China's Development Path, https://doi.org/10.1007/978-981-13-0644-0_3

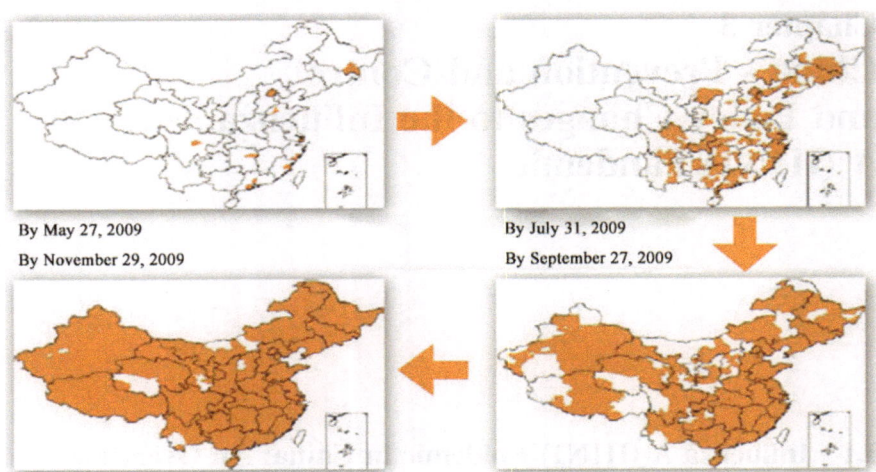

Fig. 3.1 Influenza A (H1N1) Virus Circulation in mainland China. *Source of data* Influenza A (H1N1) prevention and control (Special Issue on the 2010 Plenary Sessions of the National People's Congress and the National Committee of the Chinese People's Political Consultative Conference)

monitoring system, the accessibility of health care resources, the public's medical behaviors, specimen collecting and testing policies, and the limitations due to sensitivity and specificity of laboratory tests, confirmed cases in any country— including China—were much lower than the number of actually infected cases. The number of confirmed cases reported nationwide reached its peak (12,719) in the 48th week of 2009, and dropped rapidly afterwards. From the 14th through the 34th week of 2010 (from April 5th to August 29th), except for the 31st week during which 53 cases were reported, there were no more than 30 cases reported weekly (Fig. 3.2).

The first severely ill case in mainland China was reported in Guangdong on August 8th, 2009, and thereafter severely and critically ill cases were on the rise. After reaching its peak (1297) in the 49th week (December 6th) of 2009, the number of severely ill cases reported dropped. Beginning in the 4th week (January 31st) of 2010, the number of weekly severely ill cases reported fell below 100; from the 12th to the 17th week (March 22nd–May 2nd), except for the 14th week during which no severely ill cases were reported, the weekly number of severely ill cases reported was between one and seven; from the 18th to the 34th week (May 3rd– August 29th), no severely ill cases were reported except for the 21st, the 25th, and the 33rd week where one case was reported for each week (Fig. 3.3).

On October 4th, 2009, the first fatal case from Influenza A (H1N1) in mainland China was reported in the Tibet Autonomous Region. Reported fatalities peaked (at 119) in the 49th week (December 6th) of 2009 and tapered off thereafter. Beginning

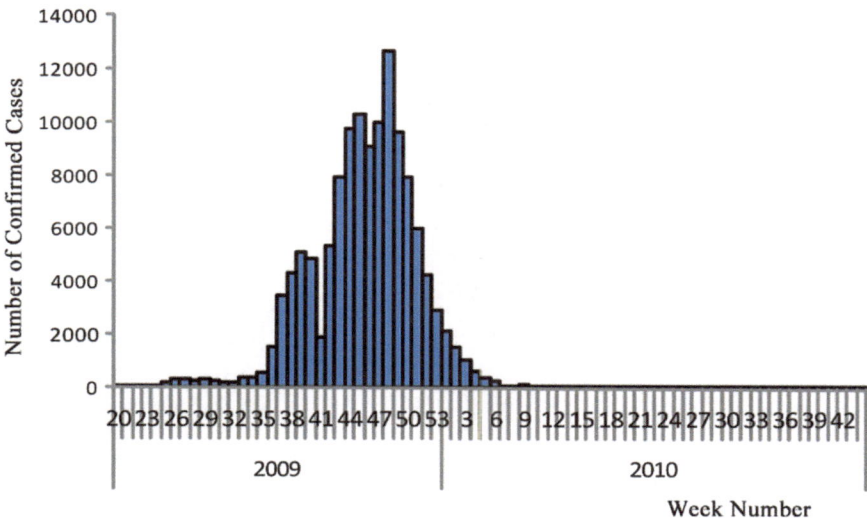

Fig. 3.2 Time distribution of confirmed cases in mainland China. *Source of data* Influenza monitoring weekly, 34th week, 2010

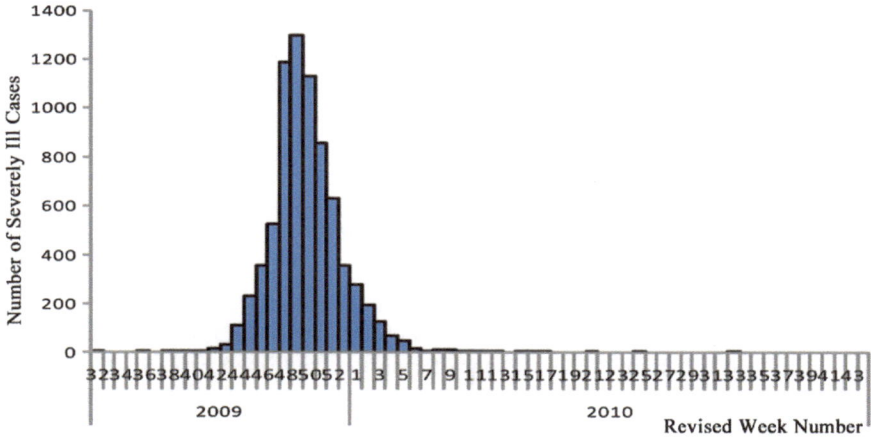

Fig. 3.3 Time distribution of severely Ill cases in Mainland China. *Source of data* Influenza monitoring weekly, 34th week, 2010

in the 6th week of 2010, fatalities reported were sporadic, ranging from zero to three cases per week. From the 19th week (May 16th) onwards, no fatalities were reported in the country for 16 consecutive weeks (Fig. 3.4).

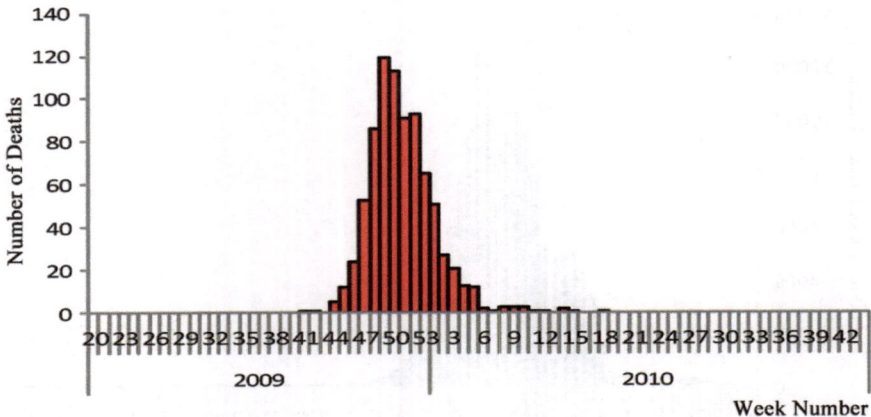

Fig. 3.4 Time distribution of fatalities in mainland China. *Source of data* Influenza monitoring weekly, 34th week, 2010

3.1.2 Age Distribution for Confirmed Cases

From the 18th week (May 3rd–9th) to the 53rd week (December 27th–31st) of 2009, a total of 118,096 laboratory confirmed cases were reported in China, over 90% of the patients aged between five and sixty-four years old. The age groups <5, 5–14, 15–64, and ≥ 65 accounted for 5.4, 42, 52, and 0.88% of the total confirmed cases.

3.1.3 Influenza A (H1N1) Fatality Rates

From the 18th to the 53rd week of 2009, the Influenza A (H1N1) epidemic in China had a case fatality rate (CFR) of 0.5%, which may have been overestimated as it was calculated by dividing the number of reported confirmed cases by the number of confirmed deaths. CFRs in this period for the age groups of <5, 5–14, 15–64, and ≥ 65 were 0.9, 0.1, 0.7, and 5.6%, respectively.

3.2 China's Response Strategies and Readjustments

At the end of April 2009, facing grim, complex situations in the wake of the global financial crisis and the outbreaks of Influenza A (H1N1), the Chinese government adopted the response principles and strategies of "focusing on, respond actively to, and coping with the epidemic scientifically and according to law through joint prevention and control mechanisms." Thereafter, specific prevention and control strategies were adopted and readjustments made appropriately in line with the different epidemic phases.

China's Influenza A (H1N1) prevention and control efforts can roughly be divided into six stages. Stage I, which occurred before April 25th, 2009 is characterized by pre-pandemic preparedness efforts. In Stage II, which lasted from April 25th to May 10th, 2009, alerts were issued and responses made, with the main strategies of containing imported cases and strengthening close contacts management. In Stage III, the initial epidemic stage which lasted from May 10th to August 30th, 2009, the response strategy was epidemic containment with anti-proliferation prevention and control measures. In Stage IV, the middle stage of the epidemic which lasted from September 2009 to mid-January 2010, local cases rose rapidly and the response strategy centered on epidemic containment and the strengthened treatment of severely ill patients. In Stage V, the post-epidemic stage which lasted from mid-January to August 9th, 2010, the number of cases fell rapidly, and the response strategy then focused on strengthening treatment of severely ill patients and stepping up etiological monitoring; evaluations on response efforts were conducted at this time. Stage VI began on August 10th, 2010, when the WHO announced the beginning of the post-pandemic period; in this stage, considering the reality of the epidemic, China readjusted its influenza monitoring strategy, optimized its influenza monitoring network, and improved overall monitoring quality (Figs. 3.5 and 3.6).

3.2.1   Pre-pandemic Preparedness Stage (Before April 25th, 2009)

After the 2003 SARS epidemic, China's public health service experienced rapid development, with a great amount of work done on influenza pandemic prevention

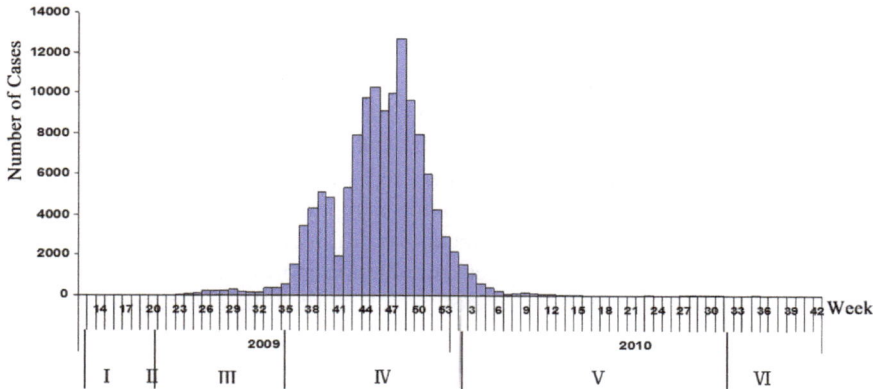

Fig. 3.5 Stages of Influenza A (H1N1) epidemic in China

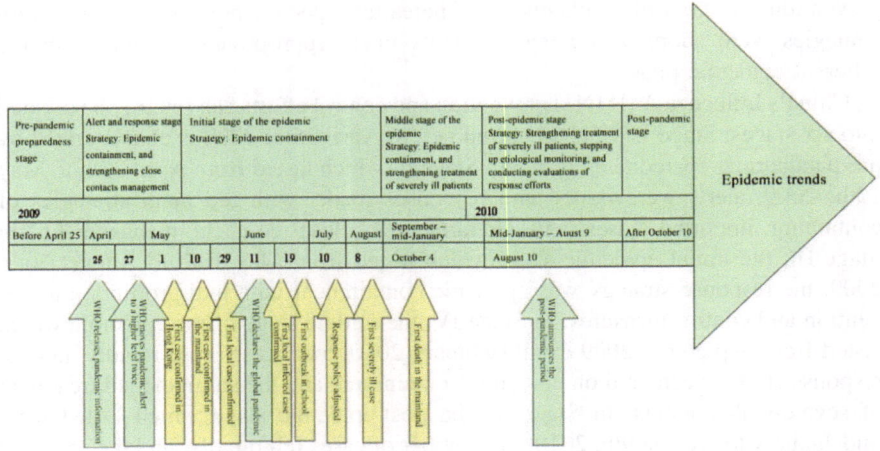

Fig. 3.6 Key epidemic developments in China

and preparedness. On the one hand, the government boosted public health development by making large improvements to the Chinese Center for Disease Control and Prevention (China CDC) and the construction of its monitoring system, strengthening field epidemiology training, developing contingency plans for public health emergencies, bolstering the leading role of the government in public health, and increasing epidemic information openness and transparency. On the other hand, pandemic preparedness efforts also became centered on contingency planning, and emergency prevention and response to the Avian Influenza, including the reinforcement of the influenza monitoring network, and the preparations to increase production capacity and materials for vaccines and antiviral drugs.

3.2.1.1   China CDC Construction and Monitoring System Development

In November 2003, the National Center for Disease Data Monitoring was built at China CDC, and on January 1st, 2004, the China Information System for Disease Control and Prevention was completed. In 2006, the MOH announced the completion of a public health information direct reporting network system. By the end of December 2008, centers for disease control and prevention (CDCs) in all regions of the country, 97% of county level and above health care institutions, and 82% of township-level health care centers were all able to report online infectious disease outbreaks and public health emergencies, which marked the completion of a basic public health emergency monitoring and reporting system. This newly constructed influenza monitoring network covered the entire country, and 63 network laboratories and 197 sentinel hospitals (including 31 rural sentinel points) were completed. Figure 3.7 shows the network structure.

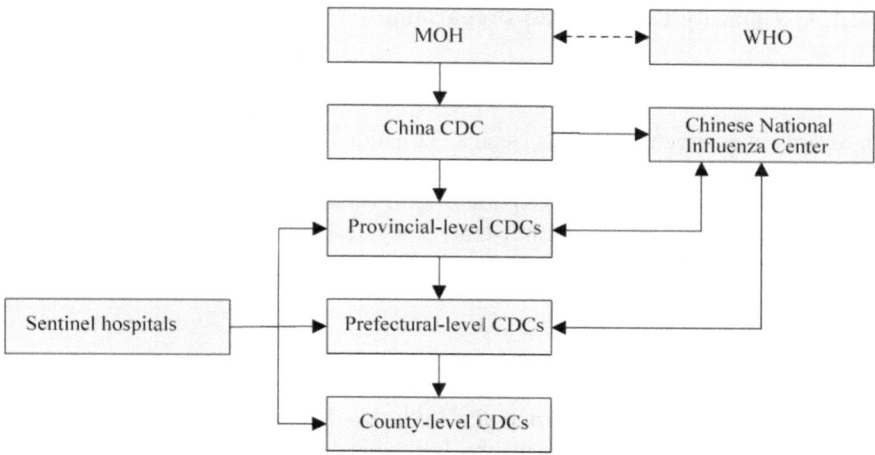

Fig. 3.7 Structure of China's influenza monitoring network

3.2.1.2   Preparedness for Pandemic Contingency Plans

During the 2003 SARS epidemic, the State Council urgently formulated and implemented the *Public Health Emergency Response Regulations*. In February 2004, it formulated and issued the *National Response Plan for the Highly Pathogenic Avian Influenza*, and in 2005 issued *the National General Response Plan for Public Health Emergencies* along with two specific emergency response plans—the *Public Health Emergency Response Plan* and the *National Health Emergency Plan for Public Emergencies*. On September 28th, 2005, the MOH promulgated the *Influenza Pandemic Preparedness and Response Plan of the Ministry of Health (Tentative)*, based on the WHO *Global Influenza Preparedness Plan*, which outlined, among other things, the organization and leadership system, duties, preparedness, emergency response, and supervision for influenza pandemics. Using this plan as its foundation, the MOH soon afterwards issued two special-purpose guidance books to local health departments, the *Manual for Implementation of the Influenza Pandemic Preparedness and Response Plan of the Ministry of Health (Tentative)*, and the *Publicity Manual on the Influenza Pandemic Preparedness and Response Plan of the Ministry of Health (Tentative)*. Also, the MOH developed sector-specific contingency plans in collaboration with the Ministry of Agriculture (MOA), the General Administration of Quality Supervision, Inspection and Quarantine (AQSIQ) and evaluated its 2005 influenza pandemic preparedness and response plan. The MOH also formulated the *Plan for Monitoring, Prevention and Control in Different Phases of an Influenza Pandemic*, and inspected the national health care system's response capabilities. Therefore, from the perspective of contingency planning, China had basically built an emergency response system consisting of overall planning, special-purpose planning, sector-targeted planning and single event planning.

3.2.1.3   Capacity Building and Preparation

Strengthened Emergency Response Teams

In regards to emergency response teams, 32 national-level specialized public health emergency management teams and anti-terrorism health emergency response teams, roughly 300 people under 6 categories, were established. At the provincial, prefectural, and county levels, health emergency response teams were also formed consisting of healthcare and disease prevention and control personnel.

Established an Expert Group

In 2004, the MOH Expert Group for Influenza Prevention and Treatment was established, and was charged with the following responsibilities: providing technical guidance, training, and supervision for national influenza monitoring; directing onsite response efforts to epidemic outbreaks; drafting national technical plans and documents; providing supervisory guidance for health departments and disease control and prevention departments at all levels; providing advice and recommendations on national response plans for influenza pandemics; and offering technical consultations on national influenza prevention and control efforts.

Strengthened Training

In October 2001, the MOH and China CDC launched a two-year Chinese Field Epidemiology Training Program (CFETP) course under the support of such international organizations as the WHO, the United Nations Children's Fund (UNICEF), as well as domestic and foreign parties. By April 2009, this program had recruited 100 people from national, provincial, and municipal disease control and prevention institutions and health supervision agencies, 68 of whom had graduated top in their class. These professionals were groomed for China's public health industry with the skills to solve a myriad of acute, difficult, and dangerous public health emergencies. With all eyes on the possible outbreak of a pandemic, China followed suit and placed pandemic preparedness at the top of its national agenda. An important part of influenza pandemic preparedness is that when a pandemic occurs, there must be adequate and effective resource management for treating large numbers of severely ill patients in a short period of time. Employing the Flu Surge Model which was developed by the United States CDC, CEETP students discovered that in the case of an influenza pandemic, Beijing could face severe shortages of important resources like intensive care units (ICUs) and respirators, an evaluation result which was immediately reported to the Beijing government and attracted a lot of attention from related departments. At the same time, the MOH and the China CDC organized yearly national training courses on influenza epidemiology and laboratory monitoring technology; in 2007, three such training courses were held for 307 people.

Key provincial laboratories also carried out hands-on training, where 10 professionals in networked laboratories received training. In 2007–2008, the MOH Office of Health Emergency provided prefectural and municipal health officials across the country with four rounds of special training in health emergency management, including risk preparedness and pandemic response.

Supported Capacity Building for National Influenza Centers

In 2005, the China CDC established an influenza pandemic preparedness and response technical group, which was responsible for monitoring global and domestic pandemic trends. The Chinese National Influenza Center (CNIC) was established in 1957 to provide technical support for national influenza prevention and control efforts. The CNIC joined the WHO Global Influenza Surveillance Network in 1981 and since then has provided the WHO with isolated influenza strains each year, because of this China has been recognized worldwide for being an integral part in providing material for potential influenza vaccines. In early 2007, WHO experts conducted an onsite assessment of the CNIC. In early 2008, the MOH submitted an official application to the WHO for designating the CNIC as a WHO Collaborating Center for reference and research on influenza and on November 1st, 2008, the CNIC began a trial period for it.

3.2.1.4   Vaccine and Antiviral Preparedness

Vaccine and antiviral preparedness included revising the *China Guidelines on Influenza Vaccination*, expanding the usage of vaccinations against seasonal influenza, boosting vaccination capacity, encouraging all localities to formulate preferential policies, and lastly expanding coverage of vaccinations against seasonal influenza.

In 2008, with the support of the WHO and the Asian Development Bank (ADB), the China CDC conducted a national survey of seasonal influenza vaccine production and usage, which provided background information and helped the country formulate strategies for the application of seasonal influenza and pandemic vaccines.

In April 2008, a pre-pandemic vaccine against the H5N1 virus was approved by the China Food and Drug Administration (SFDA), and the government invested capital and ensured an annual production capacity of roughly 20 million doses. If the pandemic strain was H5, then vaccines could be produced within three months, and if the strain mutated, it would take six months in total from strain separation to vaccine production. In regards to antiviral preparedness, in addition to a national Tamiflu stockpile of 500,000 doses and a local Tamiflu stockpile of 37,900 doses, production from two Chinese manufacturers—with an annual capacity of about 15 million courses of treatment, and a production cycle of about 3 months (which Roche licensed to produce Tamiflu) were incorporated into the country's strategic stockpile for influenza pandemics. The China CDC stockpiled 20,000 doses of the vaccine for avian influenza control.

3.2.1.5 International and Regional Collaboration

China signed the 2005–2010 Influenza Monitoring Collaboration Program with the WHO, and the China-U.S. Emerging and Re-emerging Infectious Disease Program with the United States. At the same time, China advocated establishing a ASEAN "10+3" Infectious Disease Information Communication Mechanism, which provided ASEAN countries with training in laboratory monitoring of influenza, and collaboration between Japan, South Korea, and Australia occurred through the development of pandemic response tabletop exercises.

3.2.2 The Alert and Response Stage (April 25th–May 10th)

In light of the country's actual pandemic trends, the Chinese government in this phase adopted the strategy of "containing the importation of Influenza A (H1N1) and strengthening management of close contact with infected patients." The purpose of this strategy was to "buy more time for pandemic response by preventing cross-border transmission, delaying the rate of transmission, lowering the peak of transmission, and mitigating the harmful impact per unit of time."

3.2.2.1 Policy Background

On April 25th, 2009, the WHO held the first Emergency Committee Meeting, declaring that the swine flu outbreaks in Mexico and the United States had constituted a "public health emergency of international concern," and recommended that all countries strengthen monitoring and alert concerning irregular outbreaks of flu-like diseases and serious pneumonia. On April 27th, 2009, the WHO elevated the pandemic alert from Phase 3 to Phase 4, and again to Phase 5 on April 29th. The WHO advised that all countries immediately launch their response mechanisms as per pandemic emergency response plans and to take the following effective measures: strengthen surveillance, detect and treat cases as soon as possible, and actively treat and control nosocomial infections, all of which would help prevent the outbreak and spread of the pandemic. The fact alone that the alert levels increased twice in three days indicated the urgency and severity of the pandemic situation.

3.2.2.2   Main Response Measures

Established the "8+1" Joint Prevention and Control Mechanism

On April 30th, 2009, China established a multi-departmental joint prevention and control mechanism headed by the MOH. Under this mechanism, 33 departments (which later increased to 38) and institutions constituted 8 work groups—general, port, healthcare, support, dissemination and communication, foreign collaboration, science and technology, and animal husbandry and veterinary—and an expert committee on the prevention and control of Influenza A (H1N1), forming an "8+1" structure for joint prevention and control efforts. Roles and standard operating procedures were defined for the joint prevention and control mechanism, the work groups, and the expert committee. A plenary and liaison meeting system was also established. Problems which a work group encountered would in principle be solved by the work group itself, and those which the work group found difficult to solve would be settled through coordination under the joint prevention and control mechanism—general affairs would be solved by regular liaison meetings, and major issues decided by plenary meetings.

Strengthened Entry-Exit Inspections and Quarantine and the Management of Close Contact with Infected Patients

On April 30th, 2009, after the No. 8 Proclamation issued by the MOH, the Chinese government incorporated Influenza A (H1N1) into Category B infectious diseases under the *Law on Prevention and Treatment of Infectious Diseases*, adopted prevention and control measures of Class A infectious diseases, and incorporated them into the Frontier Health and Quarantine Infectious Disease Management as stipulated in *the Frontier Health and Quarantine Law of the People's Republic of China*. The principle measures adopted included the following: ports executed a strict health declaration card system, body temperature screening, and medical inspection systems; professionals were dispatched to inform those who had entered China that they must seek medical attention and report to the related government department when having flu-like symptoms; and disease control and prevention institutions searched communities for those in close contact with infected patients, isolated them, and kept them under observation. Investigations were conducted on the places and people related to those in close contact with the virus, and effective prevention and control measures were taken for those with fever and other symptoms. Designated hospitals were prepared to receive and treat influenza patients (See Fig. 3.8 for specific measures and procedures).

As shown by the epidemiological curve of reported cases in China (Fig. 3.1), cases didn't spike until well over three months after the emergence of the first case, the peak remained at a relatively low level, and compared with other countries, the pandemic curve of this stage for the country was relatively flat (Fig. 3.9). This evinces that the country's early containment strategy did in fact reach its goal of

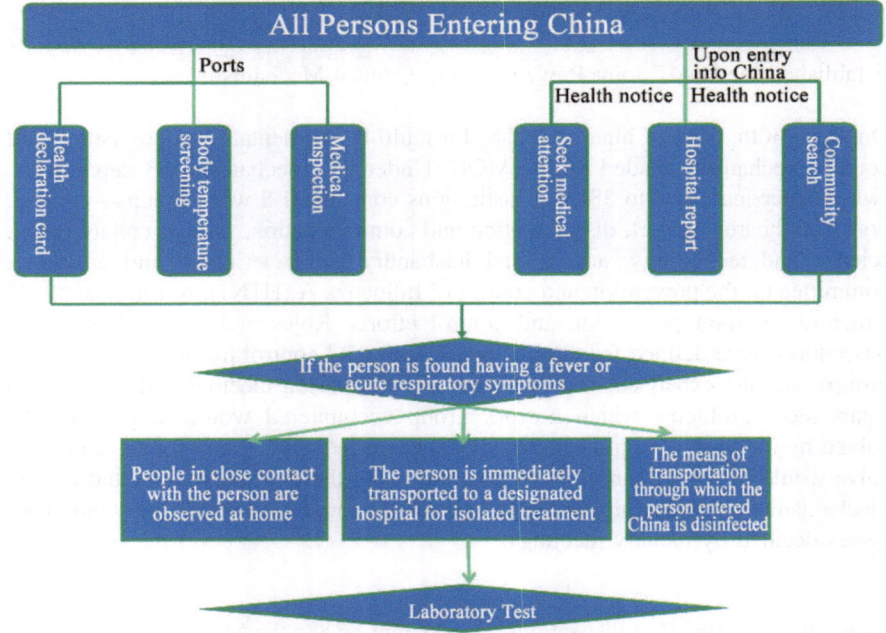

Fig. 3.8 Detection measures for traveling into China

"delaying the pandemic's transmission rate." According to the WHO's analysis of data on thirteen countries and territories in the Western Pacific, the median interval between the time the first confirmed case and the pandemic peak was 13 weeks (the average was 16 weeks), with Laos having the shortest interval (7 weeks) and China and Japan having the longest interval (30 weeks) (Fig. 3.10). This also suggests that China's early "containment strategy" was effective and provided more time for response preparation and efforts.

Strengthened Virus Monitoring and Conducted Thorough Investigations

In order to keep up to date on epidemic trends and monitor possible mutations of the virus in the wake of the outbreak, China invested nearly 400 million RMB on testing large amounts of specimens and expanding the influenza monitoring network to include 411 influenza monitoring laboratories and 556 sentinel hospitals—a network which covered all prefectural-level cities and some priority districts and counties. All of these facilities were required to begin operation in September.

The China CDC provided technical support and services for national response efforts. These services included the following: upgrading the China Information System for Disease Control and Prevention; incorporating Influenza A (H1N1) into the Disease Monitoring Information Reporting Management System, the China

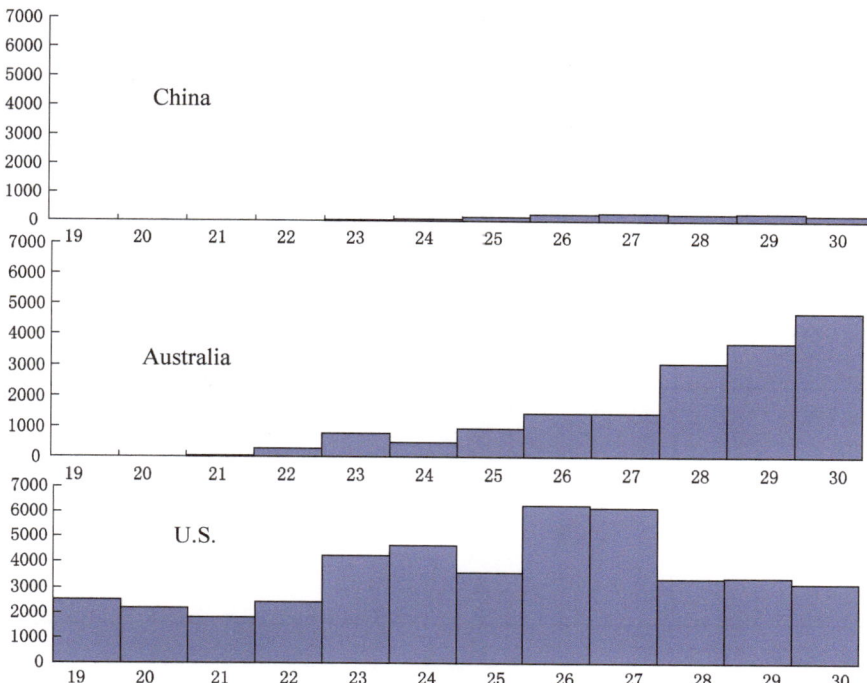

Fig. 3.9 Distribution of reported cases of Influenza A (H1N1) in China, the United States, and Australia from the 19th to 30th week of 2009

Influenza Monitoring Information System, and the Public Health Emergency Information System; specifically establishing an Influenza A (H1N1) information management system; tracking and analyzing domestic influenza epidemic trends through the National Infectious Disease Network Reporting System and the National Influenza Monitoring Network System; collecting and analyzing information on the condition, treatment and outcome of Influenza A (H1N1) cases; providing analysis reports and information support needed to improve prevention and control strategies and measures; mapping global epidemic distribution and the distribution of isolated personnel by provinces; integrating individual cases and community outbreaks into the national infectious disease and public health emergency information systems for direct online reporting; enabling timely submission of questionnaires, statistical, and analytical reports on severely ill cases; monitoring domestic and foreign epidemic information; optimizing information systems and platforms; ensuring the collection and analysis of information on mass vaccination; and monitoring any side effects of the vaccination.

The country's proactive efforts in the alert and response phase of this influenza pandemic are in stark contrast to the 2003 SARS outbreak where the epidemic was not clearly defined and there was a lack of information. The development of the

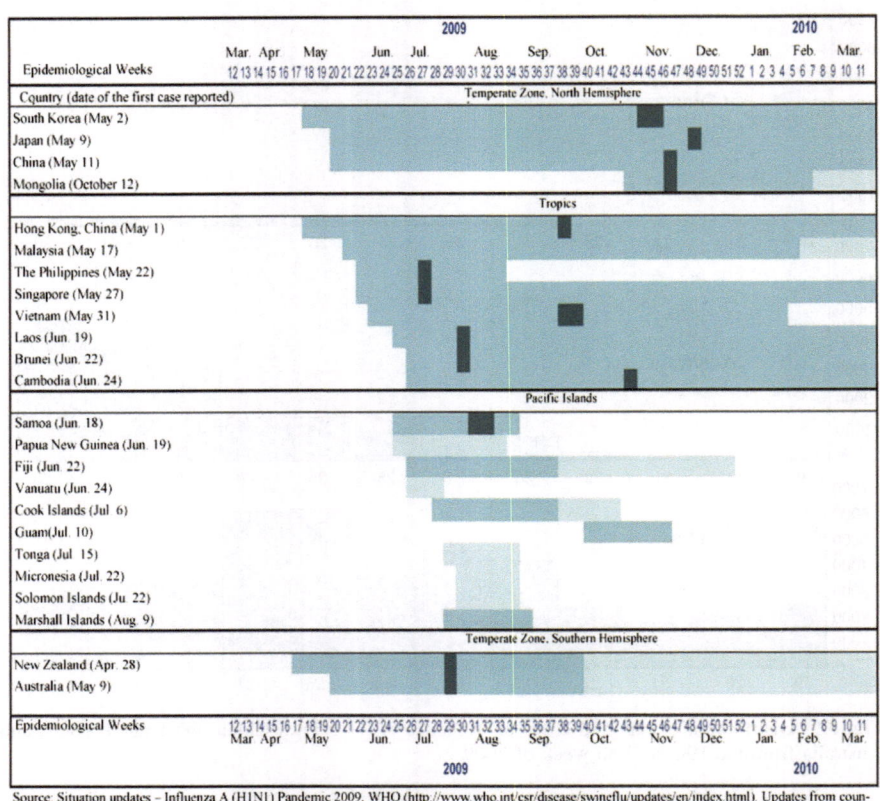

Source: Situation updates – Influenza A (H1N1) Pandemic 2009, WHO (http://www.who.int/csr/disease/swineflu/updates/en/index.html). Updates from countries are different in form: some countries provided a pandemic curve by dates of occurrence while others provided ILI (influenza-like illness) inquiry rates and virus isolation results.

■ Pandemic peak (Note: Not all countries and regions had a peak period)   ▨ Cases found   ▨ Sporadic cases found

Fig. 3.10 Peak dates of laboratory-confirmed cases reported to the WHO by Western Pacific countries and territories in the first year of the Influenza A (H1N1) Pandemic

national disease monitoring system and the capacity of the CDCs withstood this epidemic, which points to the rapid progress made in recent years in national public health emergency system and capacity building.

Nevertheless, the national prevention and control efforts for this pandemic also revealed some unusual phenomena; for instance, provinces with the best performance in combating the pandemic reported the most cases, but those provinces which reported the fewest number of cases were not necessarily performing up to par in the response efforts.

Initiated Research and Development of Diagnostic Reagents and Antiviral
Drugs

Upon learning about the Influenza A (H1N1) outbreak in Mexico, as per instructions,
the CNIC immediately began the development of testing kits. On April 27th, the
National Institute for Viral Disease Control and Prevention (IVDC) of the China CDC,
obtained information on genetic sequences of the Influenza A virus from the U.S.
CDC and immediately engaged in sequence alignments and the design and testing of
nucleic acid detection techniques. On April 29th, after receiving information on the
primer of nucleic acid detection from the WHO, the IVDC promptly compared a
variety of seasonal Influenza A (H1N1) viruses, synthesized the primer sequence
needed for detection, and prepared the first-generation nucleic acid detection reagent
for the human Influenza A virus—which was distributed to 84 influenza monitoring
laboratories across the country on the night of April 30th. On May 1st, the first round
of training for influenza monitoring laboratories, especially those in port cities, began.
Also, through the WHO, the CNIC provided 12 countries including Cuba, Mongolia,
and Vietnam as well as Macao with the test kit that China had independently developed. Test kits were swiftly deployed to monitoring network laboratories throughout
the country, and training was promptly carried out for test professionals. Because
China had strengthened capacity building for the CNIC in the aftermath of the SARS
epidemic, the CNIC was strong enough to play a crucial role in the national response to
the Influenza A (H1N1) Pandemic, earning it international recognition in the process.

Developed Communication and Collaboration with Foreign Countries,
Collected Information on the Pandemic Abroad, and Made Every Effort
to Handle Foreign-Related Prevention and Control Affairs

In the early days of the pandemic, in order to stay up to date on latest trends, the
MOH was proactive in contacting the WHO and the disease control departments of
other affected countries. At the earliest possible time, it obtained strains isolated in
the United States and Mexico for test kit research and development purposes, and
also helped Chinese vaccine manufacturers obtain seed strains from the WHO for
vaccination development. Also, through the WHO, the CNIC provided 12 countries
including Cuba, Mongolia, and Vietnam as well as Macao with the test kit that
China had independently developed. It is evident that as countries became more
interdependent in the wake of economic globalization, prevention and control
efforts against infectious diseases required the attention, participation, and collaboration of all countries involved. Facing the challenge of preventing and controlling
an influenza pandemic, China actively pursued international collaboration and
promoted the implementation of prevention and control strategies, the collaboration
in rapid information sharing, and extensive international exchanges, all in order to
improve capacity building for emergency response teams so that everyone could
enjoy the benefits of information sharing.

Conducted Response Preparations and Increased Emergency Material
Stockpiles

On April 29th, 2009, the National Development and Reform Commission (NDRC) jointly and urgently established an important coordination mechanism of emergency material support with the Ministry of Industry and Information Technology (MIIT) along with the Ministry of Finance (MOF), Ministry of Commerce (MOC), Ministry of Health (MOH) and China Food and Drug Administration (CFDA). On that same day, the NDRC made a request to the MIIT Department of Consumer Goods Industry to increase national health emergency stockpiles of clinical treatment materials and epidemic materials needed to respond to the Influenza A (H1N1) pandemic. On April 30th, a support group headed by the NDRC was established under the joint prevention and control mechanism. In early May, the central government provided 5 billion RMB and local governments appropriated capital as well to guarantee adequate funds for national response efforts. However, at this time it was also discovered that there had been a serious shortage of emergency material reserves in the past, which exposed the weaknesses of health emergency management.

Disseminated Prevention Awareness and Carried Out Health Education
Campaigns

In the early days of the Influenza A (H1N1) pandemic, the MOH's related departments and agencies established an expert advisory mechanism which included experts in public health, disease control and prevention, and emergency management, to meet the huge public demand for knowledge about the epidemic; media interviews were arranged with these experts in order to promulgate needed information. Central and local websites were upgraded on the subject of influenza. The 12320 Health Hotline, the MOH website, the Chinese Center of Health Education website, and other public health services provided channels for direct communication, and online interviews were conducted through Xinhuanet and China.org.cn to better reach the general public. Provincial-level spokesmen were appointed to release public health information as needed. The health campaigns were different this time around, as they published more specific content than just statistical data, including the addition of expert analysis, public health recommendations, and risk communication strategies that were continually being updated —these elements were never presented in previous disease prevention and control efforts. For example, during the peak period of Chinese students returning home from abroad, health experts wrote them a six-point recommendation letter advising them to protect themselves and others, and this proved to be quite an effective means of information dissemination. Governments at various levels, schools and some other institutions adopted also similar communication and education methods. Practice has proved that effective risk communication, trust in the government, and reliable information help to mitigate social and economic losses caused by public anxiety and worry.

3.2.3   Initial Stage of the Epidemic (May 10th–August 30th, 2009)

Most of the cases reported in this phase were imported, and the strategy adopted focused on "equal importance for containment and prevention, with the goal of lowering transmission peaks."

3.2.3.1   Policy Background

On the afternoon of May 10th, 2009, the MOH suddenly received a report from the Provincial Department of Health of Sichuan stating that Sichuan Provincial People's Hospital had treated a patient who was preliminarily diagnosed as a suspected Influenza A (H1N1) case based on clinical symptoms and laboratory test results. On the night of May 10th, the MOH declared the first suspected Influenza A (H1N1) case found in mainland China. Tests conducted afterwards by the China CDC and the Academy of Military Medical Sciences proved that it was in fact China's first case. On May 11th, the MOH declared it to be the first confirmed Influenza A (H1N1) case. Imported cases emerged in Shandong and Beijing soon afterwards.

On June 11th, 2009, the WHO declared the highest level of pandemic alert, i.e. Phase 6, which meant that the human-to-human spread of the virus was occurring in many other countries and regions outside North America. This was the WHO's first ever declaration of a global influenza pandemic in more than 40 years.

On June 11th, the first local case from unknown sources of infection emerged in China, suggesting that prevention and control efforts should be focused on curbing the domestic spread of the virus and its transmission in schools and communities.

On June 19th, the first Influenza A (H1N1) outbreak in a school was reported in Dongguan, Guangdong. From late June to early July, outbreaks continued to rise across the country. In light of the pandemic trends and Hong Kong's experience in strategic policy adjustment, the State Council held an executive meeting on July 3rd, at which discussions and arrangements were made to adjust and improve prevention and control measures, and duties and tasks were allocated. During the summer holidays, outbreaks occurred among attendees of summer camps in some provinces, putting the Chinese government on full alert at that time.

The country's first critically ill case was reported on August 8th. Thereafter, among new confirmed cases, imported cases were gradually overtaken by locally infected cases.

3.2.3.2   Main Response Measures

Building upon the previous phase, these measures included the following: strengthening the tracking and management of close contacts; ensuring designated hospitals treat patients; stepping up nosocomial infection control; expanding the network of pandemic monitoring sentinel hospitals and laboratories; strengthening and improving information collection and reporting; strengthening clinical case monitoring and epidemiological monitoring; implementing emergency research projects; accelerating vaccine development; adjusting and improving port quarantine and inspection measures; improving prevention and control plans by enhancing capacities for treatment of critically ill patients; bolstering prevention and control efforts in schools, communities, towns, hospitals, public places and other priority places; strengthening risk communication; and guiding public opinion. Specific measures were as follows:

Gradually Strengthened Strict Management of Close Contacts, and Modified Management Policy When Needed

Very strict management measures regarding close contacts were adopted in the pandemic's initial phase, and adjustments were made accordingly based on epidemic analysis. For example, from April 25th to June 20th, 2009, according to the Influenza A (H1N1) Port Health and Quarantine Procedure and Operational Specifications, close contacts were defined as passengers of the row where the patient with Influenza A (H1N1) was seated and of three rows immediately behind and in front of the patient in an airliner, or passengers inside the same ship cabin or railway carriage (including attendants that served the patient). After June 20th, the Notice on Adjustments to the Influenza A (H1N1) Port Health and Quarantine Procedure and Operational Specifications re-defined close contacts as including one passenger on each side of the patient, and three passengers of three rows both immediately behind and/or in front of the patient.

On July 8th, the MOH issued the *Notice of the MOH General Office on Further Improving Influenza A (H1N1) Prevention and Control Measures* (No. 122, 2009), which became an important turning point in the policy adjustment on Influenza A (H1N1) prevention and control. The notification discontinued the need for closer medical observation of close contacts and implemented home medical observation or follow-ups by the health authorities. According to survey results, per capita costs for tracking and concentrated observation of close contacts amounted to 5218.50 RMB, while it only cost 270.80 RMB on average to track and observe a close contact at home. The policy adjustment was instrumental in lowering social costs and avoiding an excess prevention and control measures.

Pushing Designated Hospitals into Motion, Actively Treated Patients, and Strengthened Nosocomial Infection Control

On April 27th, 2009, the MOH issued a document requiring local health departments at various levels to designate hospitals to receive and treat Influenza A (H1N1) cases. Provinces across the country then forwarded this document and made arrangements accordingly. From June 11th to early August 2009, though cases were largely imported ones, local mildly ill cases gradually increased. China reported its first severely ill case on August 8th, and the success in curing it paved the way for treatment of the many more severely and critically ill cases that came later on. The strict policies adopted in the three months from the first confirmed domestic case to the first severely ill case bought ample time for proper treatment preparation. As it became known that designated hospitals were not equipped to meet the needs of curing severely ill cases, as they lacked mechanical ventilators, ICUs and related technicians, local governments began incorporating general hospitals with decent intensive care facilities into their lists of reserve hospitals in preparation of treating severely ill patients.

Expanded Network of Influenza Monitoring Sentinel Hospitals and Laboratories

On May 20th, the MOH decided to convert 119 laboratories across the country into national influenza monitoring network laboratories, and 167 hospitals as national influenza monitoring sentinel hospitals. The MOH required that the added health-care institutions begin monitoring Influenza A (H1N1) starting on that very day, and the China CDC immediately began organizing personnel training for these institutions, as well as distributing test kits among the added network laboratories. Monitoring standardization and quality control also began immediately. By mid-June, there were a total of 566 influenza monitoring sentinel hospitals and 411 network laboratories in the country, and the China CDC mobilized staff to train teachers for these new monitoring network units.

Launched Emergency Research Projects and Promoted Vaccine Development

In early June 2009, an Influenza A (H1N1) vaccine development and production coordination mechanism was established consisting of the NDRC, the MOH, the MIIT, the CFDA, the China CDC, the National Institute for the Control of Pharmaceutical and Biological Product (NICPBP), and ten influenza vaccine manufacturers. During vaccine development, an alternative approach was employed in preparing the standard materials, and a quantitative testing method for vaccine antigens was created which shortened the time needed for vaccine development by one month. With established seasonal influenza vaccine production processes, the vaccine manufacturers successfully produced an Influenza A (H1N1) vaccine for clinical trials. The CFDA opened up a channel for fast-track approval of the vaccine to ensure qualified vaccines against the virus could be used for clinical trials with enough time to stay relevant. From July 22nd to September 18th, 2009, large-scale clinical trials were conducted simultaneously with 13,000 volunteers in seven regions of the country.

Made Timely Adjustments to Response Policies, Distributed
Community-Level Outbreak Control Plans and Mildly Ill Cases
Management Plans, and Categorized Influenza A (H1N1) Under Category B
for Infectious Disease Management

To curb community-level outbreaks and implement scientific prevention and control measures, on June 11th the MOH issued the *Work Plan for Control of
Community-level Influenza A Outbreaks (Tentative),* providing efficient and effective guidance for the country to engage in disease prevention and control efforts.
The timely introduction of this plan paved the way for coping with possible
community-level outbreaks. In the plan, in light of expert opinions, the MOH
disapproved the idea of taking "provinces, prefectural-level cities, and counties" as
units to cope with community-level outbreaks; instead the MOH was in favor of
making community-level response plans where the size of a community was to be
locally determined so as to avoid excessive measures and allow for timely policy
adjustment. Measures in the plan also included categorical case management,
strengthening treatment of severely ill cases, lowering case fatality rates, mitigating
damage caused by the epidemic, making prevention and control policies more
relevant, focusing attention and medical resources on patient treatment and the
monitoring of virus mutations, and adjusting prevention and control policies in a
way that is more science-based, efficient and cost-effective.

On the basis of expert recommendations, on July 10th, 2009, the MOH changed
its response policy from "treating Influenza A (H1N1) as a Category B infectious
disease for which prevention and control measures for Category A infectious diseases were adopted" to "employing countermeasures per Category B infectious
diseases," thus coping with Influenza A (H1N1) as "an infectious disease subject to
monitoring" instead of "an infectious disease subject to quarantine." In the document announcing the change, the MOH also affirmed that it would continue
adjusting its management policies along with discoveries and changes in the epidemic. The key issue in adjusting prevention and control measures for this epidemic
was the determining of the virus severity. During this process, related
decision-making entities not only focused on foreign epidemic information, practices of foreign governments, and related expert opinions, but also they took into
consideration their own domestic realities.

Taking into consideration the special characteristics of the epidemic and treatment options in China, combined with the experience the WHO and other countries
had in employing the newest countermeasures against the virus, a group of experts
from the MOH developed the *Management Plan for Home-based Isolation and
Treatment of Mildly Ill Patients of Influenza A (H1N1) (Tentative),* which was then
issued on July 13th. According to this plan, confirmed cases of normal influenza
symptoms, among non-high-risk groups, who hadn't developed any other complications could be isolated and treated at home, and prevention and control measures were then targeted mainly at people who were at high risk of severe illness,
including elderly people, children, and people with chronic disorders, so as to lower
costs and increase efficiency. On July 16th, the WHO adjusted its global

information disclosure on the pandemic and decided to no longer publish information on new confirmed cases. The MOH switched reporting on the epidemic to once every two days instead of once daily, signaling that China had shifted the focus of its prevention and control efforts to normal monitoring and management.

Bolstered Prevention and Control Efforts in Key Areas Including Schools, Communities, Towns, Hospitals, and Public Places

On June 19th, the Central Primary School in Shipai Town, Dongguan City, Guangdong, reported a concentrated outbreak among its students, which was the country's first outbreak of the kind, with 56 confirmed cases. This outbreak had no imported case as the definite source of infection, which sparked a turning point in the national prevention and control efforts—i.e. communities and schools now became the focal points of the countermeasures. To this end, the MOE and the MOH jointly issued the *Work Plan for Influenza A (H1N1) Prevention and Control in Schools (Tentative)*, with the goal of protecting schools from the virus. The summer holidays began in early July for primary and secondary schools as well as colleges and universities countrywide. Since various summer camp activities could have become a breeding ground for the epidemic, so the MOE once again issued a notice stressing the need for cancelling concentrated activities, and required careful reviews for planned student activities according to the principle of "no activity, if not necessary" and local epidemic situations. The MOH also stressed that the priority for the next phase of prevention and control would be to stop the aggregation of cases, especially preventing outbreaks in schools and communities.

Strengthened Scientific and Technological Research on Basic Research, Clinics, and Other Prevention and Control Mechanisms; Increased Scientific and Technological Reserves

In late May, the MOH and the MOST co-launched the "Emergency Research Project for Joint Prevention and Control of Influenza A (H1N1)" which included seven items. Apart from the development of fast diagnostic testing kits, this project covered the following seven areas: evaluation and development of biological protective equipment and disinfectant products; the evaluation and development of medications; an investigation into the genetic background of the Influenza A (H1N1) virus; an evaluation of protection effects from Chinese natural immunity and the seasonal influenza vaccination; the development of key technologies used to increase production capacity of influenza vaccine manufacturers; and the evaluation of clinical treatment methods and the research on case resource integration. The overall goal of this plan was to prepare the country for technological responses to a large scale epidemic.

3.2.4   The Peak of the Epidemic (September 2009– Mid-January 2010)

In this phase, the main strategy focused on containment and strengthening treatment of severely ill patients.

3.2.4.1   Strategic Backgrounds

Reported confirmed cases and severely ill cases rose rapidly beginning in September 2009, with severely ill cases peaking (at 1297) on December 6th. Influenza A (H1N1) cases in schools also increased considerably after the new semester began in September 2009. On October 4th, the first fatal case in China was reported in the Tibet Autonomous Region. With a significant increase in reported clustered cases, the continual rise of severely and critically ill cases in October, and the amounting fatalities, the Influenza A (H1N1) virus became the dominant strain of influenza in the country. Cases increased significantly into November, and infection remained at high levels for three consecutive weeks before reaching the peak of more than 1200 cases reported weekly. The proportion of Influenza A (H1N1) cases to seasonal influenza cases monitored by sentinel hospitals across the country peaked at the end of November. Of severely ill cases, children under nine years of age were the most affected, followed by high-risk groups such as people with chronic disorders, pregnant women, and those suffering from obesity, with complications including pneumonia, respiratory failure, acute respiratory distress syndrome, etc. A national serological survey showed that an overwhelming majoring of Chinese people were susceptible to the virus, which meant a big high-risk population base. In light of school activities and National Day celebrations, the strategy adopted in this phase was focused on "strengthening prevention measures, controlling the spread of the virus in communities, bolstering treatment of severely ill patients, and mitigating damage caused by the epidemic" so as to contain the virus and avoid adverse social impact.

3.2.4.2   Main Countermeasures

Strengthened Treatment of Severely Ill Cases

In response to the spread of the pandemic, the central government allocated five billion RMB in funds for support of Influenza A (H1N1) prevention and control efforts, and required local governments to appropriate funds for tailored prevention and control purposes. These funds were used to deploy materials such as disinfectants, purchase protective and medical equipment and sterilizing equipment, and develop and produce vaccines. The funds also included 1.085 billion RMB for national pharmaceutical stockpiles, and the increase in antiviral drugs, clinical and treatment equipment.

On October 12th, 2009, the MOH issued the *Guidelines on Diagnosis and Treatment of Influenza A (H1N1) (3rd Version, 2009)*, which included a revision in diagnostic criteria and added criteria for identifying severely and critically ill cases, with particular emphasis placed on the early identification and treatment of the two types of cases. On April 30th, 2010, the MOH issued the further revised *Guidelines on Diagnosis and Treatment of Influenza A (H1N1) (2010)*, in which the clinical characteristics and treatment principles of children and pregnant woman were added. By that time a total of five versions of the diagnosis and treatment guidelines had been published.

Hospital led response efforts focused on (a) recruiting rescue staff and strengthening professional training, and (b) the use of antiviral drugs for treatment purposes. It is worth nothing that some clinical studies on Influenza A (H1N1) treatment garnered worldwide recognition; for instance, *A Clinical Study on Symptoms and Therapeutics of Mildly Ill Patients of Influenza A (H1N1)* was published in the world's authoritative *New England Journal of Medicine*.

However, at the same time, certain issues came to light during the response efforts. Firstly, grass-roots capabilities for medical treatment were still inadequate. For example, many emergency medical centers lacked specialized healthcare personnel, ambulances, and related equipment and facilities; many pre-hospital emergency aid facilities in the central and western provinces, and even at the local level in the eastern provinces, were not fully established. In some areas, especially less developed ones with limited medical resources, local governments lacked the capital to invest in strengthening medical treatment capabilities and thus were faced with shortages in related equipment and facilities, antiviral drugs, and protective equipment. Secondly, medical treatment expenses for Influenza A (H1N1) patients were still being taken care of by the hospitals. In the early days of the national response efforts, the state stipulated that all Influenza A (H1N1) patients be treated free of charge, so designated hospitals paid medical and living expenses for the epidemic patients under their care. After the national prevention and control strategy was adjusted, four ministries including the MOH and the MOF jointly issued a document regarding treatment expenses which required the local governments to cover the costs for current or previous cases, and future cases would be settled through the urban employee insurance, the urban resident insurance, and the new rural cooperative medical care system. Nevertheless, obstacles arose during the implementation of this policy and some provinces to this day have yet to settle expenditures. Thirdly, designated hospitals, while bearing the loss in treatment expenses, also faced economic losses from the decrease in outpatients due to receiving and treating Influenza A (H1N1) patients, which produced an adverse effect on the hospital's survival and development. This phenomenon predominantly occurred in less developed regions of the central and western part of the country. Fourthly, treatment of severely ill cases was costly, involving the use of protective equipment that was not covered by medical insurance, so many patients were unable or unwilling to pay for their treatment. As some Influenza A (H1N1) patients were part of the floating population, issues arose regarding medical insurance settlements between different regions. There was no definitive policy in terms of compensation for the proper financial channel, responsible entity, procedure, and/or time limits for expenses paid by designated hospitals whom took the brunt of mitigating the pandemic through patient treatment, transportation, and rehabilitation.

Conducted Nationwide Serological Surveys

In order to understand the prevalence of the virus in the population and to timely and scientifically judge epidemic trends, in December 2009, the MOH launched serological surveys on Influenza A (H1N1) infections and on the virus itself. The MOH required twelve provinces, autonomous regions, and municipalities directly under the central government—including Beijing, Shandong, and Henan— to conduct three cross-sectional surveys according to the *Plan for Sample Surveys in Several Provinces of Infection with the Influenza A (H1N1) Virus*, in January, March–April, and August–September 2010, respectively. 4500 people were sampled in each province through multistage stratified random sampling methods, amounting to a total of 54,000 participants. All 31 provinces, autonomous regions, and municipalities directly under the central government, as well as the Xinjiang Production and Construction Corps, conducted four serological surveys according to the *Plan for Quick Serological Surveys Countrywide of Infection with the Influenza A (H1N1)*, before January 10th, January 20–28th, February 20–28th, and March 20–28th, respectively. Survey findings proved to be crucial in providing judgments on the epidemic, and it was the only large-scale serological testing of its kind domestically in the world.

Stockpiled Vaccines and Antiviral Drugs and Launched a National Vaccination Program

In late September 2009, Beijing provided the first vaccinations to people participating in the celebration of the 60th anniversary of the founding of the People's Republic of China. In early October, Shandong also allocated its first vaccinations to workers preparing for the National Games of China. On November 6th, the MOE and the MOH jointly issued the *Work Plan for Influenza A (H1N1) Prevention and Control in Schools*, which made adjustments to the classification of Influenza A epidemics, school suspension principles, and response procedures. It also required schools to actively cooperate with health departments on student vaccinations. This was followed by an orderly process towards realizing the national vaccination program.

Strengthened Epidemic Monitoring and Health Education in Schools

During the national response efforts, the MOE as part of the Influenza A (H1N1) Joint Prevention and Control Mechanism worked in close coordination with the MOH as they adjusted the *Work Plan for Influenza A (H1N1) Prevention and Control in Schools*. At a grass-roots level, health departments and schools developed and implemented corresponding contingency plans and work plans, set up steering bodies, took prevention and control measures—including training, information dissemination, and cooperated with health departments on taking required response measures in schools.

To ensure the success of the response measures, health departments put programs in place according to the guideline of "respond effectively and scientifically." The first was strictly monitoring the health conditions of students, faculty, and staff, including implementing morning inspections, absence registration and tracking systems in primary and secondary schools, and strengthening instructor-aided student attendance inspection in colleges and universities, all to ensure the timely detection, reporting, and treatment of students. The second was strengthening information and education efforts, with emphasis placed on campus-based dissemination of information about Influenza A (H1N1) prevention and control—through a combination of health education classes, bulletins, radio programs, and campus networks. The third was ensuring solid sanitary conditions in areas where students studied and lived, including carrying out health campaigns aimed to keep campuses clean. The fourth was reducing as many large gatherings as possible and exercising good epidemic prevention and control during National Day celebrations and military training sessions for students. The fifth was strictly implementing an epidemic reporting system, and in so doing, schools created the post of an epidemic reporter, established contact with local disease prevention and control departments, and adopted emergency measures. The sixth was cooperating with health departments on vaccinating students, faculty and staff as well as National Day celebration participants free of charge as arranged by local governments and the Influenza A (H1N1) Joint Prevention and Control Mechanism on the principle of "informed consent and voluntariness." The seventh was carrying out school-based epidemic response measures, including isolating confirmed or suspected cases and close contacts under the guidance of health departments, and where circumstances were serious, taking such measures as shutting down schools according to opinions from health departments as well in accordance with the *Work Plan for Influenza A Prevention and Control in Schools (Tentative)*.

Promoted Traditional Chinese Medicine

While increasing the stockpiling of antiviral drugs, the state also promoted the combination of Western and traditional Chinese medicine (TCM). The usefulness of TCM was stressed and practical clinical treatment solutions were developed in an effort to minimize case fatality rates and mitigate damage caused by the epidemic.

For example, drawing upon the long history TCM's effectiveness, Beijing introduced a formula against Influenza A, called "Jinhua Qinggan," which was then patented and officially launched for clinical treatment. The clinical trials took place at Beijing Ditan Hospital and Beijing You'an Hospital. Of the 845 confirmed cases of Influenza A (H1N1), 326 were treated only with TCM. The prescriptions and some Chinese patent medicines which clinical experts chose for treatment purposes agreed with the pathogenesis, symptomatic characteristics, and basic therapeutic methods of Influenza A (H1N1). The trials showed that TCM alone could relieve symptoms like fever, sore throat, and cough, with no side effects when using the regular dosage. All the patients who used TCM were cured and discharged. The preliminary outcomes of the clinical trials provided a scientific basis for stockpiling TCM and Chinese patent medicines in response to the epidemic for the upcoming autumn and winter.

3.2.5 The Decline of the Epidemic (Mid-January–August 9th, 2010)

Treatment of severely ill patients, etiological monitoring, as well as commissioned expert evaluations of prevention and control efforts all continued during this phase.

In January 2010, new cases reported in the country fell significantly in number, with results of the monitoring showing lower levels of Influenza A (H1N1) activity than activity of seasonal influenza viruses. This was largely because health departments strengthened treatment of severely ill cases based on strategies from the previous phase, and also stepped up etiological monitoring of viruses. Education departments continued their vaccination health campaigns, and port quarantine departments did the same while making adjustments to quarantine practices. Specific measures included the following. Firstly, the large population moving around the country during the Spring Festival period was monitored, experts were organized to judge the current epidemic situation, Influenza A (H1N1) prevention and control efforts before and during the Spring Festival of 2010 were deployed, and guidance to regions and related departments on collaboration and preparedness—including information reporting, event management, vaccination, clinical treatment, prevention and control in priority areas, and health information and education—was provided. Secondly, more effort was put towards vaccination and the monitoring of adverse reactions. By December 31st, 2009, 49.91 million people nationwide had been inoculated. Surveillance findings showed that suspected abnormal reactions to the vaccine occurred roughly 12.4 per 100,000, and severely abnormal reactions occurred roughly 0.1 per 100,000. There were two deaths among those inoculated in December which proved to be unrelated to the vaccination. The rate of occurrence for adverse reactions did not exceed what was found in the domestic clinical trials and was consistent with data reported by the WHO and other countries. Thirdly, medical treatment was further strengthened.

The central government appropriated a total of 397.56 million RMB to 17 central and western provinces as well as the Xinjiang Production and Construction Corps, which was used to strengthen the medical institutions' treatment capacities for severely ill cases, including ICU equipment such as intensive care beds, respirators, and monitors. Health departments at various levels continued to provide guidance on treatment for severely ill cases, especially regarding the protection of pregnant women from the virus through TCM practices, and at the same time tightened control over nosocomial infections. The Ministry of Industry and Information Technology (MIIT) sped up the storage and distribution of antiviral drugs such as Tamiflu, with more than 4.22 million doses of Tamiflu distributed among different regions and departments. Fourthly, case reporting, information disclosure, and public communication efforts were reinforced. This included the continued monitoring of cases with flu-like symptoms and of the Influenza A (H1N1) virus; strengthening the timely reporting of epidemic information; continued timely, open, and transparent dissemination of information and prevention and control efforts; as well as the continued exchange on epidemic knowledge and vaccinations among the public, especially high risk groups such as migrant workers, students, pregnant women, patients with chronic disorders, and tourists. The overall goal of these measures was to help guide the public in strengthening their own self-protection against the virus.

In lieu of global pandemic trends and characteristics as well as ample preparation, the National Joint Prevention and Control Mechanism and the Emergency Management Office of the State Council officially commissioned the School of Public Policy and Management (SPPM) of Tsinghua University in May 2010 to organize a multidisciplinary group of experts for a comprehensive, third-party evaluation of the national response to the Influenza A (H1N1) epidemic in China.

3.2.6 Post-pandemic Phase (Post-August 10th, 2010)

The focus of this phase centered on adjusting the influenza monitoring strategy and optimizing the monitoring network to better improve its quality.

On August 10th, 2010, the WHO announced the shift into the post-pandemic period, stating that Influenza A activity had returned to normal seasonal levels. The virus didn't disappear completely in this phase as localized outbreaks were still considered likely. The WHO recommended, therefore, that countries continue to strengthen their influenza surveillance and play close attention to changes in influenza activity.

3.3   Evaluation and Analysis of China's Major Response Strategies

Third party sources combined with our research data and analysis showed that the China's response strategies were appropriate to the epidemic situation, policy implementation was successful, and policy adjustments also commendable— though some could have been executed in a timelier manner.

Firstly, the Chinese government zeroed in on the imported epidemic and responded proactively by implementing strict countermeasures at the onset of the outbreak. Main considerations included: (1) China's national conditions: With a population of more than 1.3 billion people, over 700 million living in rural areas, China had quite a large floating population, which made prevention and control problematic; the floating population in 2009 was estimated at about 180 million people, and in 2008 there were 350 million people entering and leaving the country, all of which evinces the enormous complexity of coping with such a sudden outbreak. (2) Uncertainties about mutation of the emerging strain: As an emerging, unknown strain, the Influenza A (H1N1) virus was likely to mutate while in circulation and even evolve towards higher case fatality rates. (3) Compared with other countries, China's emergency stockpiles and resources were heavily inadequate. By June 2009, the U.K. had stockpiled enough antiviral drugs for well over half of its population, German states each had a stockpile of antiviral drugs for 20% of their populations; but China's national stockpile only contained 500,000 doses of Tamiflu, in addition to a local stockpile totaling 37,900 doses. (4) The WHO's guidance as well as strict measures taken by affected countries: The Influenza A (H1N1) pandemic was the first public health emergency of international concern which the WHO had declared since the implementation of the *IHR 2005*. As an important member state of the WHO, China was obligated to abide by this international convention, through active epidemic response and reporting. Additionally, countries such as the U.S., Mexico, and Singapore adopted rather strict prevention and control measures both in the early days and at the peak of the pandemic, which provided groundwork for China's own efforts.

Secondly, China's Influenza A (H1N1) response strategies were adopted giving full consideration to the impact of the global financial crisis. China was also greatly impacted by the 2009 global financial crisis, and to deal with it effectively, its countermeasures not only had to be strict to protect normal economic and social operations from the possible spread of the virus, but at the same time the response efforts couldn't be too severe otherwise they would adversely affect the economy. More importantly, as China's economic development was crucial for global economic recovery, the state's response strategies drew worldwide attention, and any action taken affected not only the people at home but also global economic and social development. Thus, China's response policies had to take into consideration both the health and livelihood of its citizens, as well as domestic and international demands. In light of the above, from the perspective of safeguarding human lives, the Chinese government was determined to minimize damage, and so immediately adopted rather strict response strategies—which were adjusted as appropriate based on discoveries and changes in the epidemic—while striving to lower the impact of measures taken on normal economic and social operations. It turned out that such prevention and control measures were quite effective. As described in the foregoing analysis, the success in the country's early containment strategy, and the school holidays that lasted from July to August, considerably delayed the advent of the epidemic's peak, buying precious time for the nation to better prepare appropriate countermeasures.

It should also be noted that because there was a lack of understanding in the early phases of the epidemic in regards to the characteristics of the Influenza A (H1N1) virus, our strategic policy adjustments were not timely enough. The Influenza A (H1N1) virus had three prominent characteristics: First, transmission was quick; second, we slowly learned that the virus was mild in nature during the course of transmission; and third, its transmission, as was shown by expert studies, was mainly via respiratory droplets. Therefore, the adjustment of prevention and control measures could have been timelier had the epidemic situation been better judged and findings from local virological analysis and epidemiological surveys had been translated more swiftly into concrete prevention and control strategies and measures when the first wave of local cases occurred.

On the other hand, as situations differed from region to region owing to the vast territory of the country, further improvement was still needed in terms of coordination—under the guidance of national strategies—between different departments and between strategies of these departments and local governments. As stated above, on July 10th, 2009, the MOH changed its response policy from "treating Influenza A (H1N1) as a Category B infectious disease for which prevention and control measures for Category A infectious diseases were adopted" to "handling it with prevention and control measures for Category B infectious diseases," coping with the virus as "an infectious disease subject to monitoring" instead of "an infectious disease subject to quarantine." However, due to coordination problems between central departments and between central and local departments, some local level entry-exit inspection and quarantine departments still treated Influenza A (H1N1) as an infectious disease subject to quarantine.

Moreover, it must also be noted that chance also played a role in the success of the public health emergency response strategies. As part of its response effort, China shortened time to market for Influenza A (H1N1) vaccines, becoming the first country in the world to complete clinical trials for an Influenza A vaccine and the first country to launch a mass vaccination campaign. Although the vaccination campaign was a success, we cannot overlook the risks involved in this process.

The process from the discovery of a new influenza strain to vaccine production and marketing authorization takes at least 3–6 months, and if time for mass production is included, the process stretches out even further. As China still lagged behind developed countries, its vaccine production capacity, even though it was considerably increased for this epidemic, could only cover 10% of the population, while the previous seasonal influenza production capacity only covered 2%. Additionally, because an influenza virus is constantly mutating, it is highly possible that the vaccine strain being researched doesn't match the pandemic strain, and that vaccine research and manufacturing simply can't keep up with the speed of the virus' mutation. Fortunately, the influenza pandemic virus didn't mutate, which, adding to that the research results from the early phases, made it possible for the country to successfully develop a vaccine and use it for the masses. It should be noted, therefore, that in response to any future influenza pandemic, we should continue to actively carry out social intervention measures while simultaneously stressing medical interventions like vaccinations. Only then will our response strategy be both effective and reliable.

Chapter 4
China's Institutional Mechanisms for Influenza A (H1N1) Prevention and Control

Innovation in institutional mechanisms is a fundamental issue in effectively dealing with public health emergencies. In the wake of the 2003 SARS Epidemic, China initially established a public health emergency management system and an emergency organization and management network, placing emphasis on "government leading, unified command, local management, responsibility on all levels, management by classifications, and inter-departmental coordination," which strengthened the existing health emergency preparation system. The state also implemented overall arrangements and various measures concerning health emergency management and these efforts boosted the country's capabilities in dealing with public health emergencies. Facing the global Influenza A (H1N1) pandemic, China played to its socialist strengths by "bringing together forces to accomplish big things" and by establishing a joint prevention and control mechanism spearheaded by the government. Roles and responsibilities were defined, and collaboration and communication between departments were strengthened. This mechanism provided the Influenza A (H1N1) prevention and control efforts with organizational guarantee, systematic support, and process specifications. Taking into consideration domestic realities and conditions, this chapter provides an analysis of the establishment and operation of Influenza A (H1N1) prevention and control mechanisms, and of the social involvement of these mechanisms at national and local levels. Some reflections are presented based on experiences and lessons learned from this pandemic, in the hope of providing ideas for innovation in future emergency management institutional mechanisms.

4.1 China's Current Public Health Emergency Institutional Mechanisms

The unexpected outbreak of the 2003 SARS epidemic revealed some of China's shortcomings in the field of emergency management, including: weak institutional mechanisms, lack of organizational communication, inefficient flow of information,

© Social Sciences Academic Press and Springer Nature Singapore Pte Ltd. 2019
L. Xue and G. Zeng, *A Comprehensive Evaluation on Emergency Response in China*, Research Series on the Chinese Dream and China's Development Path,
https://doi.org/10.1007/978-981-13-0644-0_4

and insufficient preparedness. China's fight against SARS, as it were, not only posed a great challenge to the nation's socialist modernization, but at the same time offered an important opportunity for the country to improve emergency management, especially in the field of public health.

4.1.1   Construction of a National Emergency Management System

In the wake of the SARS Epidemic, the Chinese government began pushing for a national emergency management system in a systematic, planned and gradual manner, and made remarkable progress in emergency management structured on the "one plan three systems (contingency plans, institutions, mechanisms and legislation)."

In regards to contingency planning, the country formed a system consisting of contingency plans at central, local, departmental, and enterprise levels as well as plans for major events, and this system played an important role in dealing with public emergencies.[1]

In regards to institution building, a national emergency management system consisting of general emergency management offices as well as of special emergency management bodies were established. The Emergency Management Office of the State Council and emergency management bodies of provincial (regional and municipal) governments were set up in succession,[2] in addition to emergency management systems in specific fields such as health. In comparison with the pre-SARS environment where "departments played a dominant role, and coordination was inadequate," these new institutions showed the permanent, comprehensive, and specialized nature of emergency management,[3] and laid an organizational foundation for the future. In addition, society as a whole began getting involved with the emergency management process, including: further strengthening military emergency system construction and local assistance[4]; giving full rein to experts in

---

[1]In March 2005, the third session of the 10th National People's Congress (NPC) reviewed and adopted the *Report on the Work of the Government*, which stated that "... We have formulated the national contingency plan for public health emergencies, as well as 105 special-purpose and department-specific contingency plans concerning natural disasters, accidents, public health, social security, etc.; provinces (regions and cities) also have completed their own work on the development of overall contingency plans. Breakthroughs have been made in building a government by the rule of law and in fully fulfilling government functions." see: *Report on the Work of the Government*, delivered by Wen Jiabao at the third session of the 10th National People's Congress on March 5–15, 2005.

[2]On April 10th, 2006, the General Office of the State Council issued the Notice on Setting up the Emergency Management Office (General Duty Office) of the State Council.

[3]Lang and Wang (2007).

[4]On November 14th, 2006, the Central Military Commission announced the General Response Plan for the Military to Deal with Emergencies.

emergency management[5]; and developing and implementing local emergency management plans that targeted "communities, rural areas, enterprises and schools."

Looking at mechanism construction, progress was also made in research on a science-based emergency management system, and an emergency management mechanism characterized by "unified leadership, responsiveness, orderly coordination, and efficient operation"—which enabled the interconnection of early warning, mass mobilization, quick response, and emergency handling—was gradually established to effectively mitigated public health emergencies.

In regards to legislation, the *Emergency Response Law* was took effect on November 1st, 2007.

4.1.2 Establishment and Development of China's Public Health Emergency System

China bolstered construction on their public health emergency management system according to the general requirements for such a mechanism. On May 12th, 2003, the State Council promulgated the *Regulations on Preparedness for and Response to Emergent Public Health Hazards* which stressed the need in building a public health emergency management system that could ensure "unobstructed information, rapid response, effective leadership, and definite duties." At the May 14th Executive Meeting of the State Council, chaired by Premier Wen Jiabao, members discussed building a mechanism for national response to public health emergencies, and the principles for such a mechanism were determined: "ensure unified central leadership with levels of responsibility; impose regulations and management in accordance with the law to ensure rapid response capabilities; improve the monitoring system to increase early-warning capabilities; and boost infrastructure to secure sustained operation." On June 4th, at another Executive Meeting of the State Council chaired by Premier Wen Jiabao, he once again stressed, referring to the SARS response and economic impact, that efforts should be made to "accelerate the construction of the public health emergency management mechanism; forge ahead with developing an information network system, the disease prevention and control system, and the emergency rescue system; and ensure readiness and preparedness for any emergency."

At the National SARS Work Conference held on July 28th, 2003, Premier Wen Jiabao ensured the construction and improvement of the public health emergency response mechanism, the disease control and prevention system, and the health legislation enforcement and supervision system in three years' time. Building on that, he promised to improve the country's rural health system, urban basic medical service system, environmental health system, and funding security system for the

---

[5]On December 31st, 2006, Launching Ceremony of the State Council Expert Panel of Emergency Management and the First Plenary Session was held.

long term. Efforts would be made also to strengthen the disease control and prevention system, increase public health emergency management capabilities, boost rural health development, improve healthcare for the rural population, strengthen environmental health system, and implement national health campaigns.

In February 2007, the MOH outline the following overall goals for public health emergency work in the 11th Five-Year Plan: establish and improve health emergency management legislation and the health emergency contingency planning system; build an emergency management mechanism characterized by "unified leadership, responsiveness, orderly coordination, and efficient operation" with "predominantly local management, hierarchical responsibility, and comprehensive coordination;" bolster health emergency management recruitment; improve the public health emergency monitoring and warning system; strengthen capacity for quick and effective response to health emergencies; and shape an environment of health emergency management characterized by inter-departmental coordination, collaboration, and social participation under the leadership of central and local governments.

4.1.2.1   The Formulation of a Top-Down System for Public Health Emergency Planning

During and after the 2003 SARS Epidemic, China continued to establish and improve public health emergency legislation, regulations and contingency plans, and initially formed a national system for public health emergencies contingency planning (see Fig. 4.1).

On August 28th, 2004, the Standing Committee's 11th Meeting of the 10th National People's Congress amended the *Infectious Disease Prevention and Treatment Law*. In January 2005, Premier Wen Jiabao chaired an Executive Meeting of the State Council where *the National Overall Contingency Plan for*

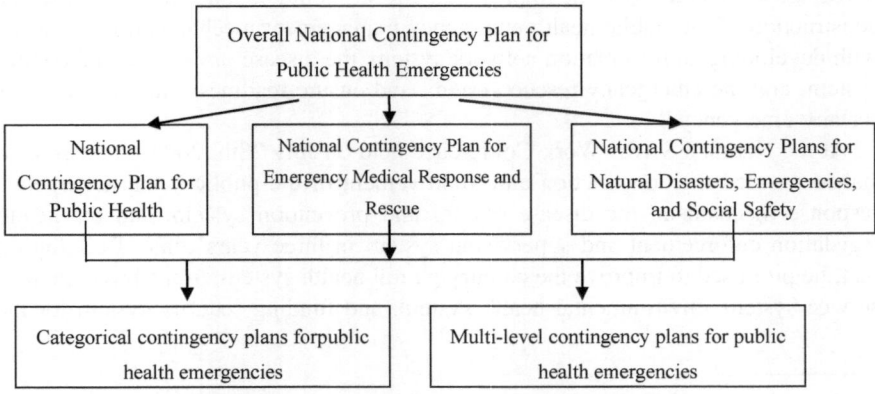

Fig. 4.1 China's hierarchical system for public health emergencies planning

Public Health Emergencies with twenty five special contingency plans and eighty departmental contingency plans were adopted in principle (a total of 106 plans). In 2005–2006, the State Council successively formulated and promulgated the *Overall Contingency Plan for Public Health Emergencies* (January 8th, 2006), the *National Contingency Plan for Public Health Emergencies* (February 26th, 2006), and the *National Contingency Plan for Medical and Health Rescue in Case of Public Health Emergencies* (February 26th, 2006). The State Council issued the *National Contingency Plan for Major Animal Disease Emergencies* (February 26th, 2006), the *National Contingency Plan for Major Food Safety Accidents* (February 26th, 2006), the *National Contingency Plan for Nuclear and Radiation Accidents,* and others. The State Council organized the drafting and revision of such health emergency response plans such as the *National Contingency Plan for Medical and Health Rescue,* the *Contingency Plan for Community-level Public Health Emergencies,* and the *Contingency Plan for Food Poisoning Emergencies.* Local governments and health departments also formulated health emergency response plans in accordance with their local conditions.

In preparation for an influenza pandemic, the MOH formulated the *Influenza Pandemic Preparedness and Response Plan of the Ministry of Health (Tentative),* which was issued on September 28th, 2005. On July 12th, 2006, the MOH issued the *Emergency Response Plan for Highly Pathogenic Human and Avian Influenza,* which, as a departmental contingency plan under the *National Overall Contingency Plan for Public Health Emergencies,* provided systematic organization and leadership against an influenza pandemic, and it outlined important factors for response efforts including division of labor, preparedness, emergency response, and supervision.

4.1.2.2 The Establishment of Public Health Emergency Management Bodies

As arranged by the State Council, in March 2004 the MOH set up the Health Emergency Office (Public Health Emergency Operations Center) which became responsible for the organization and coordination for managing emergency preparations and countermeasures. The MOH Health Emergency Office (Public Health Emergency Operations Center) established sub-offices responsible for integrated coordination, monitoring and alert, emergency response guidance, and emergency countermeasure management. The duties for this operations center include: directing and coordinating national health emergency efforts; developing health emergency and medical rescue plans, systems, contingency plans and measures; directing health emergency activities such as public health emergency preparedness, monitoring and alert, response and rescue, and analysis and evaluation; providing guidance on local implementation of prevention, control, and medical rescue measures in response to public health and other emergencies; establishing and improving health emergency information and operations systems; publishing public health emergency response information; directing and organizing health emergency response training and exercises; keeping records and plans on the national stockpile and providing recommendations on their usage; managing the National Expert Advisory Committee on Public Health Emergencies as well as public health emergency experts; directing and organizing preparation and response measures against acute infectious diseases; organizing medical rescue efforts in case of serious natural disasters, terrorist incidents, food safety emergencies, and nuclear radiation accidents; organizing and coordinating health emergency response services for major national events; organizing health emergency research and health education programs; responsible for the organization and coordination of domestic implementation for the *International Health Regulations*; coordinating the implementation of the *Biological Weapons Convention* in the health industry; and carrying out routine work for the Office of the MOH Leading Group for Disaster Relief and Disease Prevention.

At the same time, a health emergency management system was established, which included the following seven subsystems—Emergency Response Security, Command & Decision-making, Emergency Response Workforce, Monitoring & Alert, Emergency Response Management, Risk Communication, and Science, Technology & Education (Fig. 4.2).

Currently, health departments (bureaus) in 30 provinces (autonomous regions, and municipalities directly under the central government) have established health emergency response offices and the China CDC along with some provincial CDCs also have established special emergency management departments. For example, Beijing established a public health emergency operations center in March 2006, and Shanghai did as well in early 2009 to strengthen its capacity for pubic health emergency management. See Fig. 4.3 for a detailed chart of the national health emergency response command system.

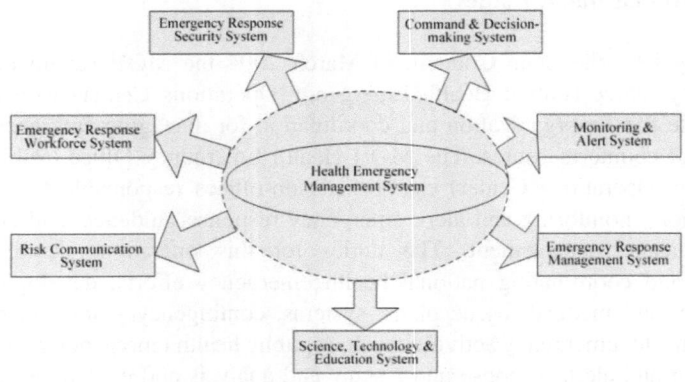

Fig. 4.2 Composition of the health emergency systems

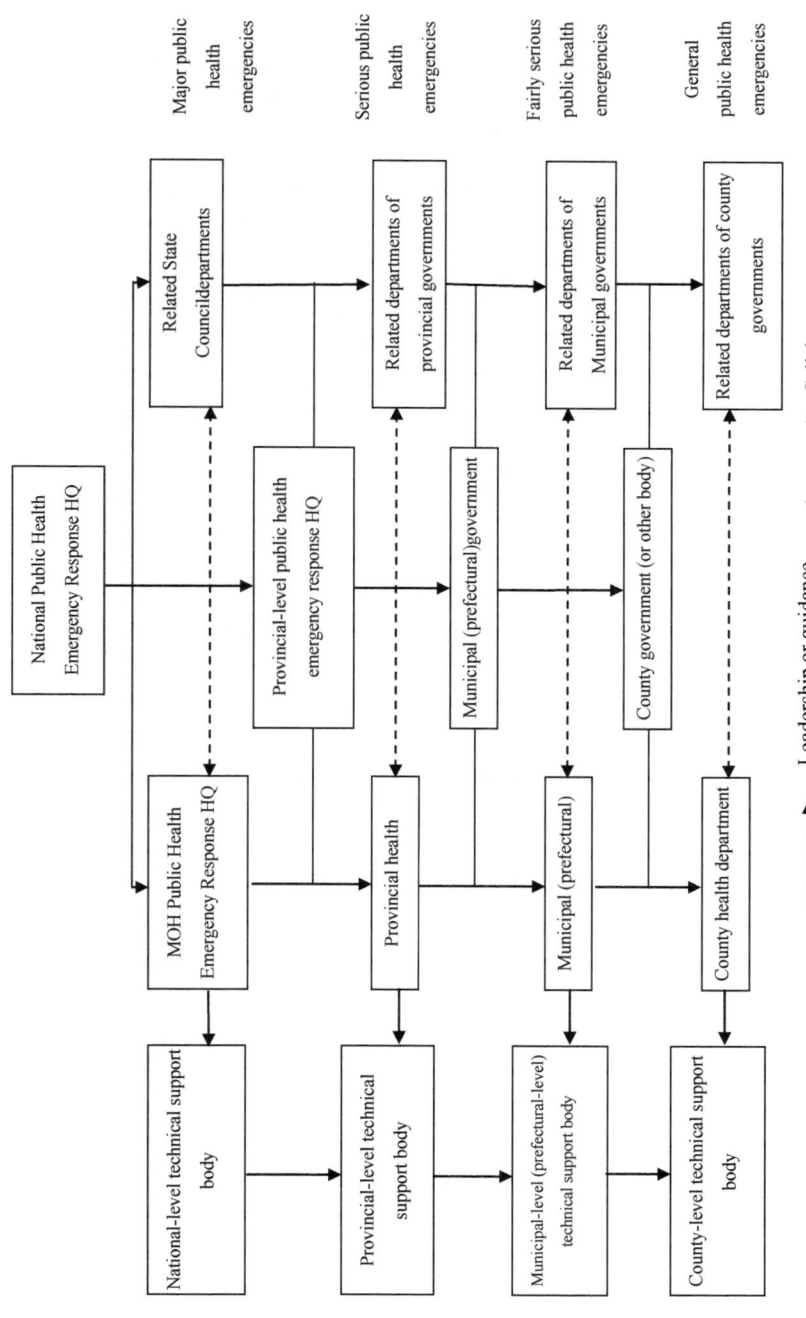

Fig. 4.3 Framework of China's public health emergency response system

4.1.2.3   The Establishment of Cross-Region, Cross-Department Public Health Emergency Coordination Mechanisms

The MOH established a public health emergency coordination mechanism with thirty one central and national departments to deal with inter-departmental collaboration, which effectively strengthened communication and coordination between departments dealing with public health emergencies. The national government and the Special Administrative Regions of Hong Kong and Macau entered into a three-party emergency response collaboration agreement and decided upon implementation regulations, and established a linkage mechanism for information communication and health emergency response. Additionally, the MOH established a joint prevention and control mechanism with the Ministry of Agriculture (MOA) to protect against highly pathogenic zoonotic viruses such as avian influenza and *Streptococcus suis*; the MOH established a coordination mechanism for joint prevention and control of public health emergencies at ports with the General Administration of Quality Supervision, Inspection and Quarantine (AQSIQ). In collaboration with the Ministry of Railway (MOR), the Ministry of Transport (MOT), and the AQSIQ, the MOH issued notices on the prevention and control of the importation of infectious diseases from abroad; and together with the MOE, issued a document requiring schools to appoint part-time or full-time teachers to identify and report infectious diseases or other health emergencies at the school. This time marked the initial formation of a working inter-departmental mechanism positioned to combat health emergencies through "paying equal attention to both prevention and response, and instilling continued collaboration for any event."

4.1.2.4   The Focus on Team Building for Public Health Emergency Experts

In early 2006, the National Expert Advisory Committee on Public Health Emergencies was established in Beijing, with the Vice Health Minister serving as its chairman. Consisting of 105 members, the Committee's routine management work was conducted through the MOH Health Emergency Office. Its main duties included: provide recommendations on appropriate response levels and countermeasures for confirmed public health emergencies; give advice on public health emergency preparation; participate in formulating and revising contingency plans and technical solutions to public health emergencies; provide technical guidance on public health emergency mitigation; advise on the termination of health emergency countermeasures; provide post-emergency evaluations; and undertake other assignments from public health emergency operations and management bodies.

4.2 The Establishment, Composition and Operations of the Joint National Influenza A (H1N1) Prevention and Control Mechanism

4.2.1 The Establishment of the Joint National Influenza A (H1N1) Prevention and Control Mechanism

The MOH responded immediately upon receiving a disease outbreak notice from the WHO on April 25th, 2009, as the MOH General Office launched the working mechanism comprised of the MOH Leading Group and Expert Panel for Influenza Pandemic Prevention and Control [in accordance with the *Influenza Pandemic Preparedness and Response Plan of the Ministry of Health (Tentative)*]. The MOH also issued a *Notice on Strengthening Preparedness for and Response to Human Swine Influenza* to health departments requiring the following: medical and disease control and prevention institutions at various levels to strengthen cases monitoring and reporting; and prepare for Influenza A (H1N1) in terms of processing, technology, manpower, and material resources. At the same time, the MOH immediately forwarded related information to the MOA and the AQSIQ.

On April 26th, Health Minister Chen Zhu convened a meeting of the MOH Leading Group and Expert Panel for Influenza Pandemic Prevention and Control, at which the attendees analyzed swine influenza situations in the United States and Mexico, predicted epidemic trends, and deliberated on domestic strategies and measures to cope with a swine flu pandemic. Health Minister Chen also held an inter-departmental meeting with the MOA, the AQSIQ, and other ministries to analyze epidemic trends and discuss response strategies and measures. Immediately after the meeting was over, the MOH reported in writing that very night to the State Council on the progress of epidemic prevention and control work.

On April 27th, following the emergency meeting held in Geneva, the WHO elevated the pandemic alert level from Phase 3 to Phase 4, stating that the "swine flu" was widespread and was being transmitted by humans in different ways. General Secretary Hu Jintao issued instructions to place prevention and control against this virus as the nation's top priority.

On the same day, Vice Premier Li Keqiang convened the State Council Meeting regarding the Human-Swine Influenza Prevention Working Mechanism, resulting in the decision to establish a multi-departmental working mechanism for joint prevention and control of the human-swine influenza. As required by the State Council meeting, the MOH called together the Publicity Department of the Communist Party of China (CCPPD), the Ministry of Foreign Affairs (MFA), the NDRC, the MIIT, the MOF, the Ministry of Transport (MOT), the MOA, the MOC, the AQSIQ, the China National Tourism Administration (CNTA), the Civil Aviation Administration of China (CAAC) among other departments on that very night for a meeting to deliberate on Influenza A (H1N1) prevention and control; the meeting established the multi-departmental working mechanism for joint prevention and control of human-swine influenza and the *Notice on Strengthening Human-Swine*

Influenza Prevention and Control was drafted and published on the night of April 27th after State Council review. The MOH issued the *Notice of the MOH General Office on Strengthening Preparedness for and Response to Human Swine Influenza*.

On April 28th, Premier Wen Jiabao convened a State Council Executive Meeting which deliberated on how to strengthen national response to human-swine influenza; at the meeting they defined the overall prevention and control principles and strategies of "taking threats to public health seriously, responding actively, and coping with the epidemic in a scientific manner according to law through joint prevention and control efforts."

On April 29th, the WHO raised its pandemic alert level from Phase 4 to Phase 5.

On April 30th, at a press conference held at the State Council Information Office, the MOH declared the establishment of a multi-departmental working mechanism for joint prevention and control against the human-swine influenza, which would be spearheaded by the MOH. Under this mechanism, 33 departments and institutions (which later increased to 38) constituted 8 work groups—General Office, Ports, Healthcare, Support, Dissemination and Communication, Foreign Collaboration, Science and Technology, and Animal Husbandry and Veterinary—and an expert committee, forming a "8 + 1" pattern for joint prevention and control efforts.

On the afternoon of May 1st, the joint prevention and control mechanism held its second joint conference, renaming the human-swine influenza which was occurring in Mexico and the United States to "Influenza A (H1N1)." The former wording of "multi-departmental work mechanism for joint prevention and control of human-swine influenza" was changed to the "Joint National Influenza A (H1N1) Prevention and Control Mechanism" and roles and responsibilities were outlined for the mechanism, work groups, and the expert committee. At the same time, a meeting system for all members and liaisons was established. Problems in principle which a work group encountered would be solved by the work group itself, and those which the work group struggled with would be settled through coordination under the joint prevention and control mechanism—general affairs would be solved by regular liaison meetings, and major issues decided by plenary meetings.

4.2.2 The Composition of the Joint National Influenza A (H1N1) Prevention and Control Mechanism

4.2.2.1 Organizational Structure

Health Minister Chen Zhu and MOH Party Group Secretary and Vice Health Minister Zhang Mao chaired the Joint National Influenza A (H1N1) Prevention and Control Mechanism, and the mechanism was comprised of eight working groups—General Office, Ports, Healthcare, Support, Dissemination and Communication, Foreign Collaboration, Science and Technology, and Animal Husbandry and Veterinary—and an Expert Advisory Committee. The heads of the work groups, the leaders of the Health Department of the People's Liberation Army General Logistics Department (GLD), the Logistics Department of the Chinese People's Armed Police Force (PAPF), and the chairman of the Expert Advisory Committee, served as members of the joint prevention and control mechanism.

The work groups, the GLD Health Department and the PAPF Logistics Department each designated one or two departmental-level officials as liaisons for routine communication purposes.

4.2.2.2   Main Responsibilities and the Division of Labor

The main duties of the Joint National Influenza A (H1N1) Prevention and Control Mechanism included: meet regularly to evaluate epidemic trends and determine prevention and control strategies; formulate prevention and control policies, response plans and major measures; coordinate and provide guidance on the implementation by all related departments and in various regions of prevention and control measures; and organize supervision and inspection activities concerning the implementation of prevention and control measures. See Table 4.1 for the main responsibilities of the work groups and the Expert Advisory Committee.

4.2.3   The Operation of the Joint National Influenza A (H1N1) Prevention and Control Mechanism

Thirty three meetings were convened under the Joint National Prevention and Control Mechanism, in which regulations were formulated, signed, and issued for local implementation. Implementation issues would be reported in real time to related State Council departments for instructions.

The establishment of the Joint National Prevention and Control Mechanism played a crucial role in the scientific and orderly response to Influenza A (H1N1), in that (1) the mechanism raised the priority level for Influenza A (H1N1) prevention and control for related departments and local governments, (2) clarified and divided responsibilities, (3) addressed investment issues, and (4) enhanced inter-departmental cooperation.

4.2.3.1   Working Consultation System

A consultation system and a liaison meeting system were established under the Joint National Prevention and Control Mechanism, which were designed to ensure effective implementation of prevention and control measures. Specific issues in prevention and control work would be resolved through consultation at liaisons meetings, and major issues decided by plenary meetings. Each working group established a fixed meeting system where they could provide timely progress

Table 4.1 Composition of the work groups and the expert advisory committee for the joint national influenza A (H1N1) prevention and control mechanism

Work group	Leading organization	Members	Duties
General office group	MOH	CCPPD, MFA, NDRC, MOST, MOA, AQSIQ, GLD Health Department, PAPF Logistics Department, Expert Advisory Committee	Comprehensively coordinate routine affairs among departments of the joint prevention and control mechanism; organize regular meetings of the joint prevention and control mechanism and oversee the handling of top agendas; collect, sort out, and report to higher-ups about progress in prevention and control efforts; prepare progress reports on the joint prevention and control mechanism; publish information on epidemic situations and response efforts; ensure the consistency in style of writing for documents intended for outside use; and shoulder other assignments from leaders
Ports group	AQSIQ	MFA, Ministry of Public Security (MPS), MOT, MOR, MOA, MOC, MOH, General Administration of Customs (GAC), CNTA, State Council Information Office (SCIO), CAAC, and State Post Bureau (SPB)	Carry out health quarantine, surveillance, health supervision and management at entry-exit ports; collect, sort out and report on information regarding epidemic developments, response measures, etc. abroad; ensure the quality and standardization of emergency materials
Healthcare group	MOH	State Administration of Traditional Chinese Medicine (SATCM), AQSIQ, GLD Health Department, PAPF Logistics Department, and China CDC	Organize the formulation and revision of technical solutions to the diagnosis, treatment, prevention and control of Influenza A (H1N1), and oversee the implementation of those solutions; provide guidance on nationwide monitoring, reporting, and epidemiological surveys of epidemic situations, specimen collection and testing, epidemic management, etc.; direct national medical treatment plans of Influenza A (H1N1); send experts, as needed for epidemic prevention and control, to go and help with epidemic handling and medical treatment in priority regions; provide recommendations on strategies and measures for improving response efforts; and undertake other assignments from leaders

(continued)

Table 4.1 (continued)

Work group	Leading organization	Members	Duties
Support group	NDRC	MIIT, MOF, MOT, MOR, MOC, MOH, AQSIQ, CAAC, SFDA, and GLD Health Department	Plan as a whole the support logistics for emergency materials, and deliberate on and coordinate major issues involved in the process; have a full grasp on nationwide support, respond to the demand for emergency materials as well as their production, circulation, storage and allocation, and coordinate affairs concerning supply and demand, production, storage, transportation, etc. of emergency materials; coordinate and arrange funding for production, purchase (import), storage, etc. of emergency materials (including instruments and equipment); oversee the implementation of support measures in regions and by departments concerned, and closely track progress in the process; monitor market situations regarding supply and demand of basic living supplies and cleaning supplies; maintain the market order through market supervision and management, price stabilization and punishment of business violations, and where needed, deliberate on and take related measures; provide feedback on support work and summarize such information in a timely manner; complete other assignments from leaders
Dissemination and communication group	CCPPD	International Communication Office, State Administration of Radio, Film, and Television (SARFT), General Administration of Press and Publication (GAPP), and main central news media	Report in a timely fashion on Influenza A (H1N1) situations and on progress made in major efforts under the joint prevention and control mechanism, and guide public opinion positively and correctly; arrange news releases on the joint prevention and control mechanism, and where necessary, organize press conferences; track public opinion at home and abroad, and clarify facts in a timely fashion; strengthen management and guidance on the release of

(continued)

Table 4.1 (continued)

Work group	Leading organization	Members	Duties
			online news; assist related departments to disseminate knowledge about protection against Influenza A (H1N1), to increase the population's self-protection capabilities; collect, sort out and report information on public opinion monitoring, etc. in real time
Foreign collaboration group	MOF and MOH	MOC, AQSIQ, CNTA, and the Hong Kong and Macao Affairs Office, Taiwan Affairs Office, and Overseas Chinese Affairs of the State Council	Handle foreign affairs related to Influenza A (H1N1) prevention and control; coordinate the handling of major foreign affairs in terms of Influenza A (H1N1) prevention and control, and coordinate affairs related to Influenza A (H1N1) prevention and control in the regions of Hong Kong, Macao and Taiwan; collect and report information on, and coordinate, affairs of collaboration and communication with international organizations such as the WHO, regional organizations, foreign governments, as well as with Hong Kong, Macao and Taiwan; collect and report information on national organizations and epidemic situations abroad; provide guidance on and oversee influenza response efforts by Chinese staff sent abroad, as well as the protection of overseas Chinese; promote related departments' external communication about China's response efforts and measures; urge related departments to track experience and practices of other countries and international organizations with regard to coping with Influenza A (H1N1); work with related departments to track and survey impacts of the virus on the country's diplomacy, economy and trade, tourism, and people migration, and make policy recommendations accordingly; oversee foreign aid and receive international donations; and complete assignments from the State Council

(continued)

Table 4.1 (continued)

Work group	Leading organization	Members	Duties
Science and technology group	MOST	MOH, MOA, MOE, AQSIQ, GLD Health Department, and Chinese Academy of Sciences (CAS)	Decide on plans for technical research into Influenza A (H1N1) prevention and treatment; organize research projects aimed to tackle technological difficulties in response to the virus; coordinate and solve technological issues involved in the development and application of monitoring technologies, drugs and vaccines on a unified basis; collect, sort out and report on such information as latest research developments in a timely fashion
Animal husbandry and veterinary group	MOA	NDRC, MOF, MIIT, MOT, MOC, State Administration for Industry and Commerce (SAIC), AQSIQ, GLD Department of Military Supplies, Materials and Oils, and PAPF Logistics Department	Closely monitor, test, prevent, and control animal epidemics; provide scientific judgments on epidemic trends; adjust prevention and control measures on a continued basis; and strengthen swine management through integrated epidemic prevention and control measures, with emphasis placed on swine epidemic monitoring and epidemiological surveys and on ensuring stable swine reproduction
Expert advisory committee	MOH	Experts from MOE, MOA, AQSIQ, GLD Health Department, CAS, as well as local health departments	Provide recommendations on appropriate response levels and countermeasures for confirmed public health emergencies; give advice on public health emergency preparation; participate in formulating and revising contingency plans and technical solutions to public health emergencies; provide technical guidance on public health emergency mitigation; advise on the termination of health emergency countermeasures; provide post-emergency evaluations; and undertake other assignments from public health emergency operations and management bodies

reports, discuss and address problems, and push ahead with prevention and control work within their fields. The establishment and improvement of the coordination mechanism remarkably increased the efficiency of inter-departmental coordination and response efforts. This success evinces the importance of a multi-departmental coordination and collaboration mechanism based on risk communication for effective epidemic prevention and control.

Firstly, documents were issued jointly by related departments under the new Joint National Prevention and Control Mechanism. For example, on June 22nd, 2009, the MOE and the MOH jointly issued the *Work Plan for Influenza A (H1N1) Prevention and Control in Schools (Tentative)*; the two ministries also jointly issued *the Urgent Notice on Strengthening the Management of Vaccination to Students against Influenza A (H1N1)* on November 4th, and the *Notice on Strengthening Influenza A (H1N1) Prevention and Control in Rural Schools* on November 26th.

Secondly, members were supplemented to the Joint Prevention and Control Mechanism to improve efficiency. On November 23rd, 2009, based on the demands of the nation's prevention and control efforts, the MOH Office of Health Emergency sent letters to the General Office of the Supreme People's Court, the Ministry of Supervision (MOS), the Ministry of Civil Affairs (MCA), the Ministry of Human Resources and Social Security (MOHRSS), and the Legislative Affairs Office (LAO) of the State Council, adding them all as members of the mechanism.

Thirdly, horizontal collaboration between related departments was strengthened. For example, on April 29th, 2009, the MOH Office of Health Emergency sent a letter to the MIIT Department of Consumer Goods Industry recommending an increase in the national stockpile of supplies necessary for Influenza A (H1N1) prevention and control including medical supplies and response gear. In another example, the Office of Health Emergency, Department of Medical Affairs, and Bureau of Disease Control and Prevention of the MOH, the China CDC, and the Chinese Medical Association, jointly formulated the *Technical Guidance on Prevention and Control of Human-Swine Influenza*, and the *Plan for Diagnosis and Treatment of Human-Swine Influenza (2009)*. One more example occurred on July 30th, when the Foreign Collaboration Group for the Joint Prevention and Control Mechanism, along with the NDRC, the MIIT, and the SFDA met to discuss donating Influenza A (H1N1) prevention and control materials to the WHO and developing countries affected by the pandemic.

4.2.3.2   Information Reporting System

During the course of the epidemic response efforts, risk evaluation, and risk management, it was necessary to build unobstructed information exchange channels to ensure the accurate transfer of data and information. Under the Joint Prevention and Control Mechanism, each of the lead departments for the work groups and the Expert Advisory Committee appointed people to collect, sort out, tabulate and analyze their work groups' epidemic information and latest progress on a daily basis, and to report in writing daily data collected by 18:00 to the General Group prior to 20:00 p.m. The General Group would then prioritize epidemic information and progress reports, and submit it representing the entire Joint Prevention and Control Mechanism to the General Duty Office of the State Council. Strengthened coordination and communication between the work groups and their members ensured an unobstructed flow of information as the working groups were informed of major issues as they happened. The General Group was also charged with publishing information crucial for the public's knowledge on epidemic prevention and control.

Updates on Influenza A (H1N1) prevention and control were submitted via four reporting systems: the Disease Monitoring Information Reporting Management Subsystem of the China Information System for Disease Control and Prevention, the Public Health Emergency Reported Information Management System, the China Influenza Information Monitoring System, and Administrative Reporting System for Health Departments. Reported information mainly included: ongoing epidemic situations, monitoring results from sentinel hospitals and network laboratories, progress in vaccination and results of side effects monitoring, and ongoing regional and departmental response efforts.

With Influenza A (H1N1) cases rising rapidly, issues with epidemic information reporting began to occur, such as overlapping reports, large discrepancies between confirmed reported cases and actual cases, and the circulation of ambiguous epidemic information. To better and more accurately reflect national epidemic situations and trends, the MOH General Office issued the *Notice on Strengthening Work of Reporting Deaths from Influenza A (H1N1)* on November 4th, 2009, and the *Notice on Adjusting the Work of Reporting Information on the Influenza A (H1N1) Epidemic* on November 13th, 2009.

By April 7th, 2010, the General Group had submitted more than 700 work reports regarding Influenza A (H1N1), and compiled and published over 200 *Response Progress to Influenza A (H1N1) under the Joint Prevention and Control Mechanism* reports. Information on epidemic trends and response efforts was released in a timely, open, and transparent manner, and by this time eight news conferences and nine press briefings had been held regarding the latest progress in Influenza A (H1N1) prevention and control.

4.2.3.3 Supervision and Inspection System

To ensure that prevention and control measures were implemented effectively and efficiently, the work groups each established a supervision and inspection system by which to examine routine work on a regular basis, identify existing deficiencies and problems, and supervise and inspect response contingency plans and procedures, operational capacities, epidemic monitoring, epidemiological investigations, designated hospitals and their isolated areas, medical observation, material supplies, staff training, and information dissemination on prevention and control.

4.3   The Establishment, Composition, and Operation of Local Influenza A (H1N1) Prevention and Control Mechanisms

In the course of Influenza A(H1N1) prevention and control efforts, local governments, as instructed by the central government, examined their own conditions and established local bodies to command and coordinate response measures. The local departments worked together to implement disease prevention and control measures in priority areas and among targeted groups, and ensured continued epidemic monitoring and treatment.

4.3.1   The Establishment of Local Influenza A (H1N1) Prevention and Control Mechanisms

The following three modes mainly represent actual prevention and control measures adopted by local governments.

The first work mode was similar to the National Joint Prevention and Control Mechanism. For example, Shaanxi set up a leading group for Influenza A (H1N1) prevention and control, whose office was located inside the provincial Department of Health and their local structure followed the "8 + 1" joint prevention and control mechanism model. Guangdong established a joint prevention and control mechanism with the participation of thirty two departments, and nine work groups and three panels of clinical, disease prevention and control, and etiological experts functioned under the mechanism. On April 30th, Fujian established an Influenza A (H1N1) prevention and control work group, headed by a provincial government official; the office was located inside the building of the provincial Department of Health whose emergency management office was charged with performing routine work for the group. The *Emergency Guidance on Influenza A (H1N1) Prevention and Control in Fujian (Tentative)*, issued on May 10th, 2009, outlined response guidance as "prevention first through joint prevention and control, timely management, and level-by-level responsibility."

The second work mode was the emergency operations center or leading group. After discovering their first confirmed Influenza A (H1N1) case, some provinces and cities upgraded their existing disease prevention and control mechanisms and established an Influenza A (H1N1) response leading group or emergency operations center. Beijing was the first in the country to establish a municipal-level public health emergency operations center in May 2006, and had earlier (April 25th, 2009) launched a public health emergency response mechanism after the WHO declared the outbreak of swine influenza in Mexico; an Influenza Prevention and Control Office (at the general office of the municipal government before it relocated to the Municipal Bureau of Health) was established under the emergency operations center, whose members included twenty two committees, eighteen district and county governments, and the GLD Health Department. This Control Office established a public health emergency response and medical rescue collaboration mechanism with the China CDC, the Academy of Military Medical Sciences, and other institutions. It established a mutual fixed epidemic communication system with local agricultural, educational, industrial, and commercial departments. A joint command response mechanism was also created with other special operations centers in Beijing. On May 13th, Shandong established a provincial public health emergency leading group and started Level-II response measures after discovering its first—and the country's second—confirmed imported case of Influenza A (H1N1). On June 2nd, Hubei established an Influenza A (H1N1) emergency operations center after the province's first case was confirmed. Immediately after the country's first Influenza A (H1N1) case was confirmed on May 11th in Sichuan, Sichuan initiated Level-II public health emergency response measures and set up a provincial response leading group as per the State Council's requirement of handling the virus as a Category B infectious disease.

The third work mode was the joint conference system. Some provinces and cities established a joint conference system in response to the Influenza A (H1N1) outbreak. For example, Henan established an Influenza A (H1N1) joint conference system on April 30th, and on the same day Guangxi established a 12-department joint conference system for its own prevention and control efforts.

While establishing provincial-level joint prevention and control mechanisms, health departments also set up internal expert panels. For example, Fujian Provincial Department of Health set up a provincial-level Influenza A (H1N1) prevention and control expert supervision panel; Guangdong Provincial Department of Health established three expert panels for clinics, disease prevention and control, and etiology; Sichuan Provincial Department of Health established a leading group, a technical guidance expert panel, and a medical rescue panel on April 30th.

4.3.2 The Composition of Local Influenza A (H1N1) Prevention and Control Mechanisms

The composition of local mechanisms for Influenza A (H1N1) prevention and control basically followed the framework of the National Joint Prevention and Control Mechanism, with an office and several work groups collaborating under a leading group or operations center. For example, Beijing's public health emergency operations center was responsible for the city's influenza prevention and control, and it was comprised of eight work groups plus an office, these groups included: immigration inspection, healthcare, epidemiological survey, material security, dissemination and communication, information, animal husbandry and veterinary, and social prevention and control supervision (referred to as "one office and eight groups"). Fujian's Influenza A (H1N1) prevention and control leading group consisted of thirty one departments and organizations, including the Provincial Department of Health, a press office, and a development and reform commission.

Sichuan's Influenza A (H1N1) prevention and control leading group (operations center) included departments from emergency management, public security, development and reform, transportation, immigration inspection and quarantine, tourism, civil aviation, foreign affairs, and publicity. The office of Sichuan's Influenza A (H1N1) prevention and control leading group was originally located in the Provincial Department of Health, which was then moved to the provincial government's General Office Building as the epidemic worsened. Its work groups consisted of emergency coordination, general support, information secretaries, epidemic prevention and control, medical rescue, supervision and inspection, press and communication, and health education.

4.3.3 The Operation of Local Influenza A (H1N1) Prevention and Control Mechanisms

Local Influenza A (H1N1) prevention and control mechanisms adopted a similar communication and coordination mechanism to the Joint National Prevention and Control Mechanism, and operated in with joint offices, conferences, etc.

Sichuan is one example of this. The provincial operations center and the provincial leading group (headquarters) shared offices in order to strengthen the province's joint prevention and control against Influenza A (H1N1), and its seven work groups were comprised of highly capable professionals from the emergency management office, third secretariat office of the general office, and the Provincial Health Department. The Health Department met regularly with the departments of public security, civil aviation, immigration quarantine, economy and trade, animal husbandry, as well as PLA and People's Armed Police troops stationed in the province. Adjustments were made in real time in according with latest local epidemic situations. Latest information on epidemic updates across the province were reported daily to members and related departments, and where cases were discovered, the departments of health, public security, foreign affairs, railway, transport, and others worked closely to track close contacts and ensure they were medically observed. Through close collaboration between departments at various levels on joint prevention and control, Sichuan ensured that cases were discovered, reported, isolated and treated at the earliest possible time, which delayed the spread of the virus and lowered epidemic intensity.

4.4 Social Participation in Local Influenza A (H1N1) Prevention and Control Mechanisms

Government departments, enterprises, institutions, communities, and nonprofit organizations (NPOs) all play important roles in prevention and control of an infectious disease. With the country's response efforts entering its second phase, the

13th Meeting of the National Joint Prevention and Control Mechanism, held on June 10th, 2006, proposed further improvements of existing mechanisms, in particular establishing accountability systems and mass prevention and control mechanisms with participation from urban communities, schools, enterprises and villages. These mechanisms could better implement tailored measures, disseminate self-protection knowledge for families and individuals, and improve measures that maintain the status quo and normal economic operations.

4.4.1   Community Participation

When confronted with a public health emergency, under the guidance of the government, the society can effectively avoid or reduce potential damage by achieving preliminary prevention and control targets at local levels through community involvement and solidarity along with raising public awareness in self-protection. In its 1989 Work Report, the WHO mentioned two types of community participation, i.e. participation as a means, and participation as a goal, and analyzed effects of the two. In the course of China's Influenza A (H1N1) prevention and control efforts, communities, the most basic social units, played an important role in knowledge dissemination and health education, the tracking and isolation of close contacts, and epidemic supervision.

When uncertainties still surrounded the pathology and virulence of Influenza A (H1N1) in the early days of the epidemic, local communities launched information dissemination and health education campaigns, playing a crucial role in stabilizing public opinion and raising awareness of scientific disease prevention and treatment methods.

In the case of community-level outbreaks, affected communities generally adopted comprehensive response measures, which emphasized managing the sources of infection in order to contain and control the transmission of the influenza virus. Measures mainly included the following: (1) Sub-district offices or town governments mobilized social forces—as per laws, rules, and regulations—to provide support for isolated cases, including logistical service to personnel engaging in medical observation; (2) Close contacts were medically observed centrally or at home, and healthcare workers reported daily on patients' progress; (3) Patients with influenza-like symptoms were recommended to rest at home and not participate in unnecessary public gatherings or travel; (4) Schools, nurseries and kindergartens, nursing homes, and construction sites were required to conduct health inspections, and enterprises with a concentrated amount of personnel or those who provided social services were required to perform morning health inspections; (5) Information on epidemic trends and response measures were published in real time, and efforts were made to strengthen information disclosure within communities; and (6) Health education and risk communication were carried out through multiple channels.

When the virus broke out in communities, healthcare departments managed cases categorically and adopted comprehensive measures for strengthening the treatment of severely ill cases, lowering case fatality rates, and mitigating epidemic damage. With prevention and control measures in place against community-level outbreaks, response measures for priority areas mainly included the following: (1) As per related laws, rules, and regulations, local governments mobilized social forces to ensure the logistical support of measures like home-based treatment of cases with influenza-like symptoms; (2) Migration was cut or restricted, recreational areas were temporarily shut down, and large-scale gatherings were canceled or postponed. Enterprises and institutions within communities were permitted to grant time off for all or some of their employees; (3) Schools, nurseries, and kindergartens were closed per related regulations; (4) Enterprises and institutions as social services providers with large workforces implemented a health reporting system, management was enhanced where there were large flows of people, and people with influenza-like symptoms were recommended to rest and receive treatment at home; (5) When necessary, outbreak points were put under isolated control, and quarantine measures were taken in epidemic areas. At the same time, measures were taken to organize and encourage volunteers to participate in prevention and control activities, to help maintain the normal operation within communities, and provide mental health interventions to avoid adverse effects on public health.

These measures, which were designed based on real community conditions, effectively guaranteed the protection of the status quo, and laid a strong foundation for local Influenza A (H1N1) prevention and control efforts.

4.4.2   Enterprise Participation

4.4.2.1   Drug Stockpiling Enterprises

In the course of Influenza A (H1N1) prevention and control efforts, drug stockpiling enterprises responded actively to the government's call for material reserves and production. Because influenza drugs weren't prevalent in clinical use, they were traditionally stockpiled through loans, government subsidies, business opportunities and moderate enterprise compensation.

Problems arose during the implementation of this mechanism such as subsidy inaccessibility and unreasonable compensation. For example, the current 10% subsidy policies regarding corporate loans and government subsidies hardly met the needs of enterprises, and the problem of unreasonable compensation to pharmaceutical enterprises still existed, partly because specific mechanisms were lacking. At the same time, more than 80% of emergency response drugs were not on the standing list of medications, and so it was necessary to build a long-term relationship between the government and enterprises to specify respective duties, and link stockpile funding with corporate social responsibility to balance compensation.

4.4.2.2   Reagent Manufacturers

Reagent manufacturing was one of the government's top priorities during the entire course of its Influenza A (H1N1) prevention and control efforts. Some reagent manufacturers which had developed and produced reagents for biological agents such as anthrax during the 2008 Olympic Games already had experience in emergency response. For example, Beijing Kinghawk Pharmaceutical Co., Ltd., the country's first to obtain approval for an Influenza A (H1N1) testing kit, signed a strategic alliance agreement with the China CDC during the Influenza A (H1N1) Epidemic. The enterprise also provided its laboratories voluntarily when there was no clear policy on state funding, doing its best for society as a corporate citizen. With its technology reserve, seven production platforms and ninety approved products, Kinghawk was able to perform research and development on product standardization during a critical time of the epidemic. The China CDC had access to international resources for preliminary research and development and successfully obtained information and strains from the WHO. This collaboration between the two parties made it possible to develop preliminary products in 72 h and thus ensured that considerable demand for clinical diagnosis was met. This played a positive role in case diagnosis during the early phases of the Influenza A (H1N1) Epidemic and was also quite meaningful in terms of drug use guidance.

The government provided active support to research and development efforts. Take Kinghawk as an example. After Kinghawk signed the agreement with the government on May 4th, 2009, both the Beijing Economic-Technological Development Food and Drug Administration and the Beijing Food and Drug Administration provided recommendations. Kinghawk had developed a rapid test kit by May 11th, received approval from the CFDA on June 17th to launch the emergency response system, and got approved for manufacturing the reagent for 250,000 people on September 25th. Kinghawk had collaborated with the China CDC in the past and had experience in reagent development and manufacturing. The development of the reagent fully demonstrated the efficiency in collaboration between the government and a commercial enterprise, and also guaranteed the timeliness of preliminary disease diagnosis.

4.4.2.3   Areas Provided for Isolated Cases

In the containment phase, hotels and other requisitioned enterprises across the country showed full support for the response measures by providing isolation zones of Influenza A (H1N1) cases. Many hotels suitable for isolation purposes were private firms and thus could not be requisitioned through administrative orders, which put a certain amount of pressure on local governments. However, coordination efforts by local governments did earn support and assistance from these hotels.

4.4.2.4 Infrastructure Enterprises

Transport enterprises shouldered the heavy task of implementing disease prevention and control for the floating population. Civil aviation, railways, road and related enterprises implemented strict prevention and control measures, including disseminating knowledge about disease prevention and control, and providing necessary infrastructure support for emergency response efforts targeting the floating population. All in all, a healthy transportation environment helped lower the transmission of the disease. Facing the unexpected onset of Influenza A (H1N1), these transportation enterprises all established prevention and control groups. For example, the CAAC North China Regional Administration established a Capital Airport Influenza A (H1N1) Prevention and Control Leading Group, which was based on the former Capital Airport Public Health Emergency Leading Group; Beijing Capital International Airport Company Limited, Air China Limited, China Southern Beijing Company, China Eastern Beijing Company, Hainan Airlines Beijing Company, CAAC Air Traffic Management Bureau all set up their own epidemic response teams to ensure the orderly implementation of prevention and control measures.

Telecommunications enterprises did their duties as corporate citizens and actively cooperated in Influenza A (H1N1) prevention and control efforts. China Mobile Group Beijing Company Limited, China Telecom Group Beijing Company Limited, China Unicom Beijing Company Limited, among other telecommunications operators, suspended their normal user notification group-messaging services and mustered network resources to send messages on epidemic updates while increasing maintenance staff, strengthening network monitoring, and closely watching the impact of group messaging on their systems.

4.4.3 Participation of NPOs

Nonprofit organizations, or NPOs, are organizations that fulfill particular social causes or missions without seeking profit for their efforts, and NPOs represented a crucial social force in the course of the nation's Influenza A (H1N1) prevention and control. For example, the Beijing Red Cross established a public health emergency operations center which consisted of a general information group, a rescue response group, a fundraising and aid group, a publicity group, and a public relations group. This organization actively engaged in response efforts in accordance with the *Beijing Red Cross emergency contingency plans for public emergencies.*

4.4.4 Public Participation

The entire nation was involved in epidemic prevention and control, including its citizens. During the response to the virus, volunteers played an important role when multiple departments suffered emergency manpower shortages. For example, medical and healthcare students in colleges and universities volunteered to work on the front lines of epidemic prevention and control. In Beijing, 170 student volunteers from Capital Medical University assisted with response efforts at Capital Airport, and similar volunteering also occurred in Fujian. The public actively supported the government's Influenza A (H1N1) prevention and control measures, and voluntarily took part in the process via the Internet and other media channels; for example volunteers called those who had just returned from abroad and informed them of potential isolation measures. At the same time, increased public health awareness was also instrumental in successfully dealing with the disease.

4.5   Analysis and Reflections on Influenza A (H1N1) Prevention and Control Mechanisms

4.5.1   Experience in Mechanism Building for Influenza A (H1N1) Prevention and Control

4.5.1.1   The Timely Establishment of Influenza A (H1N1) Prevention and Control Mechanisms

At the beginning of the Influenza A (H1N1) Epidemic, China established a national level emergency management mechanism directly under the leadership of the State Council that enabled cross-departmental joint prevention and control collaboration, which provided an effective organizational support and operation mechanism for the response efforts. Though the MOH had formulated the *Ministry of Health's Influenza Pandemic Preparedness and Response Plan (Tentative)* before the epidemic broke out, this document focused only on the duties of the MOH and didn't encompass more complex coordination and collaboration with related government departments. The joint prevention and control mechanism remedied this flaw by providing a platform for coordination and collaboration between the MOH and other related departments. Also, because this mechanism was not like the State Council's operations center, it allowed some space for strengthening the State Council's leadership and collaboration once the epidemic worsened.

During the prevention and control efforts, local governments adapted and innovated central policies and their implementation in light of local epidemic situations, public health trends, and demographic and economic conditions. Some areas established prevention and control mechanisms with local characteristics. The main features of these mechanisms are as follows:

The first was the establishment of a strong leadership system. In the process of prevention and control, local governments established their respective public health emergency leadership systems based on local epidemic situations, geographic features, and public health resources.

The second was the innovation in ideas and methods. Local epidemic prevention and control bodies closely monitored trends and reengineered their methods based on existing departmental systems in order to better target obstacles encountered in operations. For example, in the early days of the epidemic, the Beijing government issued a *Notice on Further Specifying Duties and Prioritizing Operations to Strengthen Influenza A (H1N1) Prevention and Control*, which articulated the new public health notion of "responsibility of four sides" (government, departments, enterprises, and individuals). This clarification brought about effective collaboration between the government and the society in public health emergency management. The Beijing Immigration Inspection and Quarantine Bureau employed risk analysis methods in its prevention and control efforts and ensured electronic transfer of information on inbound passengers, which not only increased quarantine and inspection efficiency but also scientifically and efficiently improved response measures. Fujian was the country's first province to implement temporary isolation measures through its local Health Department. Henan created an epidemic prevention and control network of "three horizontal fronts"—arrangements at a government level, measures at enterprise (institution) level, and protection at a local level; and "three vertical fronts"—government supervision, inter-departmental collaboration, and public opinion guidance. These institutional innovations proved very effective in the response efforts.

The third was the establishment of an inter-provincial support mechanism. On November 13th, 2009, the MOH General Office issued the *Notice on Strengthening Medical Treatment of Influenza A (H1N1) Patients (No. 245, 2009)*, announcing the decision to establish an inter-provincial support mechanism for medical treatment of Influenza A (H1N1) patients as per the *Notice of the State Council on Strengthening the Ongoing Work on Influenza A (H1N1) Prevention and Control (No. 23, 2009)* and as needed for patients. The form of assistance was technical support, especially in regards to medical treatment of seriously and critically ill patients.

4.5.1.2 The Active Implementation of an Expert Decision-Making Mechanism

Throughout the entire duration of the prevention and control efforts, governments greatly heeded experts in various fields, which aided governments in creating more scientific policy adjustments and technical plans, and consequently reduced blindness and uncertainty in policy implementation. Experts from CDCs, hospitals, publicity departments, and other departments took part in the decision-making process, and their input was adopted in real time. Some experts even took the initiative to provide police recommendations directly to decision makers.

At the same time, governments sought out expert opinions through different methods and channels, i.e., consultation at joint prevention and control meetings or direct consultation with the experts. Expert recommendations ensured scientific policies and more targeted and effective policy formulation.

4.5.1.3 Policy Adjustments Based on a Local Context

In regards to policymaking, some local governments formulated policies and adjustments based on local conditions and epidemic trends. For example, Jiangmen experimented with a home-based isolation policy, while Shenzhen created corridors at ports specifically for foreigners and a separate one for students commuting between Shenzhen and Hong Kong for school. Also, in terms of policy adjustment, some local departments were able to adjust related policies in time to better suit local epidemic situations. As for issues that necessitated policy coordination, local departments also made strategic adjustments as early as possible. For example, the Guangdong Immigration Inspection and Quarantine Bureau, at experts' suggestion, transferred persons who required isolation and medical observation to health departments for categorical management, which thus ensured the efficient use of epidemic prevention and control resources.

4.5.1.4 The Gradual Realization of Widespread and Diverse Societal Participation in Disease Prevention and Control

Over the course of Influenza A (H1N1) prevention and control efforts, the government cultivated an environment of widespread social participation under the leadership of the party and government, with enterprises, communities, volunteers and other social actors playing crucial roles in the response efforts.

4.5.2 Reflections on Influenza A (H1N1) Prevention and Control Mechanisms

4.5.2.1 The Legal Status of the Joint National Prevention and Control Mechanism

The Joint National Prevention and Control Mechanism was essentially a command and decision-making mechanism established according to the potential amount of damage Influenza A (H1N1) could inflict upon society. On the one hand, Influenza A (H1N1) response required inter-departmental collaboration, and relying solely upon health departments for countermeasures wouldn't be enough; on the other hand, because the virus was not as virulent as to merit the establishment of a State Council Operations Center (or Headquarters), the State Council instead instructed the MOH to establish a multi-departmental joint prevention and control mechanism; and this new organization represented a relatively flexible and effective response mechanism.

Although local governments were already aware of the epidemic at its onset and were actively engaging with different departments in their response efforts, because there were no explicit provisions in related laws and contingency plans for the Joint

National Prevention and Control Mechanism at the central level, no corresponding normative documents were available for its implementation at a local level. No unified standards on the name, content, form of establishment, and system structure for local governments' prevention and control bodies existed. Although local governments adapted as they went, it was still an environment that incited disorder and confusion.

4.5.2.2   Issues with Emergency Command Responsibilities, Authority and Administrative Levels

On the one hand, participating departments fully endorsed the Joint National Prevention and Control Mechanism. This mechanism, they thought, possessed several advantages: Firstly, the joint consultation system made it possible to directly formulate and sign policies at joint prevention and control conferences, which saved time for everyone; Secondly, the joint briefing system required the work groups to send daily reports to other units and departments, thus facilitating both inter-group and inter-departmental communication; And finally, internal collaboration within groups was solid, and the briefing system allowed an unobstructed flow of information. However, the Joint National Prevention and Control Mechanism based upon consultation and communication had its limitations. On issues involving departmental interest, division of duty, and so on, this horizontal collaboration was less efficient than regulation and control by a single, high level leadership department.

One contested issue dealt with the location of the local joint prevention and control office: should it be set up in the comprehensive emergency management office of the local government or in the emergency management office of a local specialized department. Some provincial emergency management offices insisted that for an emergency event like the ongoing Influenza A (H1N1) epidemic, a joint prevention and control office should be located in a specialized department so as to leverage the department's expertise and increase response flexibility, convenience and efficiency. In this scenario, the provincial emergency management office would be tasked with solving issues that the specialized department could not. On the other hand, some provincial health department's emergency offices argued that if the office was located in the local government, the joint prevention and control office would enjoy greater authority and more efficient collaboration.

4.5.2.3   The Transition Between Peacetime Mechanisms and Emergency Response Mechanisms

Achieving a smooth and effective transition between peacetime and public emergency, and establishing mechanisms that combined crucial components from both systems, was a new challenge that arose in the Influenza A (H1N1) Epidemic.

After the 2003 SARS Epidemic, local governments established permanent public health emergency response departments and corresponding working mechanisms to deal with future public health emergencies. These departments and mechanisms should have been employed upon the onset of the Influenza A (H1N1) Epidemic. However, most provinces established completely new leading groups only after the central government established Joint National Prevention and Control Mechanism. In one example, a provincial health department already had a permanent public health emergency operations center, but, after the central government established the Influenza A (H1N1) Joint National Prevention and Control Mechanism, this province created an entirely new prevention and control leading group and a port leading group. At the same time, the Health Department also established new eternal mechanisms, including: the provincial CDC established an emergency response department with leaders from major sections like emergency management and vaccination planning (starting in 2005, this provincial CDC implemented a "3 in 1" meeting system with participation from emergency management, disease control, and the disease monitoring department).

The main reason for this redundancy was because the central government did not provide specific conditions or qualifications for contingency planning and management for the transition period between peacetime to emergency. Thus, local governments lacked a clear transition mechanism that they could utilize. It was the reason that many local governments chose to re-establish emergency management bodies when Influenza A (H1N1) broke out.

4.5.2.4   Problems with Inter-departmental Coordination

As public health emergency management involved multiple collaboration systems from the central government down to local governments, regions, and departments, inter-departmental collaboration in the response efforts was intrinsically complicated. The response to this epidemic revealed problems that existed both in horizontal and vertical coordination.

In regards to horizontal coordination between central departments, the health, education, security, transportation and many other departments were involved in the Influenza A (H1N1) response efforts, which created an environment where responsibilities could easily overlap and grey areas would occur in management. There was also a lack of coordination and standardization between central-level ministries' policy documents for Influenza A (H1N1) countermeasures. For example, in regards to content standardization, the health authorities felt that using the temperature of 37.3 °C as the sole standard for sending people to the hospital was unreasonable and would cause an unnecessary burden on hospitals. In regards to time standardization, on December 2nd, 2009, one province stipulated that only patients with a temperature of 38 °C or higher must be sent to a hospital, and it took the country two more weeks to follow suit. In regards to inter-departmental work, port laboratories in some provinces had begun testing in the early days of epidemic, but stopped after provincial health departments decided that ports were not fit for such work. Obstacles also arose in horizontal coordination and collaboration between local departments. A lack of information communication between local departments due to the unavailability of complete information in the early stages of prevention and control made it nearly impossible for effective collaboration.

In regards to the division of labor and coordination between the central and local governments for disease prevention and control, some local governments held that the central government should have presented broader goals and authorized provinces and cities greater autonomy in their response measures. Some felt that the central government should not have made Influenza A (H1N1) prevention and control an issue of political significance but should have been objective in understanding the differences between executive leadership and scientists' opinions. While the main duty of administrative leaders should have been to organize and mobilize social resources needed to cope with the epidemic, scientists should have been the ones to handle technical issues such as epidemic analysis and response measures. At the same time, more efficient communication should have been present between central and local departments tasked with specific operations. For example, some local management departments felt that the entire process was quite political, making some documents difficult to fully implement; in the two most volatile months that lasted from April 28th to June, documents were issued frequently, and in some cases were in conflict with one another and lacked integrity and continuity. In regards to adjustment of prevention and control strategies, some regions' health departments reported the following issues: higher-level departments frequently adjusted technical guidance and strategies for prevention and control, there was a wide variety of information reporting methods and they were constantly in flux, different departments formulated their own response requirements, and differences occurred in measures and standards; all of which greatly complicated local response operations.

Certain communication and coordination issues also existed within the Health Department's internal system. The MOH internal horizontal collaboration needs to be strengthened epidemiological investigations, clinical diagnoses, and laboratory testing to combine the medical treatment and disease prevention. For example, the China CDC played a crucial role as a central technical support body of Influenza A (H1N1) prevention and control in epidemiological information collection, monitoring, analysis, and judgment, but at the same time it also had a lot of administrative duties, and its services and duties overlapped with those of the MOH's Bureau of Disease Control and Prevention. There should be unified leadership and coordination between higher and lower-level health departments within the national epidemic prevention and control system. A certain degree of flexibility is also necessary as provinces differ in epidemic situations, medical resources, geographic features, and so on.

In regards to information reporting within the health system, though the China CDC and the MOH had established information systems relating to epidemic surveillance, including an epidemic direct reporting system, no information sharing mechanism was created between the China CDC and medical institutions; in particular, some county level medical institutions didn't even have sound data collection and reporting systems. This resulted in a single point of decision making and command, and their lack of network and information technology weakened the support they could've had in implementing response measures.

4.5.2.5   Roles of NPOs Have Yet to Be Leveraged and Improved

NPOs such as the Red Cross Society of China played important roles during the Influenza A (H1N1) prevention and control efforts. However, by comparison with developed countries, China still lags behind in terms of public participation in public health emergencies. There still remain limitations in skill and knowledge, as no emergency volunteer systems or working mechanisms were formed, and no leveraging of NPO resources really occurred.

Reference

Lang, P., & Wang, C. (2007). On Public Emergency Management Bodies of the Chinese Government. *Chinese Public Administration 11*, 104–108.

Chapter 5
An Evaluation of China's Influenza A (H1N1) Emergency Response Measures

5.1 Monitoring, Prevention, and Control

5.1.1 Epidemic Monitoring

5.1.1.1 The Expansion of the Emergency Monitoring Network

In order to stay up to date on epidemic trends and monitor possible mutations of the virus in the wake of an outbreak, China invested nearly 400 million RMB on testing large amounts of specimens and expanding the influenza monitoring network to include 411 influenza monitoring network laboratories and 556 sentinel hospitals—a network which covered all prefectural-level cities and some priority districts and counties. All of these laboratories and hospitals were in operation by September (see Fig. 5.1).

5.1.1.2 Epidemic Monitoring and Analysis

The China CDC provided technical support and services for national response efforts. Its work in this regard included the following: Upgrading the China Information System for Disease Control and Prevention; incorporating Influenza A (H1N1) into the Disease Monitoring Information Reporting Management System, the China Influenza Monitoring Information System, and the Public Health Emergency Information System; specifically establishing an Influenza A (H1N1) information management system; tracking and analyzing domestic epidemic situations through the national infectious disease network reporting system and the national influenza monitoring network system; collecting and analyzing information on the conditions, treatments, and outcomes of infected cases; providing real time analysis reports and information support needed to improve prevention and control strategies; mapping global pandemic distribution and the distribution of isolated

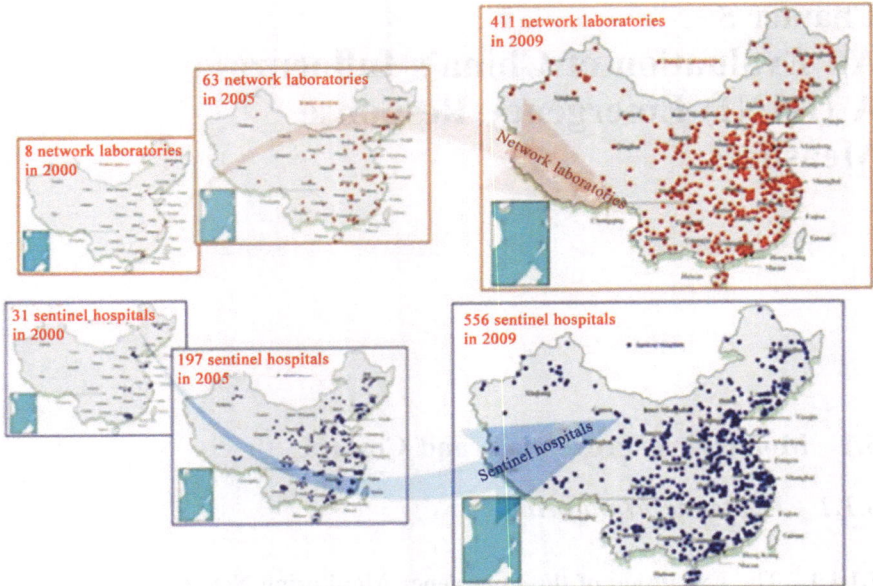

Fig. 5.1 Expansion of influenza monitoring sentinel hospitals and network laboratories in China

people by provinces; integrating individual cases and community outbreaks into the national infectious disease and public health emergency information systems for direct online reporting; enabling timely reports on severely ill cases; monitoring domestic and foreign epidemic information; optimizing information systems and platforms; ensuring the collection and analysis of information on mass vaccination, and the monitoring of side effects of vaccination.

5.1.1.3   Laboratory Testing

Upon learning of the Influenza A (H1N1) outbreak in Mexico, the CNIC immediately began developing testing kits as per instructed by the government. On April 27th, the China CDC's National Institute for Viral Disease Control and Prevention (IVDC), obtained information on the Influenza A (H1N1) virus' genetic sequences from the U.S. CDC and immediately engaged in sequence alignments, as well as the design and testing of nucleic acid detection techniques. On April 29th, after receiving from the WHO information on the recommended primer for nucleic acid detection, the IVDC promptly made comparisons with a variety of seasonal influenza viruses, synthesized the primer sequence needed for detection, and prepared the first-generation nucleic acid detection reagent for the human Influenza

A (H1N1) virus—which was distributed to 84 influenza monitoring laboratories across the country on the night of April 30th. And on May 1st, the first phase of training on influenza monitoring laboratories focusing on port-based cities began, and immigration inspection and quarantine personnel were trained later on. Also, through the WHO, the CNIC provided fourteen countries including Cuba, Mongolia, Vietnam, and Macao with the independently developed testing kit and provided training for their personnel.

The China CDC's Influenza A (H1N1) testing kits were swiftly deployed to monitoring network laboratories throughout the country, and training was promptly carried out for testing professionals. On May 10th, 2009, the Sichuan Provincial CDC tested a suspected imported case with the newly prepared reagent, with results being weakly positive. Tests conducted afterwards by the China CDC and the Academy of Military Medical Sciences proved that the case was indeed the country's first confirmed case of the virus. The testing reagent that China had independently and urgently developed proved to be a success.

In the process of coping with Influenza A (H1N1), regular etiological testing was an integral part of laboratory work. Drug resistance data obtained about the virus supported the clinical application of antiviral drugs, and knowledge acquired of the virulence of the virus and its possible mutations provided scientific support for the adjustment of prevention and control strategies and measures.

5.1.1.4   Field Epidemiology Investigations

As an important capacity that a CDC possesses to cope with public health emergencies, field epidemiology includes the detection, reporting, and response capabilities for public health emergencies, field investigation and management, emergency monitoring, survey result analysis and summation, and investigation report writing capabilities. Field epidemiology operations during this epidemic were carried out by CDCs at various levels in collaboration with related departments.

According to survey data, CDCs were able to provide real time telephone and/or online reports to their higher ups through the reporting of medical institutions, schools, nurseries, and through the active monitoring and detection of patients. This also enabled timely management of the outbreaks. CDCs at various levels had certain field investigation and management capacities, as they implemented emergency monitoring and report writing. It was also found that epidemiological survey investigators were quite able in their organization, coordination, and response, but less capable in epidemiological investigation, analysis, data interpretation, the formulation of appropriate control measures, and the assessments of prevention and control effects. Epidemiological survey investigators were able to direct or implement corresponding prevention and control measures on the spot, but they lacked sustained logistical support, personal protective equipment, and psychological counseling.

5.1.1.5   Technical Plans for Prevention and Control

On April 29th, 2009, the MOH issued the *Technical Guidance on Prevention and Control of Human-Swine Influenza (Tentative)* and the *Plan for Diagnosis and Treatment of Human-Swine Influenza (2009)*, and on April 30th, the CAAC issued the *Notice on the Work of Transporting Human-Swine Influenza Samples*. On May 7th, the MOH issued the *Work Plan for the Transport of Influenza A (H1N1) Cases* and on May 8th, it issued the *Plan for Influenza A (H1N1) Diagnosis and Treatment (Tentative, 1st Version, 2009)*. Provinces, cities, and counties organized large scale training and exercises for technical planning as per national policies, strategies, and measures.

It is worth mentioning that the 2005 *Influenza Pandemic Preparedness and Response Plan of the Ministry of Health (Tentative)* was not activated, mainly because of the following reasons: (1) this document as a departmental contingency plan only specified duties of health departments, without incorporating duties of other related departments, and (2) it was designed principally to target Influenza A virus subtype H5N1 that is highly pathogenic with high case fatality rates, and was not suitable for the Influenza A (H1N1) Pandemic.

5.1.2   Port Quarantines

After China received a disease outbreak notice form the WHO on April 25th, 2009, the AQSIQ issued the *Urgent Notice on Preventing Human-Swine Influenza from Spreading to China (No. 30, 2009)*, which made arrangements for port inspection and quarantine measures targeting people from regions with Influenza A (H1N1) outbreaks, and it also provided international travel recommendations for people traveling to such regions. Thus began the ports' battle against Influenza A (H1N1).

5.1.2.1   Port Quarantine Strategies

On April 30th, 2009, by issuing the 2009 No. 8 Proclamation, the MOH incorporated Influenza A (H1N1) into Category B infectious diseases under the *Infectious Disease Prevention and Treatment Law*, for which prevention and control measures against Category A infectious diseases were adopted, and put it under infectious disease management provided by the *Frontier Health and Quarantine Law*.

On May 2nd, 2009, the AQSIQ issued the *Notice on Restoring the Entry-Exist Health Declaration Card for People Entering China* via *Land and Water Ports (No. 37, 2009)*. On May 4th, 2009, the AQSIQ, the MPS, the MOR, the MOH, and the GAC jointly issued the *Notice on Strengthening Influenza A (H1N1) Prevention and Control in Passenger Trains Leaving China*. Up to this point in time, the country had strengthened prevention and control efforts for sea, land, and air transportation. In May and June of that year, the MOH and other departments including the MFA and the AQSIQ jointly issued, as documents under Joint National Prevention and Control Mechanism, the *Notice on Further Specifying Influenza A (H1N1) Prevention and Control Measures*, and the *Notice on Adjusting Influenza A (H1N1) Prevention and Control Measures*, raising strict requirements on prevention and control measures for aircrafts and aircrews entering China. The AQSIQ issued the *Influenza A (H1N1) Port Health and Quarantine Procedure and Operational Specifications*, which included measures targeting priority areas, groups, flights, and ports, including health declarations, body temperature testing, designated docking points, strengthened medical inspection and screening, and improved management of cases and close contacts. Airport customs X-rayed all incoming luggage from epidemic areas. In the early days of Influenza A (H1N1) prevention and control, the railway authorities implemented body temperature testing of passengers aboard trains before their entry into China, and provided berths used specifically for observing passengers with fevers; tourism authorities implemented a registration system for tourists entering and leaving the country. During this phase, China implemented an "imported case containment" strategy with strict port quarantine measures.

On July 10th, 2009, by issuing the 2009 No. 9 Proclamation, the MOH incorporated the Influenza A (H1N1) virus into Category B infectious diseases under the *Infectious Disease Prevention and Treatment Law*, for which prevention and control measures against Category A infectious diseases were adopted, and put it under infectious disease management provided for by the *Frontier Health and Quarantine Law*. One month afterwards, Influenza A (H1N1) port quarantine measures across the country gradually transitioned into a routine monitoring phase.

5.1.2.2   Port Quarantine Data

Since the outbreak of Influenza A (H1N1) in China, port inspection and quarantine departments across the country accumulatively inspected 176 million passengers entering China, detected 24,800 persons with influenza symptoms, and transferred 17,700 persons to health departments for isolated observation. A total of 10,636,200 trips of aircraft, vehicles, ships, and trains entering China were inspected. See Fig. 5.2 for details.

In the phase of strict port quarantine measures which lasted from May 2nd to July 13th, a total of 1001 imported cases were discovered at ports in mainland China. The weekly curve of cases discovered at ports and that of total cases reported were highly consistent with one another (r = 0.99), and the ratio of cases discovered at ports each week to the total cases reported across the country each week remained stable at 30–40%.

During this period, 359 imported cases were discovered at port by body temperature screening, which accounted for 36% of all imported cases reported. 46% of the cases were discovered by hospitals when they went and sought treatment after having developed symptoms upon entry into the country; 81 cases (8.1%) were discovered when they volunteered to report to health departments after having

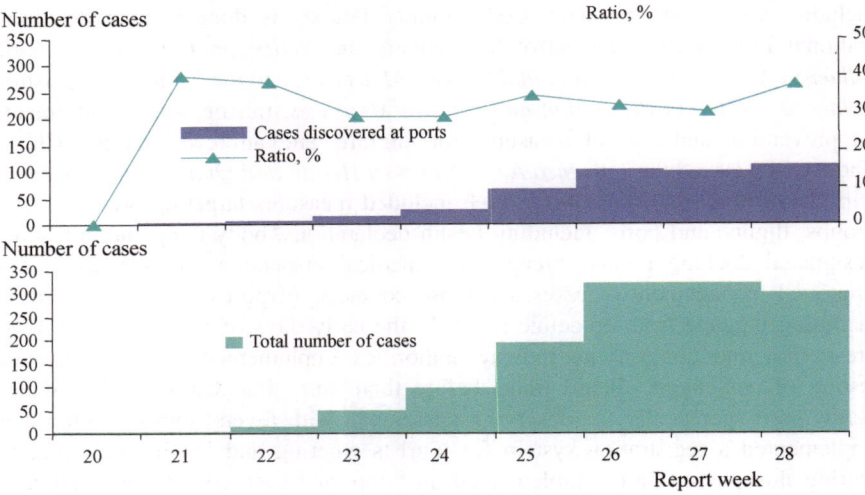

Fig. 5.2 Weekly distribution of port cases

developed symptoms on their entry; 48 cases (4.8%) were discovered when they were isolated for medical observation as close contacts; 34 cases (3.4%) declared their symptoms on port health declaration cards; and 8 cases (0.8%) were discovered in community searches upon their entry (Fig. 5.3).

5.1.2.3 Implementation of Port Prevention and Control Measures

To assess the role port quarantine measures played in the containment of imported cases, we evaluated the implementation of Influenza A (H1N1) prevention and

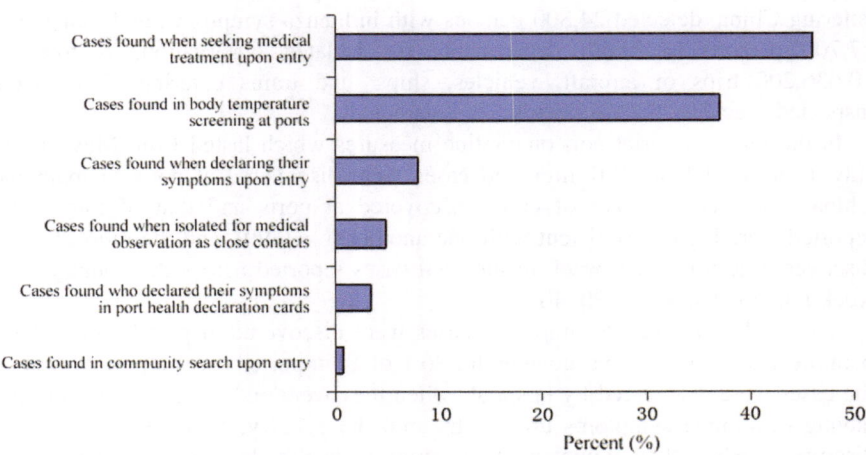

Fig. 5.3 Main detection methods for imported cases from May 2nd to July 12th, 2009

control measures by Entry-Exit Inspection and Quarantine Bureaus across the country in different phases of the epidemic, and we summarized the improvements of entry-exit inspection and quarantine strategies and mechanisms against international infectious diseases. We sampled seven Entry-Exit Inspection and Quarantine Bureaus, of Fujian, Guangdong, Sichuan, Henan and Beijing, and evaluated their emergency response efforts. These survey results served as a good representation of ports across the country.

Organization and Management

The Entry-Exit Inspection and Quarantine Bureaus and ports all established Influenza A (H1N1) prevention and control leading work groups and expert groups, with the earliest unit established on April 27th, 2009. These groups formulated response contingency plans, and implemented work responsibility and accountability systems (in which the bureau head was in command and other leaders oversaw implementation). The seven bureaus performed 186 inspections on their own Influenza A (H1N1) prevention and control work, and higher-level departments performed 78 inspections and received 476 documents; 502 prevention and control training sessions were conducted, and 686 updates were published on local media channels.

Port Prevention and Control Measures

All ports launched a health declaration card system, and set up entry passages and inspection zones specifically for passengers arriving from epidemic-stricken countries or regions; airports employed infrared thermometers and surveillance video cameras, and launched campaigns about Influenza A (H1N1) prevention and control and port quarantine requirements.

Suspected patients, once discovered, underwent epidemiological testing, and confirmed cases were strictly isolated and reported, with tracking records as complete as 95%; close contacts were strictly tracked, registered and medically observed, with records as complete as 90%. Other port countermeasures included: quarantining close contacts in designated areas; issuing clinic cards; strictly examining mail and possessions of passengers from epidemic-stricken countries and regions; disinfecting special passages and means of transport from epidemic-stricken countries and regions; environmental friendly disposition of waste generated by transport from epidemic-stricken countries and regions; crafting contingency plans and programs; and employing effective measures to protect susceptible passengers.

Personnel and Material Stockpiling for Port Prevention and Control

The seven ports surveyed deployed a total of 7533 people for Influenza A (H1N1) prevention and control work, with 6% of participants with a PhD or higher degree, 30% with a master's degree, 50% with a bachelor's degree, and 14% with a lower degree. Each month an average of 499 infrared thermometers, 91 surveillance cameras, 19 vehicles, 51 communications devices, and 19 rapid test devices were employed. The ports stockpiled 7,115,000 RMB worth of disinfectants, 5,622,200 RMB worth of protective masks, 4,327,000 RMB worth of protective clothing, and 1,574,000 RMB worth of protective eyewear. Two ports had a combined stockpile of 168,000 RMB worth of Tamiflu; six ports were equipped with 29,128,000 RMB worth of laboratory equipment; and five ports stockpiled 3,125,000 RMB worth of serological test kits.

5.1.3   Prevention and Control

In the early days of the epidemic, because of the difficulty in predicting the virus' potential damage and impact, international organizations including the WHO as well as many developed countries adopted a series of prevention and control measures. As per the WHO's response guidance, and in light of the country's epidemic trends and medical response capacity, China adopted different prevention and control strategies and measures in different phases.

As important entities for specialized disease prevention and control, CDCs played crucial roles in the nation's epidemic response. In order to evaluate the implementation and results of national prevention and control policies at a provincial, municipal, and county level for response mechanisms, we conducted research on thirty one CDCs throughout five provinces.

5.1.3.1   Close Contact Management

In the early days of the epidemic, these CDCs focused on "blocking foreign importation of the virus, containing internal transmission, and preparing counter-measures for the next wave of outbreaks." Their overall mission was to control imported cases and manage close contacts.

According to survey results, during the onset of the epidemic, 97% of the areas centrally isolated and observed close contacts, 71% tracked close contacts in their areas, 87% requested assistance from other CDCs to track close contacts, and 97% received requests from other CDCs for assistance to track close contacts.

The start of home-based isolation measures for close contacts was on May 1st, and it ended on October 8th (Fig. 5.4). On July 8th, the MOH issued the *Notice on Further Improving Influenza A (H1N1) Prevention and Control Measures (No. 122, 2009)*, which marked a turning point in policy adjustment: the Notice stipulated that

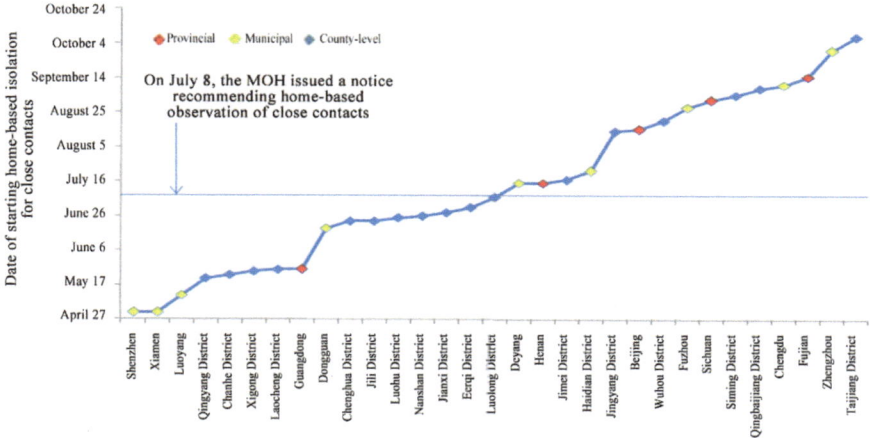

Fig. 5.4 Time distribution of close contact measures implemented in surveyed cities, regions, and counties

close contacts would no longer be centrally isolated and observed, and instead should be isolated at home with monitoring by the local health department. For people without permanent residences, medical observation was carried out either at their temporary address or at a designated area.

The earliest date among these CDCs to stop tracking close contacts was July 22nd, 2009, and the latest was January 31st. On November 6th, 2009, the MOE and the MOH issued the *Work Plan for Influenza A Prevention and Control in Schools*, and on December 10th, 2009, the MOH promulgated the *Guidance on Influenza A (H1N1) Prevention and Control by Government Organs, Enterprises and Institutions (Tentative)* and *the Guidance on Influenza A (H1N1) Prevention and Control by Towns (and Sub districts) (Tentative)*, all clearly stating that "it is in principle unnecessary to detect, track, register, and medically observe close contacts of sporadic influenza A (H1N1) cases."

The earlies date among these CDCs to stop tracking the contacts of close contacts was May 10th, and the latest was December 31st. But the country's prevention and control policies didn't expressly require tracking the contacts of close contacts of Influenza A (H1N1) patients.

5.1.3.2 Case Management

The *Notice on Further Improving Influenza A (H1N1) Prevention and Control Measures (No. 122, 2009)*, which the MOH issued on July 8th, clarified categorical medical treatment; it strengthened treatment efforts for seriously ill patients, and it pushed for potential home-based treatment for mildly ill cases. According to survey findings, 94% of the CDCs had every hospitalized case separately isolated and treated during the early stages of the epidemic; the earliest date among them to seek home-based treatment for mildly ill cases was June 24th, and the latest was November 30th. 87% of CDCs required that each case have two negative test results before being allowed a medical discharge; the earliest date among them to stop this requirement was July 13th, and the latest was November 7th. On October 12th, 2009, the MOH issued the *Plan for Influenza A (H1N1) Diagnosis and Treatment (3rd Version, 2009)*, which stopped the requirement that every case be tested negative before they could be discharged from the hospital.

In the early phases of the epidemic, the surveyed CDCs performed epidemiological testing on every single case; the earliest data among them to stop doing so was July 15th, and the latest was March 1st, 2010. All the surveyed CDCs thoroughly investigated each severely ill case or fatality.

5.1.3.3 Implementation of School Suspension

As the epidemic continued to worsen with the increase in local cases, the prevention and control strategy was adjusted to "reducing domestic cases, tightening measures against the spread among communities, strengthening treatment of seriously ill cases, and coping with changes in epidemic trends." With clusters of cases breaking out in schools, the MOH formulated work plans for Influenza A (H1N1) prevention and control in priority areas including schools, government organizations, enterprises, and institutions, with emphasis placed on concentrated groups in schools and hospitals. According to regulations and in light of experts' risk assessments, temporary school suspension was recommended by local health departments. Influenza A (H1N1) joint prevention and control mechanisms or emergency operations centers would review recommendations from experts and local education departments before their approval, announcement, and implementation.

Survey findings showed that 29 (94%) CDCs provided recommendations for school suspension in pursuant of national criteria while two CDCs did not, citing the reason that the "national criteria was too rigorous" and instead followed "local criteria." 60% of the regions surveyed completely followed national school suspension criteria, 30% did so in most cases, and the other 10% did so only in a few cases. 37% of school suspension decisions were made by governments, 43% by education departments, 10% by health departments, 7% by CDCs, and 3% by schools.

5.1.3.4 Manpower and Material Security

Survey findings showed that 90% of the CDCs suffered shortages of manpower during prevention and control efforts, mainly—in descending order—field epidemiology, epidemic management, laboratory testing, and health education. To resolve these manpower shortages, 81% of the CDCs transferred personnel from sections that were engaged in prevention and control of diseases other than

Table 5.1 CDC manpower shortages

Manpower shortage	Number of CDCs	Percentage
Field epidemiology	26	93
Epidemic management	22	79
Laboratory testing	21	75
Health education	14	50
Vaccination	11	39
Logistical services	5	18
Other	2	7

Influenza A (H1N1), and 29% borrowed personnel from other agencies for their epidemic response efforts. The ratio of personnel transferred out of their entire original sections varied from 9 to 85% (Fig. 5.1 and Table 5.1).

All CDCs received subsidies specifically for Influenza A (H1N1) prevention and control from local governments, which ranged from 50,000 RMB to 8.87 million RMB; provincial CDCs received an average of 4.29 million RMB (300,000–8.87 million RMB); municipal CDCs received an average of 2.78 million RMB (100,000–7.69 million RMB); and county-level CDCs received an average of 630,000 RMB (50,000–2.6 million RMB). The ranking of the five regions in terms of CDC funding, in descending order, was as follows: Beijing, Sichuan, Guangdong, Henan, and Fujian. 45% of the CDCs stated that they experienced a shortage of funds.

Before the epidemic, all of the CDCs had strengthened preparedness in terms of emergency materials, mostly personal protective equipment, disinfection instruments, as well as laboratory reagents, equipment and consumables; some CDCs stockpiled antiviral drugs. 26% of the CDCs stated that after the epidemic occurred, they were still faced with shortages of materials, mostly test reagents, personal protective equipment, and laboratory supplies.

5.1.4 Capacity Assessment for Monitoring, Prevention and Control

The nation's Influenza A (H1N1) monitoring, prevention, and control efforts produced some remarkable results, in which the monitoring and alert network played a vital role, with some key technologies rivaling the international market; the goal of "containing imported cases, preventing domestic transmission, delaying the spread of the epidemic, suppressing the peak, mitigating the potential harmful impact with each phase, and winning time to bolster response efforts" was achieved. Notwithstanding, problems did emerge with the monitoring system as well as with manpower and materials support, which have yet to be addressed.

5.1.4.1 The Effective Mitigation of the Epidemic's Transition and the Suppression of Its Peak

In the early stages of influenza pandemic, China adopted the strict prevention and control strategy of "containing imported cases and preventing domestic transmission," which effectively prevented the rapid development of the epidemic across the mainland. From June to August 2009, while countries in the northern hemisphere such as the United States and the United Kingdom saw the first peak of Influenza A (H1N1) cases where the virus amounted to 97% of all Influenza A viruses, Influenza A (H1N1) only accounted for 4–5% in China and no nationwide peak occurred at that time. From May 11th to August 31st, 2009, China reported roughly 3721 confirmed cases, with an average of only 33 new cases found daily. When the U.S. CDC announced on July 30th that the new Influenza A (H1N1) virus accounted for 99% of all Influenza A viruses, the ratio was only 2.3% in China. Unlike other countries in the northern hemisphere, China saw only one epidemic peak, which shows of human intervention in response efforts.

5.1.4.2 The Vital Role of the Monitoring and Alert Network

The expanded influenza monitoring network of sentinel hospitals and network laboratories made it possible to dynamically monitor, in real-time, epidemic trends and possible virus mutations (from the start of the epidemic through its spread nationwide); which enabled a comprehensive understanding of epidemic situations. This network provided a crucial foundation for scientific response measures, it provided the government with a scientific basis for decision-making, and it brought about a radical change in response by comparison with SARS in 2003 where information flow was obstructed, epidemic situations were unknown, and measures lagged in implementation. The expanded monitoring network with the advancement of information technology were iconic achievements in the investment and construction and of the public health system in recent years, and they proved their worth in this round of Influenza A (H1N1) response efforts. This network met technical requirements in epidemic management, and represented the rapid progress in capacity building for the country's public health system.

The China CDC and other specialized agencies displayed professionalism in the early phases of epidemic monitoring and alert, and the monitoring and reporting network received an upgrade in the later phases of the epidemic. The government increased the number of influenza monitoring sentinel hospitals and expanded the influenza monitoring system. Epidemic monitoring provided first-hand scientific evidence for decision-making on response efforts. In regards to Influenza A (H1N1) information monitoring and reporting, the reporting system was upgraded to the extent that it could satisfy information reporting and feedback needs in real time, which is evidence of the government's capabilities in rapid system expansion.

5.1.4.3   The Success of Rapid Testing for Influenza A (H1N1)

Within 72 h after receiving related news from the WHO, China developed a highly sensitive and specialized rapid diagnostic test kit for the Influenza A (H1N1) virus. The key probe used in the developed RT-PCR H1N1 testing kit, which was developed based on modifications made to technologies that foreign disease control and prevention centers had previously made, played a crucial role in early diagnosis of the virus. While there are no commercialized ELISA-H1N1 influenza diagnosis testing kits abroad, the SFDA has already approved seven types, which compared with their foreign counterparts, can detect the new Influenza A (H1N1) virus. Additionally, China's research and analysis of the new Influenza A (H1N1) virus' entire genome sequence garnered international recognition and played an important guiding role in the country's prevention and control efforts. At the end of 2009, after an evaluation of the CNIC, the WHO concluded that the CNIC's operations and research were on the forefront of international research, and agreed to include the CNIC as one of the five WHO Collaborating Centers for reference and research on influenza, making it the first of the kind in a developing country to earn the status.

5.1.4.4   Construction of the Monitoring and Alert System Still Needs to Be Strengthened

An imbalance still exists among provinces in terms of the development of the influenza monitoring network. Monitoring has not begun in Tibet, and some influenza network laboratories are still of poor quality. An integrated monitoring system that enables full coverage, high quality monitoring, epidemiology and laboratory monitoring has not truly been established domestically. There are still inadequacies regarding in-depth analysis and comprehensive judgments of the monitoring data, as well as a lack of related models and analysis methods appropriate to national conditions. Detection capabilities of public health emergencies are inadequate, and the existing functions of the web-based public health emergency reporting system still require expansion and improvement. Moreover, the fact that reporting for this Influenza A (H1N1) epidemic involved four information platforms - the epidemic information system, the influenza monitoring system, the emergency reporting system, and the Influenza A (H1N1) reporting system, along with the changes in the scope of information collection and reporting designs, caused trouble and confusion in local information reporting, analysis, and utilization. Multi-departmental mechanisms for information communication and integration still require further improvement.

5.1.4.5   The Inadequacy of Human, Financial and Material Resources

Influenza A (H1N1) prevention and control caused considerable pressure on human resources in local CDCs. Survey findings showed that 90% of the CDCs suffered manpower shortages, mainly in field epidemiology, epidemic management, and laboratory testing. 45% of the CDCs stated they experienced financial shortages, and 26% were faced with material shortages such as testing kits, protective equipment, and laboratory supplies after the outbreak of the epidemic.

5.1.4.6   Prevention and Control Policies and Measures Could Further Be Improved in Terms of Flexibility and Adaptability

In regards to formulating policies and countermeasures for different phases of the epidemic, many policy documents were issued providing detailed specifications of prevention and control strategies and measures, with real time policy adjustments. Our research found, however, that it was widely claimed that the national policies, strategies, and measures did not suit local epidemic situations and prevention and control capabilities, so in turn local CDCs were unable to properly adapt to them; national policies were often formulated and adjusted either ahead of or lagging behind local trends and prevention and control needs. According to survey findings, when national policies were inconsistent with local epidemic situations, nearly half of the CDCs strictly adhered to national policies, 35% formulated their own strategies and measures, and 23% didn't formulate written regulations but instead flexibly implemented measures to suit local conditions. Discrepancies existed also in the implementation of specific measures regarding to the time and process. On close contact management, for example, nearly half the local CDCs had already adopted the relatively loose measure of home-based medical observation before the national policy was promulgated, and some of them stated that they had communicated with related state departments, obtained verbal approval from them, and hence experimented with the implementation of this measure.

5.2   Medical Treatment

As a key part of Influenza A (H1N1) prevention and control efforts, the effectiveness of medical treatment has a direct impact on the livelihood of the people. Up until August 10th, 2010, of the 128,033 confirmed cases reported by the mainland's 31 provinces (municipalities directly under the central government, and autonomous regions), 31,994 cases were hospitalized—805 were fatal, with a death rate of 2.5%.

In dealing with Influenza A (H1N1), the MOH employed a comprehensive strategy, deploying limited medical resources with the integration of medical technology for the categorical treatment of patients. The MOH specified Influenza A (H1N1) diagnosis and treatment duties for medical institutions of all levels, and established national, provincial, prefectural-level expert teams, and medical rescue teams at hospitals designated for treating seriously ill patients—all with the mission to carry out categorical medical treatment. The practice of "assembling patients, experts, and resources for concentrated treatment of seriously ill patients" at designated tertiary infectious disease hospitals and general hospitals guaranteed the efficient utilization of limited and top-quality medical resources. Domestic clinical experiences were summarized on a regular basis, and multiple meetings were held to revise plans for clinical diagnosis and treatment. Additionally, international exchanges were strengthened to improve the quality of medical treatment. Meanwhile, assistance mechanisms were established between provinces, within provinces, between large general hospitals and local medical institutions, and between different departments within hospitals, all to provide regions that had inadequate medical resources with technical and material support to enhance medical treatment quality.

Medical institutions were the main fields of battle against the influenza epidemic, and their capabilities were a direct manifestation of the country's medical treatment capabilities. Medical treatment policies were under continuous adjustment as epidemic situations changed. The Evaluation Team assessed medical treatment policies and their implementation in different epidemic phases through interviews conducted with the heads of the General, Healthcare, and Support Groups under the Joint National Influenza A (H1N1) Prevention and Control Mechanism, as well as with 31 hospitals in the five representative provinces and cities. Survey results showed that these hospitals shared many similarities with their Influenza A (H1N1) prevention and control work and were definitely representative to a certain degree of the national medical treatment capabilities.

5.2.1 Medical Treatment Strategies and Measures

5.2.1.1 Time Distribution and Evolution of Influenza A (H1N1) Cases

From April 25th to June 10th, 2009, the first imported case in China was reported and subsequently a surge of imported cases followed suit. The first confirmed imported case was reported in the mainland on May 11th, 2009, and thereafter, imported cases were on the rise, mostly in provinces with air and land ports. The first domestic case was confirmed on May 29th, and on May 11th, the WHO declared a global influenza pandemic, stating that the influenza virus was spreading in seventy one countries and five continents; this was the same day the first local case from unknown sources of infection was reported, marking the start of the national epidemic response efforts. Up until June 10th, the mainland reported a total of 170 confirmed cases—including 14 locally infected cases, with no seriously ill cases or fatalities—and most of these were located in regions with more transportation ports such as Beijing, Guangdong, Fujian, and Shanghai.

From June 11th through early August 2009, mild cases increased gradually, most of them being local in nature. China reported the first severely ill case on August 8th, and the success in curing this case paved the way for later treatment of the large number of severely and critically ill cases. Up until August 10th, a total of 2348 conformed Influenza A (H1N1) cases were reported in the mainland, 2167 of them cured with zero fatalities. In the same time period, according to data published by the WHO, the Influenza A (H1N1) virus had spread to more than 170 countries and regions worldwide, with 177,457 internationally confirmed cases and a death toll of 1462.

Guangdong reported the mainland's first seriously ill case on August 8th, 2009, and from then on seriously and critically ill cases were on the rise, until two months later when only a few critically ill cases were being reported in some provinces. In September, with students returning to school after the summer holiday, cases began rising rapidly, mostly in concentrated outbreaks in schools. On October 4th, Tibet reported the mainland's first Influenza A (H1N1) fatality. With the remarkable increase of clustered cases, severely and critically ill cases continued to rise in October, alongside increasing fatalities, and at that time the Influenza A virus became the dominant strain of influenza in the country. Cases increased significantly into November, and infection rates remained high for three consecutive weeks before reaching the peak of more than 1200 cases reported weekly. The ratio of the patients infected with Influenza A (H1N1) virus to the total number of patients with influenza viruses recorded by monitoring sentinel hospitals across the country peaked at the end of November. Children under nine years old were the biggest proportion of severely ill cases, followed by high-risk groups like people with chronic disorders, pregnant women, and people with obesity, with main complications including pneumonia, respiratory failure, and acute respiratory distress syndrome.

New cases in the mainland fell gradually beginning in December. In early 2010, Influenza A (H1N1) virus activity was in decline, alongside a rapid drop in new cases. As of March 2010, only a few cases were being reported across the country, and activity gradually transitioned to seasonal influenza, dominantly Influenza B viruses.

5.2.1.2 General Requirements and Strategies for Medical Treatment

In regards to medical treatment strategies, the specific requirement, which was clarified for hospitals on April 27th, 2009, was "strengthening the monitoring and reporting of cases of pneumonia caused by unknown reasons" while maintaining the focus on medical treatment of seriously ill cases.

After the first local case caused by unknown reasons was reported on June 11th, the government reviewed its previous response efforts and revised its prevention and control strategy to "reducing domestic cases, tightening measures to prevent community-level transmission, strengthening medical treatment of seriously ill cases, and coping with epidemic changes," placing emphasis on measures aimed to control and reduce the occurrence of domestic cases and improve capabilities of medical treatment for seriously ill cases. On July 8th, the government once again issued a document stressing the strengthening of medical treatment of seriously ill cases, and specifying categorical treatment of patients.

After Guangdong reported the mainland's first seriously ill case, on September 3rd, 2009, the Joint National Prevention and Control Mechanism changed the prevention and control strategy set forth on June 12th to "reducing domestic flu cases, controlling epidemic transmission in communities, strengthening treatment of severely ill patients, protecting susceptible populations, and mitigating epidemic damage," so as to minimize the occurrence and mortality rate of Influenza A (H1N1).

5.2.1.3 Main Measures

During the phase where most cases reported were imported cases, and in order to implement measures that focused on "discovering, diagnosing, reporting, isolating and treating cases as early as possible," China, in its effort to guide and regulate Influenza A (H1N1) diagnosis and treatment operations, promulgated a total of thirteen documents and technical plans concerning monitoring and treatment in hospitals. The government also standardized monitoring plans and procedures, performed two revisions on the treatment and monitoring plans, and also made provisions concerning nosocomial infection and patient transport—with particular emphasis on cases with flu-like symptoms from epidemic-stricken regions. Health departments at various levels designated hospitals to admit and treat emerging Influenza A (H1N1) cases, and designated first aid centers (stations) to transport suspected and confirmed cases.

On July 10th, the MOH revised the *Plan for Influenza A (H1N1) Diagnosis and Treatment (Tentative, 1st Version, 2009)*, and issued the *Plan for Influenza A (H1N1) Diagnosis and Treatment (Tentative, 2nd Version, 2009)*, providing further guidance to medical institutions on Influenza A (H1N1) treatment and bolstering countermeasures against the epidemic. The second version of the Plan added diagnosis criteria and treatment guidelines of high-risk cases and seriously ill cases, stating that it was unnecessary to administer neuraminidase inhibitors (NAIs) (e.g. Tamiflu) to mildly ill cases with no complications and whose condition tended to be self-limiting, and instead provide Tamiflu to high-risk cases and seriously ill cases. The revised Plan also made provisions for medical treatment of critically ill cases, instructing that these cases be transferred to ICUs for treatment if local medical conditions permit.

On October 12th, 2009, the MOH issued the *Plan for Influenza A (H1N1) Diagnosis and Treatment (3rd Version, 2009)*, which revised diagnosis criteria from the previous version and added criteria for identifying severely and critically ill cases, with particular emphasis placed on the early identification and treatment of the two types of cases. On April 30th, 2010, the MOH issued the further revised *Plan for Influenza A (H1N1) Diagnosis and Treatment (2010)*, with the addition of clinical characteristics and treatment principles for children and pregnant patients. At that time, a total of four editions for the diagnosis and treatment plan for Influenza A (H1N1) were issued.

5.2.1.4 Hospital Preparedness and Response

The Establishment of Organizational Mechanisms

On April 27th, 2009, the MOH issued the *Notice on Strengthening Preparedness for and Response to Human Swine Influenza*, requiring local health departments to designate hospitals for the concentrated arrival and treatment human swine influenza cases. Provinces across the country forwarded this document and made arrangements accordingly. 90% of hospital directors, according to the survey, made Influenza A (H1N1) prevention and control a top priority, established a leading group before May 22nd, and were able to specify and implement response measures in the early stages of prevention and control. 38% of hospitals were so responsive that they established leading groups, medical treatment groups, and Influenza A (H1N1) prevention and control plans the day they received administrative orders.

The Formulation of Response Plans

All designated hospitals crafted preparedness plans for Influenza A (H1N1) medical treatment, strengthened organizational leadership, and arranged proper response measures. 60% of hospitals formulated response plans in the early phase of the epidemic as per state requirements, 64% had made such plans before they received their first cases, and the latest date in plan formulation for all the hospitals was September 30th.

Expert Groups and Personnel Training

Firstly, expert groups were established. 76% of hospitals set up experts group alongside their leading groups. The majority of hospitals already had experience in infectious disease prevention and control, and with their clear division of labor had no issues with rapid response once the epidemic occurred.

Secondly, personnel training was implemented. 86% of hospitals before June 10th, 2009, had launched an Influenza A (H1N1) awareness training program, which included lectures and in some cases epidemic exercises. Sichuan Provincial People's Hospital, which detected the country's first imported case, was one example. This hospital received an administrative notice on April 30th, 2009, then on May 4th sent personnel to attend provincial level emergency and respiratory medical training. On May 5th the hospital carried out hospital-wide training to disseminate knowledge about Influenza A (H1N1) prevention, control, diagnosis, and treatment, and on May 7th it participated in an exercise organized by the provincial infectious disease hospital which taught how to detect, transport, and treat patients, and how to improve the vigilance of outpatient doctors. When its emergency center received a patient with a fever from an epidemic-stricken region on the afternoon of May 9th, the hospital was able to immediately transfer the patient to a fever clinic via an isolation passage, and took proper protective measures pursuant to their response plans; the patient was determined to be China's first Influenza A (H1N1) case, confirmed by the hospital's clinical experts, epidemiological experts from CDCs, as well as by laboratory test results.

However, with the updating of the plan, personal training seemed sluggish. After the second version of the National Diagnosis and Treatment Plan was issued on July 10th, only 13% of hospitals carried out personnel training. After seriously ill cases began emerging, 39% of hospitals organized multiple training sessions; after the third version of the National Diagnosis and Treatment Plan was issued, up to 50% of hospitals carried out training with more frequency than before.

Thirdly, treatment teams for seriously ill cases were established. Multidisciplinary expert teams for the treatment of seriously ill cases were set up all over the country over a period that lasted from April 27th until December 8th, 2009, and 70% of hospitals surveyed established such teams.

Fourthly, treatment teams were supported and reinforced. 91% of hospitals tasked with treating seriously ill cases reinforced their Influenza A (H1N1) treatment forces by transferring staff members from their other sections to supplement the team, thus transferred personnel accounted for on average 30% of Influenza A (H1N1) treatment teams.

The Increase in Reserve Hospitals

According to categorical medical treatment, key hospitals and backup or reserve hospitals were designated for the treatment of seriously and critically ill patients. The MOH collected detailed information on designated reserve hospitals all over the country in order to cope with an escalating influenza epidemic, and on June 14th it issued the *Notice on Further Strengthening the Medical Treatment of Influenza A (H1N1)*, requiring all areas to designate reserve hospitals. Therefore, 406 medical institutions were subsequently designated as reserve hospitals.

Medical Equipment Funding

The central government appropriated a total of 397.56 million RMB to 17 central and western provinces as well as the Xinjiang Production and Construction Corps, to strengthen treatment capacities of medical institutions for severely ill cases, including the purchase of ICU equipment such as intensive care beds, respirators, and monitors.

Antiviral Drug Treatment

87% of hospitals surveyed used Tamiflu for the treatment of seriously ill cases. Studies show that the Influenza A (H1N1) is sensitive to the neuraminidase inhibitors in Tamiflu and zanamivir, and is resistant to amantadine and rimantadine.

The data also indicates the early use of effective antiviral drugs can suppress symptoms like fever and coughing within a few days. Controlling the reproduction of the virus both efficiently and rapidly means curbing systemic inflammatory response syndrome, reducing immunologic injury, and preventing the occurrence of multiple organ dysfunction syndrome (MODS) at the source. However, many cases were not treated early enough with antiviral drugs. According to statistics, only 28% of the cases were given antiviral drugs within 48 h of the onset of symptoms; the window was missed for the other cases and thus their prognoses were negatively affected.

5.2.2   Medical Treatment Evaluations

All in all, the national Influenza A (H1N1) treatment work was quite successful, with a high cure rate and a lower case fatality rate than in many other countries. Nonetheless, problems such as inadequate capabilities, regional imbalance in medical treatment, and unsound mechanisms for treatment compensation did exist.

5.2.2.1   The Remarkable Results of Medical Treatment

There was a three-month period within China from the first confirmed case to the first seriously ill case, which provided precious and ample time to better prepare medical treatment for seriously ill cases. As local governments became fully aware that their designated hospitals were insufficient in this regard, and especially since the hospitals lacked mechanical ventilators, ICUs, and related technicians, local governments began incorporating general hospitals with strong intensive care into their lists of reserve hospitals. Based on data collected regarding domestic cases as well as data from the WHO and other countries regarding Influenza A (H1N1) prevention and control, the National Diagnosis and Treatment Plan was revised three times to better suit treatment conditions, a move which effectively lowered fatalities caused by the epidemic.

Up until March 31st, 2010, 31 provinces had reported more than 127,000 confirmed cases, including 126,000 domestic cases and 1228 imported ones; 122,000 patients had been cured, including 4859 patients cured at hospitals and 46 at home, with a total of 800 fatalities.

According to the WHO, as of March 28th, 2010, 213 countries and/or regions had reported more than 500,000 laboratory-confirmed Influenza A (H1N1) cases, including at least 17,483 fatalities, with a global average case fatality rate of over 3%—nearly five times higher than that in China. On August 10th, 2010, the WHO announced that the pandemic had transitioned into the post-pandemic period, and listed Influenza A as seasonal influenza. By this point in time, there were 805 fatalities related to Influenza A (H1N1) in China, indeed a very low death toll compared with at least 18,449 deaths reported by 214 countries.

5.2.2.2   Some Clinical Research on Par with Leading International Studies

A Clinical Study on Symptoms and Therapeutics of Mildly Ill Patients of Influenza A was published in the world's authoritative *New England Journal of Medicine*.[1] This medical journal in the same issue also published an op-ed on the mentioned study, titled *The Need for Science in the Practice of Public Health*, authored by Professor Nicole Lurie, Assistant Secretary for Preparedness and Response (ASPR) at the United States Department of Health and Human Services (HHS), and a world-renowned expert on medicine and public health. She stated in the article that the Chinese study proved that the country had constructed a robust surveillance and response system in a relatively short period of time, and opined that China's early detection and mitigation capabilities had significantly improved. Moreover, achievements were also made in TCM treatment of (mildly ill) Influenza A (H1N1) patients. Forty varieties of Chinese patent medicine with fever reduction and detoxifying functions, such as "Lianhua Qingwen" and "Fufang Qinggan" were developed, assessed at cellular and animal levels, and put on the list of TCM medications recommended by the MOH issued *Plan for Influenza A (H1N1) Diagnosis and Treatment (3rd Version, 2009)*.

5.2.2.3   Inadequate Medical Treatment Capabilities for Pandemic Diseases

Firstly, pre-hospital emergency care was inadequate. Many first aid centers did not possess specialized healthcare workers, vehicles, or other equipment for patient transport, and in many parts of central and western China and even in some parts of eastern China, these centers simply were not established. Secondly, hospital treatment capabilities were insufficient. Some regions, especially less developed ones, had very limited medical resources, and local governments were unable to provide the funding needed to strengthen treatment capacity against a pandemic disease. These hospitals suffered severe shortages in related equipment and facilities, antiviral drugs, protective supplies, and particularly ICU facilities and equipment, which made it difficult to meet the needs of the patients. Thirdly, specialized local capabilities for medical treatment were relatively weak. Surveys found that after the National Diagnosis and Treatment Plan had been adjusted, more than a half of local level hospitals did not carry out training, and among those who did so, few conducted a post-training assessments.

---

[1]Cao et al. (2009).

5.2.2.4   Compensation Mechanisms for Medical Services Against Pandemic Diseases Requires Improvement

Although the government clearly stipulated a free treatment policy for Influenza A (H1N1) patients, local governments adopted compulsory isolation and treatment measures in the early phases of the epidemic, and since designated hospitals could not forcibly charge patients for their treatment, the hospitals ended up paying for their medical and living expenses. After the national prevention and control strategy was adjusted, four ministries including the MOH and the MOF jointly issued a document on expenses for Influenza A (H1N1) treatment, requiring that expenses for cases which hospitals had received and treated be settled by local governments, and those cases yet to be received and treated would be solved through the urban employee insurance, the urban resident insurance, and the new rural cooperative medical care system. Nevertheless, many issues arose during the document's implementation, and some provinces still have not solved the issue of expenses that designated hospitals shouldered. 45% of the surveyed hospitals did not receive government subsidies, nearly 70% bore the medical costs themselves, and 84% paid medical expenses for patients. Because medical treatment of seriously ill cases were quite expensive and in some cases could cost up to tens of thousands of RMB for a single patient, those who were not medically insured could not afford it and became indebted to that hospital. Surveys found that 26 hospitals combined paid 14,235,500 RMB in medical expenses, averaging 550,000 RMB per hospital.

While bearing the loss of expenses paid in treating Influenza A (H1N1) patients, hospitals faced economic losses from the decrease in outpatients revenue. This in turn put great pressure on their survival and development, an issue particularly prominent in less developed regions of central and western China. Moreover, treatment of severely ill cases was costly, involving the use of protective equipment that was not covered by medical insurance, which resulted in many patients becoming unwilling or unable to pay for their treatment. As some Influenza A (H1N1) patients were of the floating population, problems in medical insurance settlement between different regions kept springing up. There was no definitive policy as to the financial channel, responsibility, procedure, and time limits of compensation to the designated hospitals for expenses they paid in transportation, treatment, and living costs when treating Influenza A (H1N1) patients.

5.2.2.5   Inadequate Local Level Stockpiles of Antiviral Drugs

Though Tamiflu proved to be an effective treatment in the early phases of the Influenza A (H1N1) epidemic, only provincial-level health departments stockpiled small amounts of the drug, which was allocated on a unified basis after the epidemic broke out. On June 19th, 2009, Shanghai Pharmaceuticals Holding Co., Ltd produced the year's first batch of Tamiflu, but its supply still fell short of the demand. According to statistics, seriously ill patients did not receive antiviral drugs in time; only 28% of the cases were given antiviral drugs within 48 h of the onset of virus, and for the rest they missed their window, thus negatively impacting their prognoses. The country has not yet established an antiviral drug stockpiling mechanism or regional drug warehouses intended for local medical institutions.

5.2.2.6 Policy Feasibility Needs Improvement

The Chinese government issued related guidance documents in real time, but those documents could have been further improved in terms of guidance, feasibility, sustainability, and comprehensiveness by providing more tailored recommendations for local prevention and control efforts, diagnoses, and treatment. One example would be strengthening the scope and intensity of training through these documents for local communities, and paying more consideration to opinions and suggestions from local agencies in the process of policy making.

5.3 Vaccine Development and Supply

Vaccine plays a big role in the human struggle against epidemic diseases, and it is one of the best ways to prevent Influenza A (H1N1). An Influenza A (H1N1) vaccine can stimulate the generation of antibodies against the virus and thus provide the body with immunity. Vaccine development and supply remained one of the top priorities of the prevention and control work since the Joint National Prevention and Control Mechanism was launched.

5.3.1 Strategies and Measures for Vaccine Development and Supply

China implemented practical prevention and control strategies suitable for the different phases of the epidemic. Work on vaccine development and supply began when the epidemic first started, and afterwards adjustments were based on local epidemic situations.

5.3.1.1 The Rapid Launch of Vaccine Development and Supply

Before China's first imported case was discovered, a support group, headed by the NDRC, had been set up under the Joint National Prevention and Control Mechanism, as envisaged by the 59th Executive Meeting and its work conference on Influenza A (H1N1) prevention. With participation of the MIIT, MOF, MOT, MOR, MOC, MOH, AQSIQ, CAAC, and CFDA, the support group established a liaison mechanism and began preparing for vaccine development and supply. According to the *Work Plan for the Joint Prevention and Control Mechanism against Influenza A (H1N1)*, the support group was charged with managing affairs regarding vaccine supply and demand, production, stockpiling, transport, and the coordination and allocation of special funds. The Science and Technology Group was tasked with coordinating and addressing scientific and technological issues in vaccine development and application, and the Healthcare Group was in charge of formulating and revising technical plans for disease prevention and control, including national vaccination planning. In addition, the Expert Committee was to oversee major scientific issues related to vaccination. Such an emergency vaccine support mechanism achieved linear emergency response coordination for the development, production, stockpiling, and application of a normal vaccine supply system (Fig. 5.5).

5.3.1.2   Preparations for Influenza A (H1N1) Vaccine Development, Production, and Stockpiling

From May 11th to late August, 2009, related departments engaged in preparations for Influenza A (H1N1) vaccine development, production, and stockpiling as per the general prevention and control strategy of "giving equal importance to virus

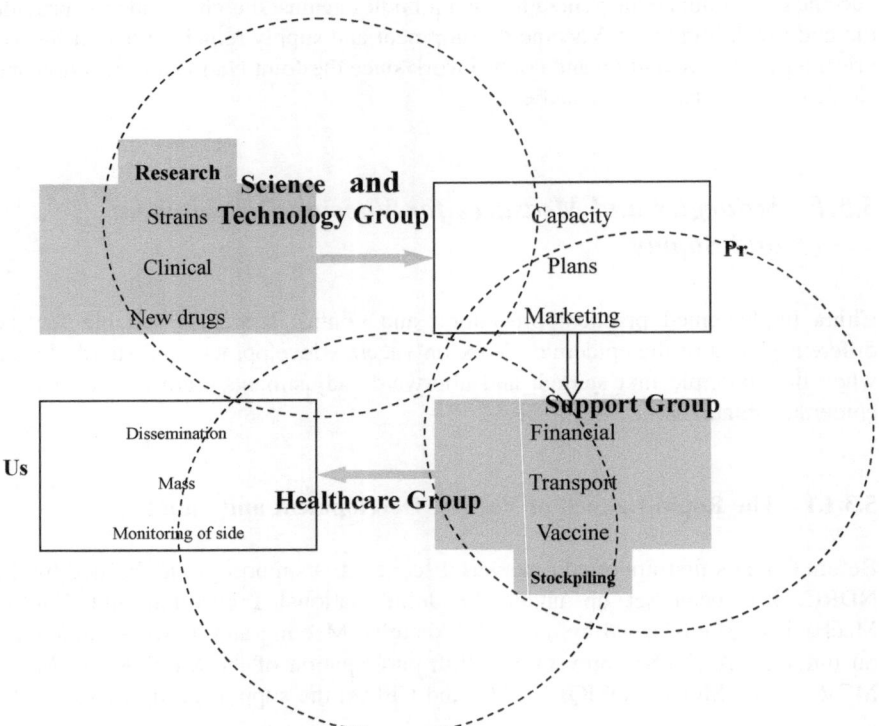

Fig. 5.5 Influenza A (H1N1) vaccine development and support system

containment and prevention with the goal of reducing peak periods." On June 2nd, the *Notice of the CFDA on Strengthening Preparations for Influenza A (H1N1) Vaccine Production* was issued. On June 25th, the MIIT began preparations for national production and stockpiling of Influenza A (H1N1) vaccine. On the same day, the MOH and the CFDA established the Influenza A (H1N1) Clinical Trials Work Committee, which consisted of experts from the China CDC, the CFDA's Center for Drug Evaluation, the Center for Drug Certification, the NICPBP, and CDCs in Beijing, Jiangsu, and Guangxi - the first CDCs chosen to conduct clinical trials, alongside related working mechanisms. Vaccine manufacturers immediately carried out toxicological experiments and clinical trials after receiving WHO-approved vaccine strains from the U.S. CDC and the British National Institute for Biological Standards and Control (NIBSC). On July 22nd, more than 13,000 volunteers in seven provinces were inoculated against Influenza A (H1N1) in the world's largest clinical vaccination trial. On August 2nd, ten Chinese vaccine manufacturers completed first-injection inoculation and serum specimen collection in seven clinics, with 12,868 people inoculated or given placebos. Observations of first-injection inoculations found no occurrences of serious side effects or incidents, and preliminary analysis showed that the Influenza A (H1N1) vaccine produced by China was safe and reliable. On August 21st, China made a global announcement that within two weeks of the vaccination, over 80% of antibodies tested positive, which demonstrated that one single injection could be enough—compared to two injections recommended by the WHO—which meant a considerable reduction in vaccine production. Trial results also demonstrated for the first time that the vaccine, after administered, manifested itself as an antigenic determinant (this was later proved by American and European scientists), indicating that case fatality rates for Influenza A (H1N1) would not be too high.

The MOH and the MOST co-launched "Emergency Research Projects for Joint Prevention and Control of Influenza A (H1N1)," which apart from the development of rapid testing kits, included the following: evaluation and development of biological protective equipment and disinfectant products, the evaluation and development of medications, the investigation into the virus' genetic background, the evaluation of cross-protection effects of Chinese natural immunity and the seasonal influenza vaccination, the development of key technologies used to increase capacity of influenza vaccine manufacturers, the evaluation of clinical treatment methods, and the research on case resource integration. These projects were launched to technically prepare the nation for a possible epidemic.

5.3.1.3 Vaccine Production and Application

Beginning in September 2009, related departments stepped up supply support for vaccinations in light of the general prevention and control strategy of "strengthening prevention measures, controlling transmission in communities, strengthening treatment of severely ill patients, and mitigating epidemic damage," which originated from the 80th Executive Meeting of the State Council. On September 2nd, the CFDA approved through a special procedure, an Influenza A (H1N1) vaccine developed by the Beijing-based Sinovac Biotech Ltd., which was the world's first of its kind to be approved and applied. On September 10th, the MIIT and the MOF officially launched allocation and distribution of the Influenza A (H1N1) vaccines from the national drug stockpile, with the hopes of strengthening development, production, and management to ensure vaccine quality and safety. On September 14th, the CFDA issued the *Notice on Strengthening Supervision over Safety of Influenza A (H1N1) Vaccine.* On September 15th, the MOH issued the *Guidelines on Vaccination against Influenza A (H1N1)for the Autumn and Winter of 2009,* ensuring the scientific, standardized, and effective distribution of the nation's vaccinations and also to ensure prevention and control efforts stayed current during the autumn and winter seasons. Up until November 24th, 2009, plans had been announced for producing 114,28 million doses of the vaccine. As of December 2nd, the SFDA had approved the allocation of 57.18 million doses in 320 batches, 50.70 million doses were received, and 29.11 million people were vaccinated against Influenza A (H1N1). On December 9th, the MOH, joined by the CCPPD, NRDC, MOE, MIIT, MOF, and MOA, issued the *Notice on Stepping up Vaccination against Influenza A (H1N1).* On January 7th, 2010, the MOH issued the *Notice about the Guidelines on Vaccination against Influenza A (H1N1) for Children Aged between 6 Months to 35 Months (No. 3, 2010).*

5.3.1.4   Emergency Vaccinations

Starting in 2010, China's general prevention and control strategy shifted to focusing on the treatment of severely ill patients, etiological surveillance, and interim evaluations of response efforts. On January 15th, the MOH held a national vaccination work symposium, conveying gratitude from the ministry's leaders to health workers across the country engaged in Influenza A (H1N1) prevention and control and vaccination. The MOH also analyzed global and domestic epidemic trends, briefed the attendees on progress in vaccinations and their side effects from the previous phase, and discussed the further improvement of the vaccination program. On February 5th, the MOH issued the *Action Plan for Mass Vaccination against Influenza A (H1N1) in Rural Areas in the Spring of 2010* so as to increase immunity coverage for priority groups in the country's rural areas. At the same time, the Healthcare Group under the Joint National Prevention and Control Mechanism stepped up communication efforts in order to accelerate vaccination for priority groups such as pregnant women, infants, children aged six months and older, patients with chronic disorders, and migrant workers employed by labor-intensive enterprises. The Healthcare Group also sped up the allocation of the country's fourth batch of the vaccine. The Support Group coordinated export affairs of the vaccine, and decided that after the seasonal influenza vaccine came into rotation, there would be no need to separate the Influenza A (H1N1) vaccination in terms of production, storage, or purchasing. As of the end of June 2010, 102.09 million people had been vaccinated.

5.3.2 *Evaluations of Vaccination Supply*

The work on influenza A (H1N1) vaccine supply was quite fruitful on the whole. All in all, the supply work for the Influenza A (H1N1) produced positive results. On the one hand, it played a big role in containing the spread of the virus and on the other the adequate amount of stored vaccines bolstered public confidence and stabilized social expectations. However, on the issue of vaccine safety, there was a certain amount of public concern, which challenged the nation's risk communication.

5.3.2.1 China First to Succeed in Developing Influenza A (H1N1) Vaccine

Influenza A (H1N1) strains a week later than other countries, Jiangsu Provincial CDC among other CDCs, as commissioned by ten Chinese vaccine manufacturers, conducted timely vaccine clinical trials, and performed scientific, rational, and effective evaluations on their safety and efficacy, which lead to legitimate and credible research results. These clinical trials were among the first of their kind in the world. Research results showed that the domestically developed vaccines against Influenza A (H1N1) were highly safe and immunogenic to different groups of people, and that the optimal immunity dose for the adjuvant-free Influenza Vaccine (Split Virion), inactivated, was 15 µg. A single injection would be enough to combat the virus through—as was indicated—a memory immune response—which some experts believed was caused by a certain overlap in antigenicity in the seasonal H1N1 influenza virus and the new Influenza A (H1N1) virus. This provided a crucial foundation for the national Influenza A (H1N1) immunization strategy, and invaluable experience for global vaccine development and promotion.

5.3.2.2 Incredibly Shortened Time to Market for Vaccine

From the time the first Chinese vaccine manufacturer obtained strains from the WHO that could be directly applied in vaccine development on June 8th, 2009, to the time the vaccine was officially approved for production on September 2nd, after the research and development, pilot production, clinical trials, field investigation, registration inspection, evaluation and review were completed, only took 87 days. This amount of time is far shorter than average process of two to three years for a new drug to pass through technical evaluation and administrative approval, which won precious time for China's prevention and control efforts. Meanwhile, the CFDA launched a special drug review and approval procedure, which formulated detailed approval plans and required technical points. The CFDA achieved synchronization in three areas while adhering to the principle of "protecting all procedures and standards": the Center for Drug Evaluation synchronized its technical evaluation with interim applications filed by enterprises, the Center for Drug Certification synchronized its field production inspection with production processes, and the NICPBP synchronized its batch inspections of clinical samples with enterprises' self-inspection procedures. Related provincial-level food and drug supervision departments tightened supervision and completed required tasks with limited time through early intervention, comprehensive coordination, proactive response, and field inspections.[2]

At the same time, the NRDC and the MOF worked closely to provide specialized vaccination research and development funds early on to domestic vaccine manufacturers', ensuring adequate preliminary preparations for the rapid development of Influenza A (H1N1) vaccine. The Support Group under the Joint National Prevention and Control Mechanism accomplished the following tasks: coordinated the rapid handling by the GAC and the AQSIQ of customs clearance formalities for vaccine strains, closely followed domestic influenza vaccine manufacturers' progress in research and development, actively coordinated the material supply (chicken embryos, etc.) for vaccine production, and organized the development of vaccine batch approval procedures for rapid verification. The Expert Committee under the Joint National Prevention and Control Mechanism, worked with related MOH departments, the China CDC, MOST, CAS and other departments and institutions, and provided integral support and assistance for drug evaluation and approval tasks. The NICPBP launched organized research into quantitative measurement of vaccine antigens, which provided technical support for vaccine development and saved the one month it would've taken in waiting for WHO standards. The China CDC organized clinical trials for the developed Influenza A (H1N1) vaccines, including the recruitment, vaccination, observation, and blood sampling for over ten thousand participants, which produced considerable data in support of vaccine evaluation and approval.

5.3.2.3 Overall Vaccine Is Safe and Effective

Results from the clinical trials showed that the domestically developed Influenza A (H1N1) vaccines were both safe and effective. The injection of a 15 μg dose of Influenza Vaccine (Split Virion), inactivated, could reach or exceed a certain serum

---

[2]Specifically, the CFDA formulated support guidance on emergency prevention and control, such as the *Emergency Work Plan for Special Review and Approval Procedure of Vaccine against Pandemic Influenza*, the *Work Plan for Review and Approval of Vaccine against Influenza A (H1N1)*, and *the Technological Considerations for Influenza A (H1N1) Vaccine Research and Development*, as per Special Procedure for Drug Evaluation and Approval of the China Food and Drug Administration. While ensuring safety and effectiveness, the CFDA launched the special drug review and approval procedure, which provided an effective means of epidemic prevention and control and accumulated invaluable experience in terms of evaluation and approval of emergency drugs.

antibody titer (1:40), with a serum protection rate of over 85% among the subjects and of over 80% among those aged 60 and older; the trials proved that the vaccines were safe, and side effects were mostly mild reactions such as local inflammation, pain and fever. Results of clinical trials carried out in other countries also supported China's research findings. At the same time, according to monitoring results of suspected uncommon side effects from mass vaccination, up until November 30th, 2009, the country had reported 2867 cases of suspected uncommon side effects from vaccination, including common side effects (76.6%), uncommon side effects (11.48%), coincidental symptoms (6.63%), and psychogenic side effects (3.14%). Of the uncommon side effects, 29 cases suffered serious uncommon effects, including one case of Guillain–Barré syndrome, 16 cases of anaphylactic shock, and 12 cases of laryngeal edema, with an incidence rate of about one per one million people.

Influenza A (H1N1) vaccines developed and produced by China proved to be safe and effective, and the incidence rates of suspected uncommon side effects and serious side effects were on the whole consistent with conclusions published by the WHO about global safety evaluations of Influenza A (H1N1) vaccination. Data showed that the domestic incidence rate of serious side effects from mass vaccination was quite low, with no occurrences of mass drug-related safety incidents. According to results of the clinical trials, China's Influenza A (H1N1) vaccine and seasonal influenza vaccine were consistent in safety standards with other vaccine prototypes from North American countries, the EU, and Japan. Moreover, quality standards were higher for China's Influenza A (H1N1) vaccine than for seasonal influenza vaccines, with significantly higher control standards for constituents liable to cause allergic reactions such as egg albumen; the production review and approval process also involved animal experiments, which ensured the safety and effectiveness of vaccines. A vaccine with poor quality, if widely distributed, could cause considerable negative results. With more than 100 million people vaccinated in the country, the incidence rate of suspected uncommon side effects reported up until December 31st, 2009, was roughly 12.4 in 100,000 people, and most of those effects were mild in nature; the incidence rate of serious uncommon side effects was roughly 0.1 in 100,000 people, which evinces the safety of said vaccine. That being said, some serious cases did emerge. The occurrence of coincidental incidents and serious unusual side effects from mass vaccination is unavoidable; such cases were mostly incidental, followed by anaphylactic shock which caused death due as treatment was unavailable in time. During the same period, fatalities from the vaccination were reported in several countries, including five deaths in both the United States and Sweden, one in Hungary, two in Norway, and one in Israel.

5.3.2.4   Adequate Supply of the Vaccination

As stipulated by the 80th Executive Meeting of the State Council, the Support Group set the target of stockpiling 100 million doses of the Influenza A (H1N1) vaccine in the first quarter of 2010. The MIIT tapped into the potential of domestic vaccine manufacturers' capabilities, increasing the monthly vaccine production capacity from 20 million doses in September 2009 to 45 million doses in January 2010. Sinovac Biotech Ltd. increased its annual vaccine production from 20 million doses to roughly 30 million doses; Hualan Biological Engineering Inc., the country's largest manufacturer of influenza vaccines, increased its annual production to 90 million doses; Zhejiang Tianyuan Biological Pharmaceuticals Co., Ltd., which had had an annual vaccine production capacity of five million, increased to 15 million doses, and possessed a monthly production capacity of five million doses.

Following the success in vaccine development, from September 2nd, 2009, to April 1st, 2010, the MIIT, joined by the MOF, the MOH and other departments, announced the *Vaccine Production Plans* to ten vaccine manufacturers, which called for the production of 151,546,000 doses in 795 batches (26 million doses for the national stockpile), covering over 10% of the Chinese population. Vaccination stemmed, to a certain degree, virus transmission in regions where people were inoculated. In November 2009, 360 clustered outbreaks were reported across the country, which was down by 39.5% from 595 outbreaks in October, suggesting that vaccination to certain groups had worked as successful deterrent against the pandemic influenza virus. Moreover, vaccination priority was also given to National Day parade troops and security guards (100,000 doses), to National Day celebration participants, and 11th National Games of China service workers (400,000 doses), which was a solid political move that engendered positive social feedback.

5.3.2.5 Industry Development for Vaccine and Diagnostic Reagents

Technological research into vaccine production capacity expansion led to considerable breakthroughs in key technologies, and the developed Influenza Vaccine (Split Virion), Inactivated, was approved as a new drug certificate. In addition, through the technical vaccine innovation alliance platform, the vaccine manufacturers involved experienced a huge boost in production capacity as breakthroughs in key technologies occurred. Up until April 13th, 2010, 151,546,000 doses in 795 batches produced by ten manufacturers were approved by the SFDA for distribution, with a proportion exported to foreign countries such as Mexico and Pakistan; multiple varieties of influenza diagnosis reagents were also authorized by the SFDA to go to market.

5.3.2.6 Vaccination Risk Communication Requires Improvement

On November 13th, 2009, the MOH declared two fatalities from the vaccination. Some websites published articles attributing the mid-November Influenza A (H1N1) outbreak in Beijing to the vaccination of primary and secondary school students; foreign media also reported the growing distrust the public expressed in the vaccines. According to results of a nationwide questionnaire, the ratio of respondents willing to be vaccinated to those unwilling to do so was at 4:1 in

August 2009, which then plummeted to 1:1 in November; meanwhile the rate of respondents unwilling to be vaccinated for safety reasons rose from 15 to 50%. In early December 2009, it was reported that nine children diagnosed with Influenza A (H1N1) in Shenzhen were found to have brain damage, which sparked a public debate as to "when to fight the virus and when to get vaccinated." There were multiple factors to this problem. Firstly, government leaders in some regions expressed suspicion of vaccine safety, and at the same time they worried that too much advertising could cause a vaccine shortage, which would make their vaccination arrangements appear inadequate. Secondly, some provinces didn't specify targets in their vaccination plans and instead simply distributed vaccines equally, making it difficult for local departments to select targets for the vaccination and hence compounding organization of the program. Thirdly, failure to clarify compensation for local workers engaged in the vaccination program was demotivating and the objective was not conducive to effective promotion of the vaccine. Moreover, media coverage of individual deaths from vaccination, coupled with unfavorable comments from well-known experts on the safety of the vaccines, and some home and foreign manufacturers' acts of recalling problematic vaccines, produced certain psychological effects on the general public. Risk communication in the early phases of the epidemic mobilized the public and projected confidence in "preventing, controlling, and curing" the virus, which in turn made the vaccination look unnecessary. Risk communication that followed was so inadequate that the public lost all confidence in the program and some even expressed an "anything that is free can't be good" mentality. Therefore, issues such as how to strengthen public affairs and risk communication, how to stress the pertinence and flexibility of vaccination programs, and how to avoid the awkward situations such as "people with access to vaccination don't want to be vaccinated, and people who want to be vaccinated have no access vaccination," are all worth further reflection.

5.3.2.7 Industry and Local Initiatives Need Further Strengthening

It is the government's duty to foster good market conditions and guide business practices of vaccine manufacturers. The particularities of the vaccine industry mean it can neither be monopolized by the government nor be left to liberal market competition; a government monopoly could lead to low efficiency, and liberal market competition is not in the interest of the country's security and social justice strategies. Presently, both national policies that encourage influenza vaccine research and development, and policies on financial compensation to vaccine manufacturers, are flawed in some way or another. Research capacity, development, and vaccine production against new subtypes or new strains are still not up to par, which poses a barrier to the early supply of vaccines against new influenza viruses. Vaccine application strategies and strategies regarding targeted priority groups also need refinement. At the same time, vaccine manufacturers should be encouraged to pursue influenza vaccine development and capacity building as part of their social responsibilities. Departments all over the country need be more active in their vaccine supply efforts. It is important to note the duty of the government at various levels to fund vaccine storage and inoculation which in turn will greatly help less developed regions establish dynamic influenza vaccine storage systems, and help craft reasonable plans for the allocation of influenza vaccines. Surveys found that as of the summer of 2010, that local governments still had roughly 50 million doses of Influenza A (H1N1) vaccines in stock, and some regions and departments saw those unused vaccines as "a loss," a sentiment that was shared across the board by many others.

5.4   Emergency Funding and Material Support

Dealing with a public health emergency requires adequate storage facilities and sound mechanisms for emergency materials storage, and involves the allocation of funds and materials needed for staff training, communication and education, epidemic monitoring, medical treatment of patients, inspection and quarantine, emergency management, and so on. In influenza A (H1N1) prevention and control, the availability of adequate funds and materials was crucial for the victory over the influenza pandemic.

5.4.1   Funding Support

5.4.1.1   The Central Government's Specialized Funds for Influenza A (H1N1) Prevention and Control

In response to the spread of the pandemic, the central government allocated five billion RMB in funds for support of Influenza A (H1N1) prevention and control efforts, and required local governments to appropriate funds for tailored prevention and control purposes. These funds were used to deploy materials such as disinfectants, purchase protective and medical equipment and sterilizing equipment, and develop and produce vaccines.

In 2009, the central government provided an appropriation of 4.328 billion RMB for the stockpiling of drugs and materials, and for prevention and control support efforts. To minimize the number of imported cases of Influenza A (H1N1), in implementing its "virus transmission containment" strategy, the central government appropriated 580 million RMB in special-purpose funds, allocated for inspection and quarantine, civil aviation, public security and other frontline departments to purchase body temperature measurement instruments, equipment sterilization and disinfectants, protective supplies and testing kits, inspection and quarantine devices, and eco-friendly treatment equipment. The strengthened immigration inspection and quarantine measures created a "firewall" against Influenza A (H1N1) and effectively accomplished the following: mitigated the pace and intensity of the domestic transmission of the virus, won precious time to bolster response measures, it protected public health interests and safety, and greatly lowered adverse social and economic effects. The aforementioned funding included 1.085 billion RMB in national pharmaceutical stockpile funds used to purchase antiviral drugs, clinical treatment equipment, etc.; 896 million RMB in vaccination subsidies to western and central regions; and 1.26 billion RMB in national vaccine stockpile funds.

With the WHO raising the alert level to its highest measurement and with domestic cases on the rise, the central government appropriated funds in active support of epidemic surveillance, including the following: 301 million RMB in two installments to local health departments, allocated for expanding influenza monitoring sentinel hospitals and laboratories; 31 million RMB to the MOA, used for animal epidemic surveillance, stockpiling emergency materials, and vaccine evaluation; 63 million RMB to the MOH, used by the China CDC to improve its surveillance and testing capabilities, including purchasing equipment needed for Influenza A (H1N1) testing, as well as supplies and reagents necessary for large-scale rapid testing of nucleic acids, virus separation and cultivation, virus mutation analysis, and drug resistance monitoring; 37 million RMB and 43 million RMB to the MPS and the CAAC respectively; used in related prevention and control efforts; and 32 million RMB for other prevention and control purposes. In 2010, the central government appropriated 533 million RMB in subsidies for vaccine and syringe purchases.

At the same time, the MOF and the MOH, joined by other departments, issued the *Notice on the Issue of Expenses for Medical Treatment of Influenza A (H1N1)*, stipulated that medical expenses incurred by treatment in designated hospitals for Influenza A (H1N1) patients (including suspected and confirmed cases) and those with fever or acute respiratory symptoms, who were enrolled in the basic medical insurance system for urban workers, the medical insurance system for urban residents, or the new cooperative healthcare system, would be reimbursed pursuant to regulations through the mentioned systems. For patients who had not enrolled in any of those three insurance systems, and for poor patients who were still unable to afford their portion of medical expenses after reimbursement, could seek help from urban and rural medical aid programs. The MOF also issued the *Urgent Notice on Ensuring Funds for Influenza A (H1N1) Prevention and Control*, stipulating the following: make funding support for Influenza A (H1N1) prevention and control a top priority, utilize funds for vaccination and inoculations in real time, strengthen support of capacity building for medical treatment, ensure funding for paid transfer and storage of drugs, address funding for epidemic monitoring, and strengthen funds management and supervision.

5.4.1.2 Local Funding Support

Local finance departments also introduced policies and adjusted budget in time to increase funding for Influenza A (H1N1) prevention and control. For example, Beijing's finance departments appropriated over 800 million RMB for response efforts, the Provincial Finance Department of Hebei appropriated more than 40 million RMB, and the Provincial Finance Department of Guangdong appropriated 43.95 million RMB.

In addition, some enterprises also stepped up investment in support of national disease prevention and control policies. Beijing-based Sinovac Biotech Co., Ltd., for example, invested 100 million RMB (including 20 million RMB in subsidies) in building production lines for new vaccines.

5.4.2   Material Support

On April 29th, 2009, the NDRC established a major emergency material support and coordination mechanism jointly with the MIIT as well as with MOF, MOC, MOH, and SDA; on that same day, the MOH made a request to the MIIT Department of Consumer Goods Industry for the increase of national health emergency stockpiles of clinical treatment materials and anti-epidemic materials needed for response measures. The support group headed by the NDRC was established under the Joint National Prevention and Control Mechanism on April 30th.

5.4.2.1   The Stockpiling of Antiviral Drugs

After the epidemic broke out, two Tamiflu manufacturers, whom were already a part of the national strategic stockpiling organization dedicated all of their production capacities to increasing the national stockpile. China also made timely re-arrangements in the export of raw materials needed for Tamiflu manufacturing to guarantee adequate supply for domestic production. In regards to insufficient production capacity, urgent expansion measures were adopted, and 10.2 million RMB was appropriated from the central finance budget to support the two manufacturers transforming and increasing their immediate and intermediate production capacities. As of July 15th, 2009, China had stockpiled 20 million doses of Tamiflu and formed a monthly production capacity of 60 million doses. 13 million doses of Tamiflu had been stockpiled by October 1st, and the stockpiling of 26 million doses as arranged by the State Council was completed by December 22nd, 2009. Moreover, 200,000 doses of the antiviral drug Zanamivir were also imported and stored. As of April 2010, more than 4.22 million doses of Tamiflu from the national stockpile had been deployed to provinces and related departments all over the country. Overall, the stocked amount of antiviral drugs did meet emergency response needs.

5.4.2.2   Material Support for Prevention and Control

Diagnostic testing kits, reagents, disinfection instruments, disinfectants, and protective equipment were stockpiled by various departments, and preparations were made for the provision of medical equipment needed to treat seriously ill patients. In April 2009, the MIIT appropriated 27 million RMB for the launch of a quality inspection system, including the purchase of 19,069 units of equipment and 3,502,500 units of protective equipment for port quarantine measures. Ports stockpiled emergency materials such as necessary disinfectants and diagnostic testing kits. On May 2nd, the MIIT issued the *Urgent Notice on Production Supervision over Medical Equipment for Influenza A (H1N1) Prevention and Control*, initiating daily production supervision in nine medical equipment manufacturers. On May 12th, the MIIT issued the *Urgent Notice on Production and Inspection of Peroxyacetic Acid, Bleaching Powders and Rapid Hand Disinfectants*, conducting real-time supervision over the production, orders, distribution and inventories in nineteen enterprises. On May 15th, the MIIT issued the *Urgent Notice on Production and Inspection of Masks and Protective Clothing*, carrying out dynamic monitoring of thirteen enterprises to ensure effective protection of the production and marketing of key prevention and control materials.

5.4.2.3   Traditional Chinese Medicine

Traditional Chinese medicine (TCM) is an important part of China's medical and public health industry, and together with Western medicine, it serves to protect public health and it plays a big role in public health emergencies. The MOH and SATCM issued the *Notice on Strengthening the Role of Traditional Chinese Medicine in Public Health Emergency Management*, clearly stating that, "There should be necessary support given to TCM with the arrangement of emergency health funding and material storages." Chinese patent medicines were stockpiled in relatively large amounts because of the options available for clinical treatment. For example, Beijing replaced 1 million doses of Tamiflu in its original stockpile plan with 2 million doses of TCM and Chinese patent medicines, which amounted to a four million-dose stockpile of Western and Chinese medicines.

5.4.3   Funding and Material Support Evaluations

During Influenza A (H1N1) prevention and control efforts, efficient and appropriate arrangements in terms of funding and material stockpiling bolstered public confidence in national response capabilities and laid a firm foundation for orderly, effective, and powerful future prevention and control work. Funding and material support also helped beat this epidemic. Nevertheless, there is still room for improvement in emergency stockpile standards, contents and methods, and corresponding funding measures.

5.4.3.1   Central Funding and Material Support Were Adequate and Efficient

The central government's appropriation in the initial stage of five billion RMB in specialized funds provided a fundamental guarantee for the success of national prevention and control efforts.

During the process of Influenza A (H1N1) prevention and control, central funding was relatively adequate by ensuring smooth operations for response efforts. These funds contributed to the following: the completion of antiviral drugs production and stockpiling which met prevention needs; the rapid coordination and fulfillment of prevention and control materials; the application of port quarantine prevention and control equipment and materials; and the protection of market supply for daily necessities and sanitary goods. However, the procedure for emergency appropriation of central funds requires refinement so that future funds can be rapidly allocated and fully leveraged for response efforts.

5.4.3.2   Local Funding and Materials Support Capacities Remain Inadequate, with Funding Mechanisms Yet to Be Improved

Because of the healthcare disparities between regions, some local governments have yet to pay in full for purchased vaccines, and there is a lack of proper financial support mechanisms for local governments' funds. The situation is even more severe when it comes to financial and material support for schools, as the general financial budget provides no consideration to health spending on the education system.

5.4.3.3   Medical Stockpiling Mechanisms for Pandemic Diseases Require Improvement

Executive Meeting of the State Council presided by Premier Wen Jiabao on April 28th, 2009, announced the decision to increase stockpiles for protective and epidemic prevention supplies, antiviral drugs, clinical treatment equipment. Nevertheless, the process of Influenza A (H1N1) prevention and control revealed problems that exist with the implementation of drug stockpiling for pandemic diseases (i.e. pandemic influenza).

Firstly, the *Administrative Measures for National Drug Stockpiling*, which was enacted in 1999, needs revision based on public health emergency situations as well as on adjustments in departmental functions. According to the *Administrative Measures for National Drug Stockpiling* and related contingency plans, national drug stockpiling takes place at both central and local levels. For national-level stockpiling, the MOH provides recommendations on the content and amount for stockpiling based on actual demand, and the NDRC (it is now the MIIT that oversees drug stockpiling) then consults the MOF to make funds available.

Similarly, for provincial-level stockpiling, health departments propose the content and amount to be stockpiled, and economic and trade departments then request funding from finance departments and to carry out the measures.

Secondly, national drug stockpiling was not comprehensively implemented at central and local levels. National funding fell short of meeting the needs of stockpiling health emergency material. When some provincial development and reform commissions made requests to finance departments for stockpiling funds, the finance departments deducted these funds from the provincial health budget, which discouraged local stockpiling efforts. When health emergency needs arose, these health departments directly requested the MOH to draw on the national strategic stockpile, even though their emergencies didn't reach the level that necessitated the use of the national stockpile. This caused unnecessary work for health emergency management. During the state of emergency, related ministries and commissions were unable to acquire comprehensive information on national and local stockpiles.

5.4.3.4 Medical Stockpiling Standardization, Measures, and Categories Need Further Refinement

A perplexing problem which was frequently came up in related departments and local governments surveyed was the lack of standards on drug and material stockpiling. Some local governments and departments stated that the population proportion needed for vaccination stockpiling was mostly based on officials' speeches, but whether these standards were adequate, scientific, and authoritative merits further discussion. At the same time, guidelines on drug and material stockpiling should be adjusted based upon epidemic trends. In regards to the stockpiling of drugs, provinces stockpiled general items on the drug list for the national stockpile, but procedures and regulations for government procurement in a state of emergency were lacking. The five regions surveyed suggested two-stage decision-making for emergency drug stockpiling: firstly, expert evaluations are performed; secondly, health departments could then determine the size of stockpiles, and in consultation with related departments, propose appropriate stockpiles according to capabilities of provinces and cities.

On the same token stockpiling materials used in public health emergencies should have robust reporting and management mechanisms regarding the amounts and types of materials, and specific principles for the allocation of funds. During the process of Influenza A (H1N1) prevention and control, problems emerged for local stockpiles of materials such as antiviral drugs, with few varieties and inadequate amounts. Though the use of Tamiflu in the early stages of Influenza A (H1N1) proved effective, in the early days of prevention and control only provincial-level health departments stockpiled small amounts of the drug, which was then allocated on a unified basis after epidemic break out. There were only 500,000 doses of Tamiflu and a very limited amount of N95 masks in the national stockpile before the Influenza A (H1N1) outbreak. Only 37,900 doses of Tamiflu were locally stored, according to the *National Questionnaire on Material and Manpower Preparedness for Influenza A (H1N1)*, which the MOH Health Emergency Office conducted in early May of 2009 among health departments. Considering the shortage of materials in the national stockpile at that time, the MOH and the MIIT tightened the use of Tamiflu from the national stockpile. Moreover, the relationship between capacity building and material stockpiling needs strengthening, the drug bidding system needs improvement so that it matches the drug stockpiling system and guarantees that drugs and equipment to be stockpiled are safe. As for financial compensation for drugs, a regular claim system linked with stockpiling funds should be established. There should be a supporting system governing drug rotation, and both the central and local governments should move on to create a stronger stockpile system through collaboration between the government, market and the society, which would shed more light on capacity building and cyclical stockpiling.

5.5   Publicity and Risk Communication

Taking communication seriously with the public and mass media is one of the crucial components of emergency management both in theory and in practice. For a public emergency in particular, given its widespread impact, large population involvement, and risk to life and property, the people are anxious to know their situations and need to obtain facts from related departments or organizations to build confidence. In coping with Influenza A (H1N1), the Chinese government and related departments, drew upon experiences and lessons learned in the 2003 SARS crisis, and were then able to implement effective risk communication and health education campaigns. As a whole, the government launched comprehensive publicity and opinion guidance efforts in accordance with the needs of the entire prevention and control in the process.

5.5.1   Systematic Risk Communication

SARS crisis in 2003 shed light on risk communication and its importance in handling public health emergencies. For the first time, China actively employed and developed its risk communication ideas and methods to cope with Influenza A (H1N1).

5.5.1.1   The Foundation and Preparation of Risk Communication

In 2007, the MOH collaborated with the U.S. CDC on textbook compilation and nationwide training revolving around risk communication, and one year later compiled the *Guidance on Public Health Emergency Response and Risk*

Communication. This Guidance Document, intended for response practices for public health emergencies, provided a detailed and rich introduction to risk communication theories in the sphere of public health emergencies. A series of contingency plans, most notably the *Influenza Pandemic Preparedness and Response Plan (Tentative)*, as well as other related plans, enriched knowledge and information about epidemic prevention and control. Meanwhile, the MOH launched a nationwide risk communication training program for public health emergencies, which created a considerable reserve of professionals ready to handle such situations.

In regards to the construction of a risk communication system, the MOH established a press release and spokesperson system as well as communication mechanisms and relations with major news media and journalists, which played an important role in the building of risk communication channels and mechanisms. The *Notice of the General Office of the Ministry of Health on the Work of Health Publicity for 2009*, which was issued at March, 2009, by the MOH's General Office, was the first MOH document to enshrine the words "risk communication" in a public document. It stressed the importance of "strengthening risk and crisis communication" and required "the full recognition of the importance of risk communication in routine work and of the dissemination of information in emergency management." In March 2009, the MOH refined the *Guidance on Public Health Emergency Response and Risk Communication*. These systems and documents provided a policy basis for the application of risk communication in public health emergencies.

5.5.1.2 Early Warning Risk Communication

In late April 2009, when Influenza A (H1N1) started across North America but had yet to reach China, China's related health departments began taking action, including conducting epidemic analysis, making preparations, and guiding public opinion towards a proper understanding of the virus. Upon receiving an epidemic alert from the WHO, the Chinese government placed it as a top priority and began coping with new epidemic challenges in an orderly and organized manner. This included the following actions: providing the public with information on Influenza A (H1N1) situations abroad through press releases, media coverage, and interviews with experts; describing the virus' features and transmission mediums as well as potential preventive measures; and projecting a knowledgeable and authoritative voice to the public in the early phases of the epidemic. In this stage, related departments' publicity and communication efforts made through various channels and forms, enabled people in having a basic understanding of Influenza A (H1N1) and spurred the public to take preventative actions against it. This timely initiative in risk communication was conducive to raising public awareness of the virus and acted as a warning for the public.

5.5.1.3   The Reduction of Social Panic

Effective risk communication after the first imported case was reported helped the public come to terms with Influenza A (H1N1) and removed any unnecessary panic. After the first imported case was found on May 11th, and the first domestic case on May 29th, 2009, people began to feel uneasy about this new infectious disease of foreign origin. In response, related departments took swift action: On May 11th, i.e. a day after the first case was reported, related departments held a press conference briefing the media about the possible route of transmission of the first case, its diagnosis and treatment, epidemiological survey outcomes, etc. While stressing the importance of self-protection and a reasonable attitude towards the virus, the public was also told that more cases could emerge; meanwhile, experts and related professionals were requested to provide scientific, authoritative, and comprehensive knowledge about disease prevention and control, in an effort to reduce public fear and guide the people to employing rational treatments. Of course, sensationalized reporting from some news sources after early cases began to emerge may also have intensified the public's uneasiness. This suggests that proper guidance of the media and public opinion is crucial for risk communication.

5.5.1.4   Confidence Building Through Scientific Risk Communication

In the early days of the Influenza A (H1N1) epidemic, related departments made it a point to use authoritative media to disseminate scientific and dependable epidemic information to the public, with the hopes of bolstering public confidence in the departments' response capabilities, and to project the firm belief that the people could beat the virus. At the onset of the epidemic, the MOH in collaboration with the China CDC, organized a risk communication team of experts on epidemiology, emergency disease control, vaccine research and development, and international relations, to ensure the timeliness, authoritativeness, and effectiveness of risk communication. After the epidemic continued for some time, fearing that people had become complacent in their own self-protection, the public was urged now and again to stay alert and employ scientific response actions. On August 31st, 2009, for example, the MOH, joined by related departments, launched an Influenza A (H1N1) Prevention and Control Initiative, which was widely promoted through multiple channels. Its purpose was to boost public awareness, ideas, and actions against the virus, and to ensure continued response efforts from all of society.

5.5.2   Strengthened Public Health Education

Coping with a public health emergency like the Influenza A (H1N1) epidemic requires not only the maintenance of the status quo but also the employment of emergency risk communication and related measures; not only does it require comprehensive collaboration between departments and institutions, but also public participation and cooperation. One crucial way to achieve this is implementing widespread health education campaigns.[3]

Health education was placed at the forefront in the process of coping with the Influenza A (H1N1) Epidemic. On April 27th, 2009, the MOH issued the *Notice on Strengthening Preparedness for and Response to Human Swine Influenza*, requiring health departments at all levels to launch extensive public health campaigns—including disseminating prevention knowledge to the public via T.V., radio, and pamphlets. With concerted efforts and collaboration from various departments throughout the country, a countrywide health education campaign rapidly unfolded. News reports, advertisements, bulletin boards, posters throughout the country—in schools, hospitals, stations, airports, government buildings, and other crowded places—informed people that Influenza A (H1N1) was "preventable, controllable and curable." These public health campaigns were designed to provide the people with a comprehensive and accurate overview of prevention and control methods.

5.5.2.1   The Organization of Experts in Promoting Health Education

Influenza A (H1N1) Epidemic, related departments and agencies of the MOH established an expert advisory mechanism which included experts in epidemiology, public health, disease control and prevention, and emergency management, to meet the huge public demand for knowledge about the epidemic; media interviews were arranged across the nation with these experts in order to disseminate pertinent public health information. On May 8th, 2009, related departments held a health education and risk communication symposium, at which experts in health education and influenza prevention and control provided an overview of the virus to journalists, and this information including routes of transmission, symptoms, preventive measures, and hygienic habits was then given to the public to aid in their prevention and control efforts.

5.5.2.2   The Timely Dissemination of Health Education to the Public

With the continuous development of the epidemic as it morphed into different phases, it was crucial that the public possess comprehensive knowledge about Influenza A (H1N1) symptoms, body temperature measurements, prevention, isolation, treatment, vaccinations, and the use of TCM medicines. In response, related

---

[3]Health education focuses "knowledge, faith and behavior" about health, i.e. disseminating knowledge, changing people's attitudes towards some health issues and letting them develop good behavioral habits.

departments worked together tirelessly to collect and summarize related epidemic prevention and control information in order to provide timely updates to the public via effective communication channels.

5.5.2.3 The Use of Media to Broaden Health Education Channels

A prominent feature in the process of Influenza A (H1N1) prevention and control was the application of multifaceted dissemination channels by related departments. For health information regarding the epidemic, traditional mainstream T.V. channels and newspapers performed well given their advantages of wide coverage and their capabilities to present a wide range of content. In addition, a wide variety of alternative methods were applied as a complement to traditional news dissemination, including workshops, posters, cartoons, slogans, billboards, leaflets, bulletin boards, web pages, short messages, and electronic displays.

5.5.3 The Methodical Implementation Publicity and Public Opinion Guidance

Publicity and opinion guidance are of particular importance when mitigating public health emergencies. The 2003 SARS crisis taught everyone a harsh lesson in regards to this. After 2003, central and local government agencies began pushing for the establishment of a sound press release and spokesperson system, with the MOH taking the lead by creating such a scientific and effective system to cope with public health emergencies. All provincial-level health departments across the country appointed spokespersons who then published health information either regularly or irregularly. Preparations were already in place for publicity and opinion guidance in dealing with Influenza A (H1N1). These preparations were fully integrated with a high degree of coordination, including the planned release of epidemic information, and comprehensive opinion surveillance, and these concerted efforts yielded positive results for response efforts.

5.5.3.1 The Planned Release of Epidemic Related Information

Before Influenza A (H1N1) cases emerged in China, the MOH Information Office had formulated the *PRCContingency Plan for Information Release on the First Confirmed Case of Influenza A (H1N1)* in accordance with the *Infectious Disease Prevention and Treatment Law*, the *Government Information Disclosure Regulations*, the *Plan of the Ministry of Health for Information Release on Notifiable Diseases and Public Health Emergencies*, and the *Contingency Plan of the Ministry of Health for Information Communication over Emergencies*. When a suspected case was reported, according to the *PRC Contingency Plan for Information Release on the First Confirmed Case of Influenza A (H1N1)*, the MOH Information Office would publish that news, and once the case was confirmed, hold a press conference at 10:00 a.m. or 15:00 p.m. on the day of the confirmation. The division of labor was as follows: the press release script was drawn up by the General Group under the Joint National Prevention and Control Mechanism; answers to questions were prepared by the Healthcare, General, Port, and Dissemination and Communication Groups; and it was the duty of the General Group (MOH Information Office) to arrange media interviews, press conferences, and the collection of information on public opinion about the press conference.

With the Influenza A (H1N1) epidemic raging in North America, as per instructions from the CPC Central Committee and the State Council, the General Group under the Joint National Prevention and Control Mechanism, in light of epidemic characteristics and the procedures and requirements for dealing with such a public health emergency, carried out planned news publications and press releases in order to form a unified communications front for epidemic response. On May 2nd, the MOH Information Office issued the *Notice on Strengthening Publicity and Opinion Guidance with Respect to the Influenza A (H1N1) Epidemic*, which provided instructions on epidemic information disclosure, requiring health departments of all levels across the country to strengthen publicity, health education, and risk communication and respond to questions raised by the public. The Notice pushed for public opinion correction and maintenance social harmony and stability, and it required health departments to appoint—and submit the names of—press spokespersons and information office heads for Influenza A (H1N1) prevention and control efforts. Provincial health departments were required to communicate with the MOH before publishing epidemic information, and some provinces ensured horizontal risk communication for news releases between its health department and ministerial departments.

According to division of labor and work requirements, the MOH Information Office released epidemic information on a national scale, with provinces, regions and cities publishing information separately; it also coordinated press and publicity efforts among press departments, such as the CPC Publicity Department, as well as mainstream news outlets surrounding hot topics and related departments' decisions on prevention and control measures. Since April 2009, the MOH has held eight press conferences and eleven briefings, ensuring the timely announcement of important information and policy measures. The MOH also established a six-person team—whose members came from several departments—tasked with communicating with the media, analyzing media focal points, monitoring media activity, formulating communication strategies, passing timely and accurate information to media sources, and providing guidance to provincial health departments on information disclosure.

In regards to public communication, direct communication channels were provided by the 12320 Health Hotline, and MOH website, the website of the Chinese

Center of Health Education, and other public health services. Online interviews were also conducted through Xinhuanet and China.org.cn to stimulate public communication.

5.5.3.2   The Leveraging of Mainstream Media for Publicity and Communication

As per arrangements and requirements of the Joint National Prevention and Control Mechanism, member agencies of the Dissemination and Communication Group launched an epidemic press coordination mechanism for communication and publicity. With concerted efforts made on all sides, a news reporting network was swiftly created which consisted of central and local mainstream and emergency media channels—including newspapers, radio, T.V., and the web—for the accurate, timely, and appropriate reporting of epidemic information and government prevention and control measures. With the emergence of imported cases and the influx of epidemic trends, all media channels reported—as per the principles of "timeliness, and accuracy, openness, and transparency"—on measures from related departments and local governments as well as on outcomes of such efforts in various fields. All in all, a positive, orderly, and stable social atmosphere was created during response efforts from the close collaboration and painstaking arrangements on the part of the Dissemination and Communication Group, related agencies and departments. These efforts provided strong public opinion support that lasted the duration of the epidemic.

5.5.3.3   Comprehensive Public Opinion Monitoring and Guidance

A comprehensive public opinion monitoring system was created through internal publications including the State Council General Office's *Internet Information Digest*, the CPC Publicity Department's *Press Work Bulletin, Online Public Opinion Monitor* overseen by the Public Opinion Bureau of the State Council's Information Office, *CAS Bulletin*, the MOH Information Office's *Analysis and Reporting of Public Opinion about Influenza A (H1N1)*, Xinhua News Agency's *Press Proofs of Domestic Events: Public Opinion*, the Ministry of State Security's (MSS') *Express News,* and *China-related Public Opinion Bulletin* of the International Communication Office of the CPC Central Committee.

During Influenza A (H1N1) prevention and control efforts, related departments carried out opinion guidance work that was based upon scientific decision making and thorough coordination, targeting hot discussion topics about domestic and foreign events—especially online opinions expressed in online messages, blogs and posts—including: (1) Clarifying falsehoods and guiding public opinion regarding foreign media allegations that Influenza A (H1N1) had originated in China; (2) Helping the public understand national response measures like isolation and medical observation, and dispelling doubts over "excessive prevention and control" and "too harsh measures;" (3) Working with internet users who called for China to suspend relations with the United States and Mexico, and encouraging users to face the epidemic and migration rationally; (4) Encouraging the public to rationally deal with the large number of students abroad who might return for summer holidays; (5) Dispelling fear from the increase in imported cases and when the WHO raised its pandemic alert to the highest level on June 11th, 2009; and (6) Requesting the public, especially targeted priority groups, to try and understand the importance and need for vaccinations.

5.5.4 Overall Evaluation of Publicity and Risk Communication

Overall, during the epidemic, related departments put a lot of effort in publicity and risk communication; results for risk communication in particular were quite successful, and played a crucial role for over a year in epidemic management. Nevertheless, it should be noted that problems did arise in publicity and risk communication, which are worth attention.

5.5.4.1 Successful Risk Communication Ideas and Methods Employed in the Newly Built System

When the influenza pandemic was raging abroad and closing in on China, related departments meticulously and scientifically brought risk communication ideas to life, ensuring smooth and orderly operations during the entire epidemic response effort. Risk communication provided the public a solid understanding of the epidemic, removed unnecessary worries and fears, and ultimately bolstered public confidence and resolve in defeating the epidemic. The incredible outcomes of these efforts are as follows:

Firstly, successful publicity, risk communication, and health education provided the public with scientific information and necessary guidance, which helped people overcome their fears and instead build confidence and resolve, which was an important assurance of beating the epidemic.

Secondly, risk communication to a certain degree changed public perception and attitudes towards public health risks. It encouraged people to look at the epidemic scientifically and objectively, and thus ensured the continuation of the status quo.

Thirdly, by providing the media with authoritative, timely, and comprehensive information, interactions between the public and media were strengthened, which created a positive atmosphere to defeat Influenza A (H1N1).

Fulfilled the requirement of "strengthening public opinion monitoring and actively guiding the public towards participation in epidemic prevention and control" according to the principles of "timeliness, accuracy, openness, transparency, positive guidance, and moderateness in amount."

Fifthly, the epidemic represented a precious opportunity for risk communication teams, which helped them gain experience, increase knowledge, and strengthen capabilities in public health emergency mitigation.

Finally, it helped us to improve publicity and risk communication in terms of systems, mechanisms, and specific support measures.

5.5.4.2 Publicity Channels and Methods Require Further Development, and It Is Necessary to Actively Develop Information Resources and Make Full Use of New Media Channels

How, in press release and publicity, to meet new challenges that arise from the emergence of different media platforms, and innovate channels and methods for publicity and dissemination, are some of the key issues that merit further attention for present and future public emergency management. New dissemination methods and communication platforms also pose unique challenges for publicity and dissemination.

Influential news media should take the brunt of the responsibility in coping with public health emergencies. Survey results show that related health and disease control departments expected the news media to take on as much information dissemination tasks as possible while performing their normal duties in the case of a public health emergency. There was also the expectation for related departments to come forward and coordinate with the media during public health emergencies by providing potential scenarios or phases of the epidemic, to enable the rapid and widespread dissemination of relevant prevention and control information

Mainstream media represented by central media such as People's Daily, Xinhua News Agency, China Central Television (CCTV), and China National Radio (CNR) leveraged their traditional and irreplaceable advantages in dealing with the Influenza A (H1N1) Epidemic. It must be noted, however, with the recent emergence of the internet as a representative of commercial portals and other new sources, reporting and public opinion on related events—especially public health emergencies—have diversified and enriched the channels and methods by which people receive information. That being said, this diversification also presents unprecedented challenges in the work of publicity and opinion guidance. Targeting this divergence and imbalance in public opinion, related departments should, in addition to bolstering public opinion monitoring, spend more energy expanding new sources, mobilizing and utilizing new media participation, find innovative ways to integrate and lead this new trend, and provide scientific, effective, and reliable public opinion guidance. This will in turn create an atmosphere which is positive, objective, and progressive. Today, it is imperative that we explore leveraging new media spaces and channels like blogs, microblogs, social websites, and mobile media for more effective publicity, risk communication, and health education.

5.5.4.3 Risk Communication Mechanisms Require Further Improvement

In the process of risk communication in the Influenza A (H1N1) Epidemic, no solid, multi-interactive platform was established between the health departments, experts, and the public; instead information flowed predominantly in a single direction. Without a multidisciplinary and well-defined risk communication expert team and a scientific, authoritative, and systematic risk communication system, it was essential to enhance public participation and interactions with experts. Discrepancies in risk communication capabilities between central and local governments still exist, and in some cases, the differences are staggering. There was also inadequate communication content, forms, and channels (multi-dimensional) that were tailored (focused) and familiar to different groups of people. In addition, the "social mobilization" risk communication model produced some negative results. The exaggerations at the start of the epidemic about the situation abroad caused unnecessary panic. Some medical workers surveyed felt that there may have been an over-projection of confidence by prematurely declaring Influenza A (H1N1) "preventable, controllable and curable" in early May 2009, when not much was known of the virus, nor was there any rigorous scientific proof supporting that claim. These findings merit discussion. Thus, in dealing with public health emergencies, utilizing the news for effective, scientific, and appropriate risk communication, so as to avoid either unnecessary panic due to sensational reporting or the possible disinterest in the epidemic due to lack of reporting, is an issue that needs improvement for future public health emergencies.

5.5.4.4 Risk Communication Regarding Controversial Issues Still Has Room to Improve

For risk communication regarding such subjects as case fatality rate, pregnant women cases, and vaccination safety, there are still several areas which need further analysis and improvement, as there is a lack of comprehensive and planned risk communication strategies and measures. Moreover, facing uncertain epidemic trends and the overflow of complex information, people need access to scientific and authoritative knowledge and information about epidemics. In retrospect, during the Influenza A (H1N1) epidemic, the rumor circulation about prevention and control in some ways confused the public and undermined the effectiveness of health education campaigns. For example, rumors such as: "Ordinary Chinese medicine can cure Influenza A (H1N1)," "Prickly pears also can kill Influenza A (H1N1)," and "A hot pot to treat Influenza A (H1N1)" circulated constantly throughout the epidemic.

5.5.4.5 There Is an Urgent Need for Health Education to Be Regular, Standardized, and Systematic

Health education is an important part of public health emergency mitigation. However, it should be noted that when handling a public health emergency, we could achieve twice the results with half the effort if people had regular access to related knowledge and developed good health awareness and habits. It is therefore crucial to carry out regular, society-wide health education campaigns targeting related public health issues. Health education in terms of regularization and systematization needs strengthening, and vigorous improvement is required in making health education more individualized, original, and participatory. Moreover, health education expert groups should be better reinforced.

5.6 International Collaboration

The Influenza A (H1N1) Epidemic originally broke out in Mexico and the United States, places where China had close contacts. In light of this, the Joint National Prevention and Control Mechanism specifically established the Foreign Collaboration Group at the onset of the epidemic, which was tasked with international (including Hong Kong, Macao and Taiwan) affairs related to epidemic prevention and control, collecting related information, and actively participating in global efforts to fight Influenza A (H1N1). This group took the perspective of maintaining the country's national interests and international prestige, in an effort to strengthen international collaboration. Overall, China's active participation in international collaboration on the Influenza A (H1N1) epidemic garnered positive worldwide feedback and recognition.

5.6.1 Collaboration with the WHO

In April 2009, when the Influenza A (H1N1) epidemic broke out in North America and began spreading to other countries, China's related departments stayed in close contact with the WHO, reporting domestic epidemic situations and enhancing collaboration on information reporting and technology.

Moreover, China participated in WHO events and global activities in the sphere of public health. At a critical moment in Influenza A (H1N1) epidemic response efforts, on August 21st, 2009 the MOH and the WHO held an international symposium on "influenza response and preparedness," which explored public health policies and implementation strategies, where related parties shared experience and lessons learned in global efforts towards Influenza A (H1N1) prevention and control. The symposium also encouraged international communication and collaboration between specialists in related fields.

5.6.2   Collaboration with Other Countries and International Organizations

5.6.2.1   The Strengthening Scientific and Technological Exchanges and the Sharing of Epidemic Information

In dealing with Influenza A (H1N1), in addition to collaboration with international organization such as the WHO, related departments also worked with other countries and regions in multiple respects. The Chinese government followed epidemic situations and response measures abroad, and worked actively on domestic epidemic prevention and control. At the beginning of the epidemic, China stayed in contact with Mexico, the United States, Canada and other countries to strengthen collaboration on information and technology. On May 7–8th, 2009, Health Minister Chen Zhu led a delegation to the ASEAN Plus Three Health Ministers' Special Meeting held in Thailand, during which the health minister coordinated specific response measures, adopted a joint statement, signed an action plan for China, Japan, and South Korea against the influenza pandemic, and launched an epidemic reporting mechanism, all of which were part of the country's effort to strengthen collaboration with neighboring countries on epidemic response. To better understand epidemic developments and trends in Mexico—which could be of some value to China's epidemic prevention and control efforts, Chinese and Mexican health officials held a teleconference on May 27th, 2009, to share latest technological information and experiences.

Moreover, the China CDC and the U.S. CDC collaborated on virus specimens, disease resistance research, information exchange, etc., and exchanged personnel to strengthen such collaboration. China also cooperated with Canadian health authorities, and through their Global Public Health Intelligence Network (GPHIN) became acquainted with global epidemic trends and latest response efforts, which provided necessary references and a basis for the country's response strategy. The government carried out diplomatic activities in seeking support from related countries and international organizations in terms of vaccine development and storage, which was valuable in the development of the world's first Influenza A (H1N1) vaccine.

5.6.2.2   The Provision of Humanitarian Assistance to Countries Based on China's Domestic Capabilities

China was vigorous in its provision of humanitarian aid to other countries based on epidemic trends and on China's own domestic capabilities. On May 1st, 2009, days after the Influenza A (H1N1) Epidemic broke out in Mexico, the Chinese government donated five million USD worth of materials in humanitarian aid to Mexico, which was transported in a chartered airplane and was the first aid Mexico had received since the outbreak. On May 4th, China's second donation to Mexico included 70 tons in weight of masks, eyewear, gloves, disinfectants, and thermometers. In June 2009, China provided training in Influenza A (H1N1) laboratory technologies to 16 specialists from eight ASEAN countries. On September 23rd, 2009, President Hu Jintao, spoke at the 64th Session of the United Nations General Assembly, making the promise to the international community that "China is willing to offer help in its power to developing countries in dealing with Influenza A (H1N1)." At the end of 2009, when vaccine production was still inefficient in meeting the needs of 1.3 billion people, the Chinese government allocated a portion of the vaccines to help African countries plagued by the virus, highlighting China as a responsible major country. In early 2010, related government departments permitted Beijing-based Sinovac Biotech Ltd. to export Influenza A (H1N1) vaccines to Mexico.

In addition, through collaboration with the WHO, the CNIC provided fourteen countries including Cuba, Mongolia, and Vietnam, as well as Macao, with China's independently developed test kit and training for their professionals.

5.6.3   Foreign Affairs Management

Not much was known by the people regarding epidemic trends and characteristics in Northern American countries, where the epidemic was in full swing. To prevent the epidemic from spreading to China, related government departments tightened entry measures according to regulations, including: suspending flights from Mexico, placing passengers entering China under quarantine, and tightening visa policies towards epidemic-stricken countries. These measures bought precious time for the country to judge epidemic situations and prepare for it. However, misunderstandings and dissatisfaction among some foreign governments and people about China's related measures did emerge. In response to this, foreign affairs departments took a series of powerful, organized, and effective actions to communicate with these groups, and managed to resolve conflicts and yield positive results.

5.6.3.1   The Suspension of Mexican Flights

On May 2nd, 2009, the Chinese government decided to temporarily suspend Aeroméxico flights flying from Mexico to Shanghai, and reached agreement with the Mexican government that both countries would send chartered planes to return nationals. Though Chinese authorities communicated frequently with their Mexican counterparts, misunderstanding still arose in Mexico and elsewhere. In response, related Chinese ministries and embassies made concerted efforts—including multi-party communication and cooperation- to clarify the situation and strengthen cooperation. On July 2nd, 2009, Health Minister Chen Zhu, with his delegation, participated in a high-level meeting on global Influenza A (H1N1) prevention and control held in Cancún, Mexico, at which meeting he profiled China's epidemic situation and response measures, and garnered support from the participants. Through painstaking efforts, the unfavorable effects caused by suspending Mexican flights were successfully mitigated.

5.6.3.2 Placing Passengers Entering Chinaunder Quarantine

Because Influenza A (H1N1) originated abroad, isolation and medical observation measures for passengers from epidemic regions, especially ones who once had close contact with suspect or confirmed cases, became a major countermeasure with which the government dealt with Influenza A (H1N1) in the early stages of the epidemic. Therefore, the government and related departments, from the beginning, ensured careful and considerate arrangements were made. Living conditions for foreigners quarantined in China was a top priority, and standards and procedures were formulated to ensure their stay was as comfortable as possible. All related departments properly handled isolation and observation measures in accordance with the law, and provided foreigners with scientific diagnoses, living necessities, and ensured the patients were properly cared for. Meanwhile, strengthening information reporting mechanisms and channels between local foreign affairs departments and related central departments was high on the list of priorities, and related countries were informed at the earliest possible time of their nationals quarantined in China. This was to ensure smooth operations and to minimize possible adverse effects.

On May 1st, 2009, upon learning that the first confirmed case in Hong Kong had traveled via Shanghai, related departments immediately took action and tracked down all passengers who had been on the same flight (AM098). Isolation and medical observation measures were then adopted in accordance with the law. On June 8th, Ray Nagin, Mayor of New Orleans, was placed under quarantine in Shanghai after a suspected case was found on his flight. An official statement from the U.S. noted that Nagin and others quarantined were treated well in China.

Moreover, in order to effectively control the spread of the virus and lower the risk of transmission from imported cases, the Chinese government also tightened visa policies towards epidemic-stricken countries and cultivated proper support measures. Because of these measures and arrangements were well executed, the matter didn't attract any undue attention abroad.

5.6.3.3 Policy Adjustments on Visiting Delegations and Groups

With China's frequent cultural and trade exchanges, along with targeting necessary delegations to China, related governments departments ensure tailored and flexible treatment of different groups on a case by case basis. Through active collaboration, arrangements, and strict planning by related departments, local, and central governments, response measures and prevention preparedness plans were implemented, along with active communication and information disclosure. These efforts helped garner understanding and cooperation from the foreign visitors. In June–July 2009, the 2009 Chinese Bridge for American Headmasters and Summer Camp activities were carried out smoothly, safely and efficiently, which greatly promoted cultural exchange and cooperation between China and the United States, and earned praise from both sides. Moreover, with meticulous preparations, prevention and control was successful for foreign participants of the Canton Fair 2009 and the China Cross-Straits Technology and Projects Fair 2009.

5.6.3.4 Communication Over Foreign Prevention and Control Measures

Related prevention and control measures needed to be strengthened as China is the world's largest pig producer, and it was emphasized that China's related measures were all in accordance with relevant regulations and principles of the World Trade Organization (WTO) and the World Organization for Animal Health (OIE). These were temporary measures targeted to protect the health of Chinese citizens and the security of the country's livestock industry. These temporary measures were crucial since the "swine flu" was still largely ambiguous. The United States and Canada finally expressed their understanding and recognition of China's measures.

5.6.4 Evaluations of International Collaboration

Overall, through concerted efforts and close collaboration for Influenza A (H1N1) prevention and control, while related foreign departments maintained social and economic stability, they also strengthened multi-faceted international collaboration, obtained necessary international resources and support for response efforts, and resolved misunderstandings that related countries and people had about certain domestic prevention and control measures. This was the first time China had received worldwide recognition and praise for mitigating a public health emergency.

Nevertheless, in regards to specific communication and collaboration, especially the treatment of foreigners kept in quarantine, further coordination between provincial-level foreign affairs departments and national level agencies like the MFA needs to be strengthened.

Reference

Cao, B., Li, X.-W., Mao, Y., Wang, J., Lu, H.-Z., Chen, Y.-S., et al. (2009). For the National Influenza A Pandemic (H1N1) 2009 Clinical investigation group of China. Clinical features of the initial cases of 2009 pandemic influenza A (H1N1) virus infection in China. *The New England Journal of Medicine, 361*, 2507–2517.

Chapter 6
Cost-Benefit Analysis for China's Influenza A (H1N1) Prevention and Control

6.1 The Basic Framework for Cost-Benefit Analysis

6.1.1 Overarching Ideas for Cost-Benefit Analysis

The impact of a public health emergency on a society and economy depends upon two factors: one is the harmful nature of the event along with its duration, and the other is the effect of the social response and measures. Both of these factors are wrought with uncertainty. Firstly, the nature of the event itself is uncertain, for example there may be a lack of understanding regarding the virulence of the epidemic. Secondly, different intervention measures bring about varying uncertainties, such as the use of health campaigning measures to change people's actions in an epidemic and potentially reduce the number of infected cases.

In order to illustrate this problem, we constructed a decision matrix in Table 6.1. When facing the spread of a known infectious disease, decision makers will adopt "relaxed" or "strict" countermeasures based upon the virulence of the virus or bacteria, so that the measures match the losses. The final results of this decision could be A (minimal cost, minimal losses), or D (high costs, minimal losses). However, when dealing with an unknown infectious disease, such as SARS and Influenza A (H1N1), decision makers are faced with a much more difficult task. If the virus is virulent, but the measures adopted are "relaxed," then the result will be B: low cost for response measures but high losses. If the virus is more mild, but the measures adopted are "strict," then the result will be C: minimal losses but high costs. Because epidemics with unknown infectious diseases pose a potential threat to the lives of their citizens, different countries normally will lean towards adopting "strict" measures, which avoids Result B: minimal cost but high losses. If Result C occurs, the high cost can be understood as a type of insurance against the potential

© Social Sciences Academic Press and Springer Nature Singapore Pte Ltd. 2019
L. Xue and G. Zeng, *A Comprehensive Evaluation on Emergency Response in China*, Research Series on the Chinese Dream and China's Development Path, https://doi.org/10.1007/978-981-13-0644-0_6

worst case scenario[1]; however, normally a cost-benefit analysis does not take into account the benefit of paying out this high amount as a type of insurance against the worst-case scenario.

In this Chapter, we will perform a cost-benefit analysis on the prevention and control measures adopted at that time and calculate the costs and net social earnings of the national Influenza A (H1N1) prevention and control efforts. We will also estimate the social and economic benefits generated from these measures. The overarching ideas behind this Chapter's cost-benefit analysis are as follows: we will compare the difference in results by adopting or not adopting certain response measures in order to estimate the overall net benefit of the measures adopted; if the investment cost from those specific measures is less than the overall loss that could've occurred without those measures, then the net social benefits for those measures outweigh the costs. And vice versa would be the net social costs outweigh the benefits of the response efforts. However; we mustn't forget that this cost could be a type of insurance in preventing a worst-case scenario from occurring.

For the total social costs, we estimated the direct and indirect costs from government departments, public institutions, enterprises, social groups, and individuals in the Influenza A (H1N1) prevention and control efforts.

For the total social benefits, we considered the direct and indirect economic and social benefits from the adoption of these measures and the prevention of more Influenza A (H1N1) cases.

6.1.2 Cost-Benefit Analysis Index System

6.1.2.1 Total Social Costs Indicators and Calculation Methods

Indicators for Total Social Cost

We took into consideration both direct and indirect costs incurred in the prevention and control efforts for calculating total social cost. Direct costs mainly include entry/exit quarantine and inspection investment, isolation costs for close contacts of Influenza A (H1N1), inoculation development and storage costs, the China CDC testing and educational training costs, prevention and control investment by the education system, hospital diagnostic costs, and development and treatment costs of Chinese traditional medicine. Indirect costs mainly include social and economic loss due to loss of work from being infected with Influenza A (H1N1) and healthcare manpower costs. The major indicators can be found in Table 6.2.

---

[1]A prime example would be the U.S. government's decision in facing the 1976 Swine Flu virus.

Table 6.1 Virus virulence and prevention and control measures

Virus virulence response measures	Mild	Severe
Relaxed	A (low costs, low losses)	B (low costs, high losses)
Strict	C (high costs, minimal losses)	D (high costs, low losses)

Calculation Methods

For the national cost estimation for each category, we took the investment by each sampled agency and the number of targets for the prevention and control measures to calculate the average investment per person. Then we took this amount and multiplied it by the total population, which is the estimated value for the national cost. Of course, we also recognize that this estimation inevitably has its limitations due to the choice of sample provinces and the unbalance between regions.

6.1.2.2 Indicators for Total Social Benefits

For the total social benefit, we calculated the direct economic benefits and the social benefits from the implementation of these prevention and control measures.

Direct economic benefits include: one is estimating the amount of cases that could've occurred without the implementation of the prevention and control measures along with the investment that came from treatment and loss of work; second is estimating the amount of cases that were prevented from inoculating the population, and the investments that came from treatment and loss of work.

For other social benefits, we measured the impact of the prevention and control efforts on the nation's image, the disease prevention and control capabilities, the credibility of the government, and the protection of National Day celebrations. As some of these benefits are difficult to quantify, we utilized qualitative measures to analyze them.

6.2   Cost Estimation for Prevention and Control Efforts Against Influenza A (H1N1)

6.2.1   Direct Cost Estimations

6.2.1.1 Cost Estimations for Inspection and Quarantine Agencies

As of the end of December 2009, the investment ratio for prevention and control efforts by sampled inspection and quarantine agencies is illustrated in Fig. 6.1. Equipment made up the principal amount of the investment at 43.9%, with labor

Table 6.2 Cost indicators and calculations for Influenza A (H1N1) prevention and control

Cost type			Measured indicator	National cost calculation method
Direct costs	Investment from sampled inspection and quarantine agencies		Equipment investment, labor costs, protective equipment costs, health campaign and training costs, etc	Average investment for prevention and control for each entry X total number of entries
	Tracking, isolation, and medical observation costs for close contacts	Centralized isolation costs	Health campaign costs, epidemiological investigative costs, transportation costs for close contacts, material costs, accommodation, meals and daily expenses of close contacts, labor costs, etc	Average cost for tracking and centralized isolation for one case X number of cases in centralized isolation + average cost for at home tracking and isolation X number of cases isolated at home
		At home isolation costs	Health campaign expenses (costs incurred using SMS, telephone, etc. to find close contacts)	Use the ratio of at home versus centrally isolated confirmed cases to calculate number of isolated cases
			Materials (disinfectants, protective equipment, and other consumable materials); labor costs; etc	
	Inoculation costs	Inoculation costs	Vaccine purchase costs; matching injection needle costs; labor costs; printed material costs; emergency medicine and facilities costs; etc	Cost of one completed dose X number of people already inoculated + storage cost of one dose X total number of vaccines stored
		Vaccine storage costs	Cold chain costs	
	Material supporting investment	Material stockpiling costs	Production investment by enterprises for stockpiling pharmaceuticals, stockpiling costs for treatment drugs	Investment in material stockpiling by central and local governments
	Investment by the China CDC	Virologic detection costs	Laboratory construction costs, reagent supplies costs	Cost for one virologic test X total number of domestic virologic tests
		Health education costs	Health education costs	(Health education investment costs per 10,000 people at the provincial level X same costs per

(continued)

Table 6.2 (continued)

Cost type		Measured indicator	National cost calculation method
	and training costs		10,000 people at the municipal level +same costs per 10,000 people at the county level) X total population (10,000 people)
	Other activities	Influenza monitoring investments, epidemiological survey costs	
	Investment by the educational system	Disinfectant and protective equipment costs, equipment purchasing costs, overtime fees, training costs, health campaign costs	Average prevention and control investment per sampled school X total number of students in the country X coefficient of correction (ratio of schools affected by epidemic)
	Diagnostic investment by hospitals	Cost of treatment for a case: treatment costs for suspected, mild, severe, critical and death cases	Treatment costs for all types of cases X total number of cases
		Hospital influenza A (H1N1) prevention and control investment: new influenza control equipment investment and ward transformation and supporting facilities costs; experts and labor costs; Tamiflu and other drug purchasing costs, protection and disinfection expenditures, etc.	Average hospital investment in one case X total number of hospitalized cases in the country
Indirect costs	Treatment costs for non-hospitalized confirmed cases	Treatment costs for non-hospitalized confirmed cases	Treatment costs for non-hospitalized patients X (total number of cases in the country—hospitalized patients)
	Labor costs from missed work of patients with latent infections	Patients with latent Influenza A (H1N1) infections on average missed 7 days of work, and by deducting that from their future income the resulting loss can be calculated	Number of patients with latent infections X average social daily wage X 7 days
	Nursing labor costs for infected patients	On average, each patient with a latent case of the virus needed the care of 0.5 nurse and would miss 3 days of work, deducting that	Number of patients with latent infections X 0.5 nurse X average social daily wage X 3 days

(continued)

Table 6.2 (continued)

Cost type	Measured indicator	National cost calculation method
	from the future income the losses incurred from missing work can be calculated	
Labor costs from missed work of infected patients	According to the number of cases and days hospitalized for severe to critically ill patients, deducting that from their future income the losses incurred from missing work can be calculated	Number of hospitalized cases X number of days admitted X average social daily wage
Nursing cost estimations for infected patients	The average patient required the care of 0.5 nurse, according to the average daily wage a person's daily economic contribution can be calculated; average number of days nursing is needed	Number of patients X 0.5 X average social daily wage X average number of days a person is sick

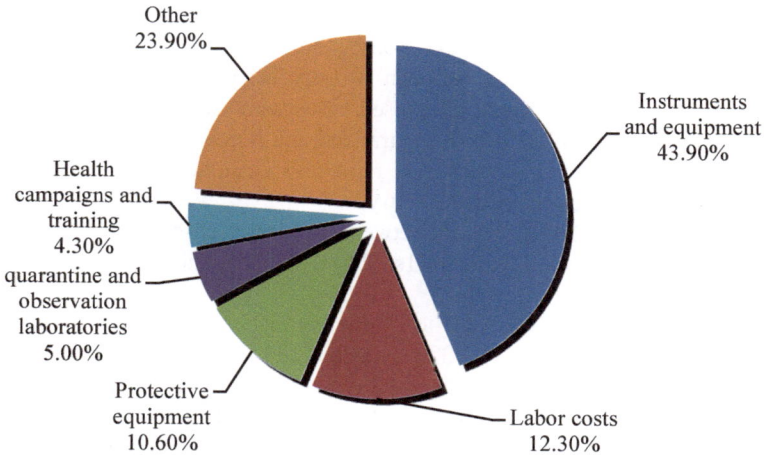

Fig. 6.1 Prevention and control investment ratio by sampled inspection and quarantine agencies in 2009

costs (12.3%) and protective equipment costs (10.6%). Other areas such as drug procurement and laboratory construction accounted for nearly one fourth of the total investment.

According to the sampled data, this report highlights the estimations on national prevention and control investment by inspection and quarantine agencies using the eight-year depreciation provision for equipment. The sampled agencies spent 7.84 RMB for each entry into the country, and by December 31st, 2009, 348 million people were reported to have undergone inspection by these agencies upon entry. Therefore, the total cost spent by national inspection and quarantine agencies in prevention and control can be calculated as: 7.84RMB × 348 million people = 2.728 billion RMB.

6.2.1.2   Cost Estimations for Tracking, Isolation, and Medical Observation of Close Contacts

Isolation for close contacts of Influenza A (H1N1) can be divided into two categories: centralized and at-home care. The mean value from the valid sampled data of the evaluation study was used as the reference value, and the average cost for tracking, isolating (centralized), and observing a close contact was 5218.50 RMB. The average cost for tracking, isolating (at-home), and observing of a close contact was 270.80 RMB.

As of August 31st, 2009, 3127 Influenza A (H1N1) cases had been diagnosed across the country, and from September 1st, 2009, to December 31st, 2009, the total number of diagnosed cases reached 116,473.[2] In accordance with local

---

[2]Data from the network for epidemics of the Chinese Disease Prevention and Control Information System.

developments, strict isolation measures for close contacts were in place up until the end of August, and starting the next month, those measures were slowly relaxed. Using August 31st as a marker between two distinct phases on the epidemic, we calculated the ratio of confirmed diagnosed cases with the number of close contact cases that were being isolated (both centralized and home-based) on data from five sampled provinces. We then took this ratio and calculated the total number of isolated close contact cases in the country.

As of August 31st, 2009, the ratio between confirmed cases and isolated contacts stood at 1:10.99. Between September 1st, 2009, and December 31st, 2009, the ratio was 1:0.94.

According to this analysis, the total number of isolated close contacts (both centralized and at-home) was 143,850 people (3127 people × 10.99 + 116,473 people × 0.94). The sampled data shows that centrally isolated close contacts accounted for 41.72% of the total number of isolated cases, therefore 600,014 people were isolated in hospitals (centralized) while 83,836 people were isolated at home. The total calculated isolation cost for the country was 335 million RMB.

6.2.1.3 Cost Estimations for Influenza A (H1N1) Vaccinations

From September 2nd, 2009, to April 1st, 2010, a total of 795 batches with 151,546,000 doses of the vaccine were issued, with the government storing 26 million doses and distributing the remainder to all the regions. A total of 102 million doses were administered.[3] According to sampled data, it cost 27.43 RMB per vaccine dose, in addition to 21.22 RMB for storage costs, which amounted to 3.849 billion RMB in national vaccine investment.

6.2.1.4 Cost Estimations for Material Stockpiling

Due to the large investment gap of local governments between provinces, cities, and counties (as each area's financial and epidemic situations varied greatly), it is difficult to rely upon survey data to estimate the national average of investment in material stockpiling. According to existing data, pharmaceutical stockpiling companies invested 105.26 million RMB into production, and by December 22nd, 2009, there were 20.8 million doses of Tamiflu within the national stockpile, with the capacity to produce 5.2 million more doses Tamiflu intermediates. There were also 200 thousand doses of the antiviral drug "Zanamivir" that were imported for emergency use.[4] For example, Beijing had three million doses of Tamiflu in reserve, and Sichuan province invested ten million RMB in its medical stockpiling efforts. In the absence of sufficient data, the 1.085 billion RMB from the Material

---

[3]Data derived from the Material Management Group of the Prevention and Control Mechanism.
[4]See Footnote 3.

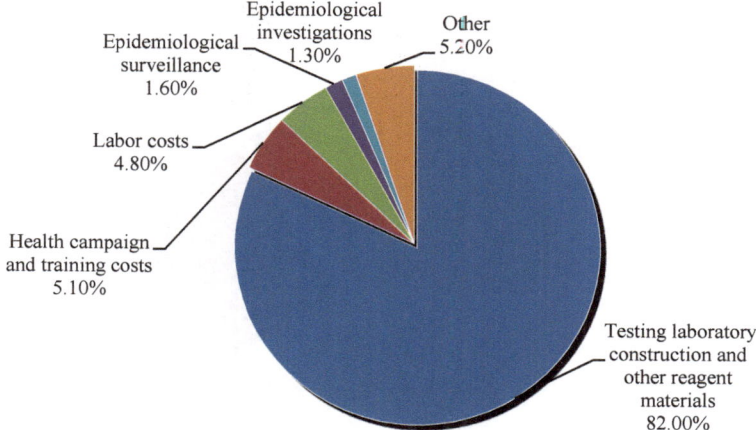

Fig. 6.2 Investment structure against Influenza A (H1N1) by surveyed prevention and control agencies in 2009

Management Group of the Prevention and Control Mechanism was used as data in this study. However, it was discovered in in-depth interviews that because there was no national stockpiling program in mitigating public health emergencies, provincial level institutions created emergency stockpiles according to their local needs. We discovered that these local stockpiles were poorly planned, costly, and wasteful.

6.2.1.5   Cost Estimations for Prevention and Control Investment for the China CDC

As shown in Fig. 6.2 Investment Structure against Influenza A (H1N1) by surveyed prevention and control agencies in 2009, laboratory construction and the use of reagent supplies constituted the principal amount invested in the prevention and control system, standing at 82% of the total. Health campaigns followed at 5.1%, labor costs at 4.8%, and other costs such as epidemiological surveys (including surveyor costs) and monitoring costs accounted for a total of 8.1%.

Virus Detection Costs

The Influenza A (H1N1) virus is virulent, and the early detection costs are quite high. Additionally, laboratory testing fees differ widely due to the different prices of domestically produced and imported reagent materials. According to sampled data, the average cost for a virology test was 415.80 RMB (including sampling,

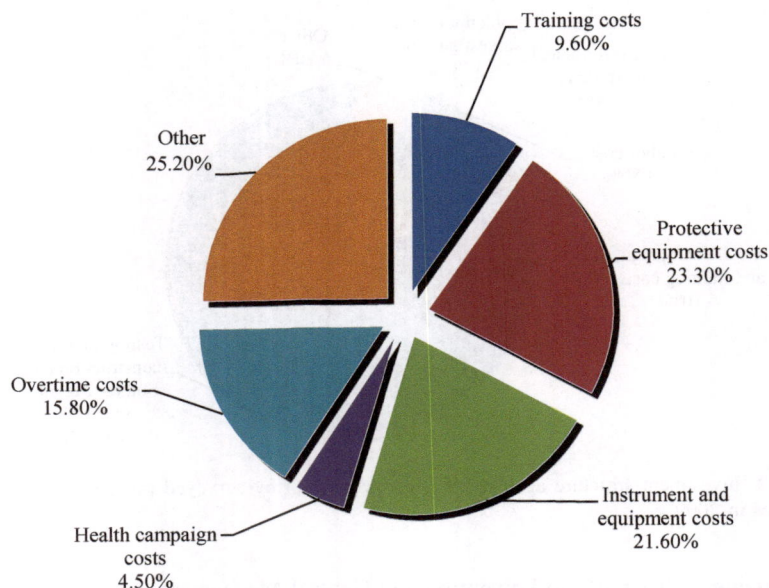

Fig. 6.3 Annual investment ratio for sampled schools in Influenza A (H1N1) prevention and control efforts for 2009

transportation, protective gear costs), and the country supplied 418,236 virology tests. Thus, we can conclude the national cost for all virology tests came to 174 million RMB.

Cost Estimations for Health Education and Training

We performed a cost analysis on the annual investment spent by provinces, cities, and counties on health education and training. According to sampled data, provinces spent an annual average of 215.09 RMB per 10,000 people on health education and training, cities invested 62.89 RMB for the same number of people, and counties spent 821.42 RMB. By the end of 2008, China's population stood at 1.32802 billion people (data derived from China Statistical Yearbook 2009). Thus, the average amount spent nationally for health education and training was 146 million RMB.

Investment Estimations for Laboratory Construction and Other Activities

According to data received on the investment into other activities by the CDC, we calculated investments estimations for the CDC on Influenza A (H1N1) prevention

Table 6.3   Costs of 441 varying Influenza A (H1N1) cases in 2009

	Suspected	Light	Severe	Critically ill	Fatal	Total
Number of sampled cases	72	168	¯13	82	6	441
Average cost (RMB)	1709.2	1710.7	8282.1	27309.2	43385.6	4561.5
Number of hospitalized cases nationwide	–	25,011	4005	1510	648	31,174

and control laboratories. Using the eight-year depreciation provision, we estimate that the total investment in laboratory construction for Influenza A (H1N1) was roughly 832 million RMB.

6.2.1.6   Cost Estimations for Prevention and Control of Influenza A (H1N1) in Educational Systems

Based on the data collected from the schools surveyed, the breakdown of different invested costs is shown in the figure below. Among these numbers, disinfectant and protective gear accounted for 23.3% of the total cost, equipment procurement 21.6%, overtime fee 15.8%, training costs 9.6%, health campaign costs 4.5%, and other fees totaled 25.2% (Fig. 6.3). The figure shows that the proportion of other costs are quite high, and from our qualitative analysis we found this was because of the costs incurred by the school in the provision of books, lunches, gifts, and toys given to students when class was suspended. These measures were taken to lessen the social impact of having to stop class. In caring for the students, schools did a lot of innovative work in counseling students and family members, and provided a strong foundation for the smooth development of Influenza A (H1N1) prevention and control efforts.

According to the 2008 Statistical Report from the Ministry of Education, as of December 31st, 2008, there was a total of 320.99 million students in school. From our sampled data, we found that as of December 31st, 2009, the total investment costs sat at 621,309 RMB for 16 schools with a total population of 32,892 students. According to the data above, the average per capita investment on Influenza A (H1N1) in these sampled schools was 18.89 RMB. Considering the sampled schools were chosen because they were affected by the epidemic, we correct our ratio in comparison with the national total investment. According to qualitative interviews and expert consultations from the Ministry of Education and other related prevention and control agencies, we have calculated the correction factor is R = 0.76. Therefore, the total national investment in schools is estimated to be 3.996 billion RMB.

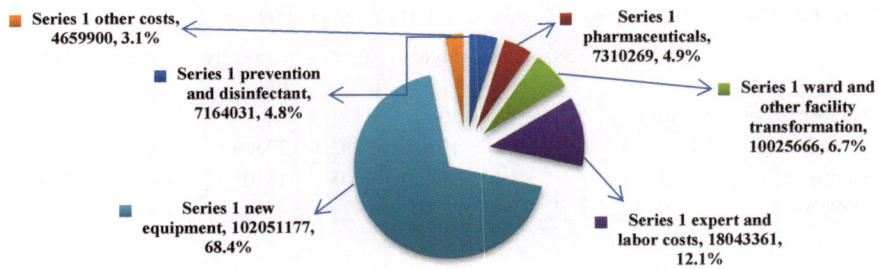

Fig. 6.4 Investment structure of 12 sampled hospitals for Influenza A (H1N1) prevention and treatment

6.2.1.7   Investment in Hospital Diagnosis and Treatment of Influenza A (H1N1) Cases

Direct Costs for Influenza A (H1N1) Diagnosis and Treatment

We collected 441 samples of suspected, mild, severe, critically ill, and fatal cases of Influenza A (H1N1) from 18 random hospitals and calculated the average cost for different levels of diagnosis and treatment of the virus (Table 6.3).

According to Table 6.3, the national direct cost for diagnosis and treatment was calculated as 159 million RMB.

Investment in Hospital Prevention and Control of Influenza A (H1N1)

As of the end of December in 2009, the total investment of 12 sampled hospitals for their Influenza A (H1N1) prevention and control stood at 149.2544 million RMB. Among that, the government allocated 33.5094 million RMB, accounting for 22.45% of the total investment, and the average amount invested per sampled hospital was 12.438 million RMB. As seen in Fig. 6.4, among the investment amount between the 12 sampled hospitals, new equipment for Influenza A (H1N1) prevention and treatment, ward transformation, and supporting facility construction accounted for almost 70% of the total costs. Expert and labor costs stood at 12.1%, and other costs like Tamiflu procurement, protection and disinfectant expenditures (including patient and specimen transport, publicity and education, and training) only accounted for less than 5%. These numbers are evidence to the fact that procurement of new Influenza A (H1N1) equipment and instruments along with ward construction were the key areas of hospital's prevention and treatment investments.

A large portion of the capital invested by hospitals in prevention and treatment of the virus went to procurement of equipment and ward transformation. After calculating the eight-year depreciation provision for the equipment used, the average investment for a sampled hospital in prevention and treatment was 50.268

million RMB, with the average amount spent on one hospitalized case at 16,761.6 RMB. Thus, the estimated total for investment by hospitals nationwide comes in at 523 million RMB.

6.2.1.8   Medical Treatment Costs for Diagnosed Patients Outside of the Hospital

According to in-depth interviews and expert assessments from the five sampled provinces, the medical cost for each diagnosed patient outside of the hospital was 450 RMB. Between August 31st, 2009, and December 31st, 2009, there was a total of 116,473 people diagnosed in China with Influenza A (H1N1), and deducting the 31,174 people that were hospitalized, the total cost for medical treatment for patients outside of the hospital totaled at 38 million RMB.

6.2.1.9   Self-medication Costs for Undiagnosed Patients

The number of total diagnosed cases in the country did not effectively represent all the patients suffering from the Acute Respiratory Infection (ARI). Looking at statistics from other countries, we see that is extremely difficult to identify the exact number of Influenza A (H1N1) cases among all ARI cases. This report assumes that patients suffering the symptoms of Influenza A (H1N1) would likely self-medicate, and the process for estimating undiagnosed patients is as follows: According to the results of serologic tests and expert assessments in 2010, 21.5% of the population tested positive in Influenza A (H1N1) serologic testing.[5] Taking away those that tested positive due to inoculation, a total of 86.7 million people (102 million × 85%), the total number of people infected in China with Influenza A (H1N1) was 198.8243 million people. Taking into account that 2/3[6] of patients showed symptoms, it is estimated that a total of 132.5495 million people was infected with the virus, and deducting the 116.5 thousand people that were diagnosed between August 31st, 2009, and December 31st, 2009, the total number of people infected with Influenza A (H1N1) that went untreated amounted to 132.433 million people. According to our in-depth interviews and expert analysis, if patients with suspected or confirmed cases of the virus were not showing any symptoms, they didn't need to be hospitalized, and the medicines used were similar to those taken for the common cold. Doctors normally recommended Banlangen or cold medicine in powder form, and other common antipyretics were also taken. These medications are quite cheap, and the average daily cost of consumption is roughly 10–20 RMB. Experts estimated that as long as the

---

[5]Derived from the China CDC monitoring data.

[6]Zhong Nanshan: Mainland report on number of Influenza A (H1N1) fatalities: "I just don't believe it." Guangzhou Daily, November 19, 2009. http://news.ifeng.com/world/special/zhuliugan/zuixinbaodao/200911/1119_6347_1442153.shtml.

Table 6.4 Framework for indirect cost estimation

Total population			
Population with Influenza A (H1N1)			
Number of diagnosed patients	Undiagnosed individuals	Number of people that avoided the disease due to the implementation of effective prevention and control strategies	Healthy people

condition didn't worsen, the average cost of care was 200 RMB.[7] According to the phone survey conducted by the China CDC's Office for Disease Control and Emergency Response after the peak of the epidemic, it was estimated that 45% of people self-medicated and from this estimation we can calculate the total self-medication expenses from undiagnosed patients: 132,433,000 × 45% × 200 RMB = 11.919 billion RMB.

6.2.2 Indirect Cost Estimations

The population in indirect cost estimations is divided into three groups. One group includes all patients diagnosed as recorded in the web-based reporting system of infectious diseases and undiagnosed individuals (including the expected number of patients due to lack of prevention and control), the second group includes the number of people that avoided the disease thanks to the implementation of effective prevention and control strategies, and the third group includes all healthy people. Missed work time and care costs were calculated for each individual group (Table 6.4).

6.2.2.1 Missed Work Costs for Patients with Influenza A (H1N1) Symptoms

According to in-depth interview data and expert assessments, the total population of patients with Influenza A (H1N1) symptoms that went untreated was 132.433 million, and 1.2% of them have missed work. As there is no data on the exact number of people that missed work across the nation as well as a stipulated national average wage, this study used the wages found in the national compensation law to estimate the cost for missed work time. Article 33 in the *National Compensation Law* stipulates that the daily compensation for infringing upon personal freedoms would be calculated according to the average daily wages of the previous year. Within the *Notice*, data from 2007 collected by the National Bureau of Statistics showed that the average annual salary for an urban worker in a non-private enterprise was

---

[7]http://blog.163.com/ch7w_yf005@126/blog/static/12760391920091122102953373/.

32,736 RMB. According to related national statistics, the average daily wage was 125.43 RMB. Thus, the total expense for missing three days of work for patients with Influenza A (H1N1) symptoms was $132,433,000 \times 0.012 \times 125.43 \times 3 = 598$ million RMB.

6.2.2.2   Missed Work Costs for Diagnosed and Isolated Patients

To calculate the losses resulted from missing work of Influenza A (H1N1) patients we used the human capital approach to estimate the present value of a person's future income. Based on the number of hospitalized cases for mildly, severely, and critically ill patients along with the number of days spent in the hospital, discounting future income can be used to calculate losses caused by missing work.

According to Article 33 of the *National Compensation Law*, the average daily wage was 125.43 RMB. As listed above, the total number of diagnosed Influenza A (H1N1) cases between August 31st, 2009, and December 31st, 2009 stood at 116,473 people, adding to that the estimated number of hospitalized patients (60,014) and patients isolated at home (83,836). If we assume that this group of people missed seven days of work, we can calculate that the indirect economic loss caused by the virus was $(116,473 + 60,014 + 83,836) \times 125.43 \times 7 = 229$ million RMB.

6.2.2.3   Nursing Care Costs for Those with Influenza A (H1N1) Symptoms

Data from the five sampled provinces showed that the care of 0.5 nurse was required for each person with the virus symptoms. The average daily wage of 125.43 RMB was used to calculate the financial contribution in a working day, and three days were accounted for the average amount of time for caregiving.

Therefore, nursing care costs were calculated as: $132,433,000 \times 0.012 \times 0.5 \times 125.43 \times 3$ days $= 299$ million RMB.

6.2.2.4   Nursing Care Costs for Influenza A (H1N1) Patients

Data from the five sampled provinces showed that 1.5 nursing care was required for each patient. The average daily wage of 125.43 RMB was used to calculate the financial contribution in a working day, and seven days were accounted for the average amount of time for caregiving.

Therefore, nursing care costs were calculated as: 116,473 people $\times 1.5 \times 125.43$ RMB $\times 7$ days $= 153$ million RMB.

Table 6.5 Total social cost for Influenza A (H1N1) prevention and control

Cost type		Cost estimation
Direct costs	Investments by inspection and quarantine agencies	2.728 billion RMB
	Tracking, isolation, and medical observation costs for close contacts	335 million RMB
	Influenza A (H1N1) vaccination fees	3.849 billion RMB
	Material stockpiling costs	1.085 billion RMB
	Investments by CDC	1.152 billion RMB
	Investments in the educational system	3.996 billion RMB
	Direct costs for diagnosis and treatment for Influenza A (H1N1) cases in hospitals	159 million RMB
	Hospital investment in prevention and control efforts against the virus	523 million RMB
	Medical expenses for non-hospitalized diagnosed patients	38 million RMB
	Self-medication expenses for those with Influenza A (H1N1) symptoms	11.919 billion RMB
Indirect costs	Missed work costs for those suffering from Influenza A (H1N1) symptoms	598 million RMB
	Missed work costs for diagnosed and isolated patients	229 million RMB
	Nursing care costs for those with Influenza A (H1N1) symptoms	299 million RMB
	Nursing care costs for Influenza A (H1N1) patients	153 million RMB
Total social cost		27.063 billion RMB

6.2.3 Calculations of Total Social Costs

Based on the aforementioned expenses, the rough calculation of the total social cost in the prevention and control of this Influenza A epidemic is found in Table 6.5.

Additionally, since there is a lack of data on the direct and indirect costs of traditional Chinese medicinal uses against the virus, this report is unable to provide any concrete statistics regarding that topic. However, according to the data provided by the National Traditional Chinese Medicine Management Bureau, the costs for using traditional Chinese medicine in treating light to mild cases was much lower than the cost of using Tamiflu and other antiviral drugs. Thus, it is estimated that traditional Chinese medicine had better cost-effectiveness in treating lighter to mild cases of the virus.

6.3   Benefit Calculation for the Prevention and Control of Influenza A (H1N1)

The start of Influenza A (H1N1) in China occurred at the same time as the U.S. subprime mortgage crisis, which triggered an international financial crisis and negative economic growth. The financial impact of this pandemic globally and domestically was a major concern for both policymakers and researchers alike. In its early stages, the spread of this unknown infectious disease wreaked havoc both economically and socially for countries such as Mexico, the United States, Ukraine, and South Korea. In terms of China, although there were some places that merited concern, it only affected the economy and society to a certain extent. For example, some schools were temporarily closed and certain social activities suspended, but as a whole, there was no serious impact on economic activities. The only areas to suffer were tourism and exhibition type industries. Moreover, the government actually had to increase its investment in areas such as vaccine and medicine production, material stockpiling, and medical treatment provisions, which in some way helped further the development of these industries.

That being said, the worst-case scenario shows us that as soon as another outbreak occurs, or even when prevention and control is lost, quite a bit of damage can be caused to both domestic and international economies. It is evident that China effectively prevented the epidemic from getting out of control, and the state also reduced the impact it could've had on GDP. Therefore, the benefits calculated from the prevention and control efforts are divided into three categories: direct economic benefits, indirect economic benefits, and macroeconomic benefits.

6.3.1   Direct Economic Benefits

According to monitoring data by the Chinese Center for Disease Control and Prevention, as of January 2010, 17.1% of the population that had not been inoculated against the virus tested positive in serologic testing for H1N1 antibodies, and only two thirds of patients of Influenza A (H1N1) showed symptoms. Therefore, the incidence of Influenza A (H1N1) among the population of people who had not been inoculated stood at 11.46%. As it is very difficult to acquire statistics on the occurrence of the virus in the natural population, this study used this statistic as the natural occurrence rate.

The literature shows that Mexico, the United Kingdom, and Hong Kong adopted a segmented "compound interest of R_0" in their relevant research, but as we were unable to obtain the data needed for such segmented calculation, we believe that in China it is closer to $R_0 = 1.5$ according to our data from five sampled provinces and expert recommendations from the China CDC.[8] Therefore, the total number of infected individuals with Influenza A (H1N1) in China's natural population is calculated as: 1,328,020,000 × 11.46% × (1 + 1.5) = 380,477,700 people.

The prevention and control measures reduced the number of infected individuals with Influenza A (H1N1), and we can calculate it as 380,477,700 people– 132,433,000 people = 248,044,700 people. By the end of 2009, there were 31,174 patients hospitalized with Influenza A (H1N1), which accounted for 0.028% of the country's total number of patients. Therefore, it is estimated that 69,453 people out of 248,044,700 people were hospitalized. With reduced number of patients, the avoided hospital costs totaled: 69,453 × 4561.5 RMB = 3.168 billion RMB. The total medical costs saved due to the reduction of patients totaled: (248044700−69453 people) × 45% × 200 RMB = 22.318 billion RMB.

6.3.2   Indirect Economic Benefits

6.3.2.1   Benefits in Preventing Loss Arising from Medical Leaves

Benefits in Preventing Loss Arising from Medical Leaves of Hospitalized Patients

Based on the fact that effective prevention and control measures prevented the hospitalization of 69,453 people, the average time gone from work was seven days, and the social daily average wage of 125.43 RMB, benefits for preventing loss of work is 61 million RMB (69,4537 days × 125.43 RMB).

6.3.2.2   Benefits in Preventing Loss Arising from Medical Leaves of Non-hospitalized Patients

As effective prevention and control measures also reduced the number of infected individuals to 248,044,700 people, and deducting the estimated 69,453 hospitalized patients, according to the 1.2% of non-hospitalized patients that missed seven days of work, the total amount saved in preventing loss arising from medical leaves of non-hospitalized patients is as follows: (24804.47−6.9453) × 1.2% × 7 days × 125.43 RMB = 2.612 billion RMB.

---

[8]Fraser et al. Science 2009, Science 19 June 2009: 1557–1561. Published online [https://doi.org/10.1126/science.1176062].

Table 6.6 Cost-benefit analysis without taking into account the impact of Influenza A (H1N1) on GDP

Estimates	Costs (100 million RMB)	Benefits (100 million RMB)	Benefits/costs
	253.99	250.82	0.98

6.3.2.3 Benefits in Preventing Nursing Care Costs

Based on the fact that successful prevention and control measures prevented 48,543 people from being hospitalized, and because each patient required 1.5 nurses with seven-day care, then according to the average daily wage of 125.43 RMB, the benefits of preventing nursing care costs is totaled at: 91 million RMB (69,453 people × 7 days × 1.5 nurses × 125.43).

From April 25th to December 31st, 2009, prevention and treatment measures for Influenza A (H1N1) is estimated at 1 RMB cost to 0.98 RMB benefit (Table 6.6).

6.3.3 Macroeconomic Benefits

According to the report *Analysis and forecast of the effects of Influenza A (H1N1) on the Chinese economy* by Taoxiong Liu et al., with a moderate outbreak of the virus where it spread through the country to a certain degree and was then effectively controlled, predictive calculations purport that this type of situation affects domestic demand, thus causing a 1.2 percentage point drop in the annual GDP.[9]

According to annual statistical analysis for 2009 of the primary, secondary and tertiary industries, the only one to be directly affected after the outbreak of the virus was the tertiary industry, as the tourism sector was hit pretty hard. After revising the data in the predictions by Liu et al., we found that after the adoption

---

[9]Taoxiong Liu, Xiaoming Wu. *Analysis and forecast of the effects of Influenza A (H1N1) on the Chinese economy*, 2009.

Table 6.7 Cost-benefit analysis taking into account the impact of Influenza A (H1N1) on GDP

Estimates	Costs (100 million RMB)	Benefits (100 million RMB)	Benefits/costs
Coefficient of consumer multiplier = 1	270.63	2029.32	7.99
Coefficient of consumer multiplier = 1.5	270.63	2933.62	10.84

of prevention and control measures, the outbreak of Influenza A (H1N1) affected GDP by 0.53–0.8%.[10]

Therefore, the cost-benefit analysis with the GDP loss avoided by effective prevention and control measures as social benefits is as follows: when the coefficient of consumer multiplier is 1, the amount of social benefits created is 177.85 billion RMB; when the coefficient of consumer multiplier is 1.5, the amount of social benefits reach 268.28 billion RMB.

From April 25th to December 31st, 2009, prevention and treatment measures for Influenza A (H1N1) at its lowest is estimated at 1 RMB cost to 7.99 RMB benefit, and its highest at 1 RMB cost to 1.5 RMB benefit (Table 6.7).

As seen above, cost-benefit analysis involves many specific assumptions and judgments regarding economy, technology, and society, and it must take into account aspects of data collection and measurement. On this matter, the assessment team put forth a lot of effort in its research and analysis. However, because of limited time and resource available, the assessment is not perfect and the exact numerical results should be used with caution. We also look forward to more efforts in the future in improving cost-benefit analysis for emergency management.

---

[10]The consumer multiplier model is based on the Keynesian theory of economics. It first takes into account the direct effects of the epidemic on consumption, for example tourism, and then through the multiplier application, it also looks into indirect effects on the economy, and together it calculates the total economic impact. After the outbreak of Influenza A (H1N1), the service industries were directly affected, especially tourism. Economists used a multiplier between 2 and 3 in estimating the multiplier effect on domestic tourism. The following analysis is based upon online data and should provide a reasonable speculation and analysis of the entire country's situation. According to data about visitors from outside China, the numbers show that in the first half of 2009, foreign exchange earnings from tourism dropped 11%, and 122.4 billion RMB was lost. According to last year's domestic flight and tourism trends along with the decreasing amount of large scale activities or gatherings, a conservative estimate shows a 10% loss in domestic tourism earnings, a loss of up to 56.45 billion RMB. Thus the total loss for both domestic and foreign tourism was up to 178.85 billion RMB. Taking into consideration that the epidemic tapered off in the fourth quarter, this study adopts the following two parameters: First, there is no multiplier effect. The impact totalled 177.85 billion RMB in 2009, China's total GDP was 33.5353 trillion RMB, so the affect accounted for 0.53%; the second is calculated in accordance with the multiplier being 1.5, and the impact was 268.28 billion RMB. In 2009, China's total GDP was 33.5353 trillion RMB, so the affect accounted for 0.8%.

Chapter 7
Evaluations from Different Parties on Influenza A (H1N1) Prevention and Control

Assessments of policy formulation and implementation by domestic and international stakeholders, especially domestic stakeholders, comprise a crucial component of policy evaluation. The end goals of the state's prevention and control efforts were: to ensure the protection of public health and safety, protect social order, and maintain the status quo in work and life. Thus, assessments on the state's responses by patients, close contacts, medical personnel, the public, and international community could reflect in many ways the degree of completion for expected objectives and the social effects of adopted prevention and control efforts.

In order to objectively evaluate the assessments on the state's response to Influenza A (H1N1) by patients, close contacts, medical personnel, and the public, this research group conducted the following data collection: questionnaires for 3262 randomly sampled residents across the country, phone interviews with 893 Influenza A (H1N1) patients and 646 close contacts from Beijing, Fujian, and Henan areas, and field interviews with 519 personnel from 31 disease control agencies and 243 medical personnel from 29 key hospitals in Beijing, Fujian, Henan, Guangdong, and Sichuan. In order to gauge the international community's assessments on China's response to the pandemic, this research group also conducted interviews and field surveys with the WHO, along with a literature review of international media.

7.1 The Public's Assessment

The public's satisfaction with the central government's response to Influenza A (H1N1) reflects their assessment of the state's overall performance in the prevention and control of the virus. The changes in the level of public trust in the state's emergency response capabilities also reflects the credibility of the government in handling emergencies, and it also gives credence to the efficient communication between government and society. The effect of individual differences in

© Social Sciences Academic Press and Springer Nature Singapore Pte Ltd. 2019
L. Xue and G. Zeng, *A Comprehensive Evaluation on Emergency Response in China*, Research Series on the Chinese Dream and China's Development Path, https://doi.org/10.1007/978-981-13-0644-0_7

satisfaction to a certain extent reflects the impact of specific prevention and control measures on different groups of people.

Based on the above presumptions, in order to objectively gauge the public's assessment on the state's response to Influenza A (H1N1), the assessment group worked with the Horizon Surveying Company to conduct door-to-door surveys with 3262 randomly sampled residents across the country. These surveys analyzed the following: the level of satisfaction regarding the central government's overall performance in its prevention and control efforts; the perceived effectiveness of the Prevention and Control Mechanism established by the central government; level of satisfaction in the local government's (including sub-district office; and government from the town and township level to the provincial level) overall performance in prevention and control; the level of trust or changes of trust in the central government's and local government's (including sub-district office, and government from the town and township level to the provincial level) emergency response capabilities (after experiencing the Influenza A (H1N1) epidemic); and information credibility provided by the central and local governments.

7.1.1   The Public's Satisfaction Assessment of the State's Influenza A (H1N1) Prevention and Control Efforts

As the outbreak of Influenza A (H1N1) constituted a national public health emergency, the central government took the lead by forming a Prevention and Control Mechanism and also by formulating an overall response strategy. Under the guidance of this strategy, local governments then adopted relevant measures to mitigate the disaster. Assessing the level of public satisfaction of the government's efforts means we must evaluate the overall performance of the government in mitigating this epidemic. The strategies made by the central government needed to be carried out by the local governments, and the extent to which measures were implemented directly affected the efficiency of prevention and control efforts. Therefore, the public's level of satisfaction of the local government's (including governments at the provincial, municipal, county, town and township level, and sub-district offices) overall performance in prevention and control is actually based upon their direct perception of how the measures were implemented in their local area.

7.1.1.1   Nearly 92% of the Public Was Satisfied with the Central Government's Performance

In mitigating the Influenza A (H1N1) pandemic, a large portion of the sampled public, nearly 92%, expressed their satisfaction in the central government's overall performance. Among these, 44.9% of respondents stated they were very satisfied

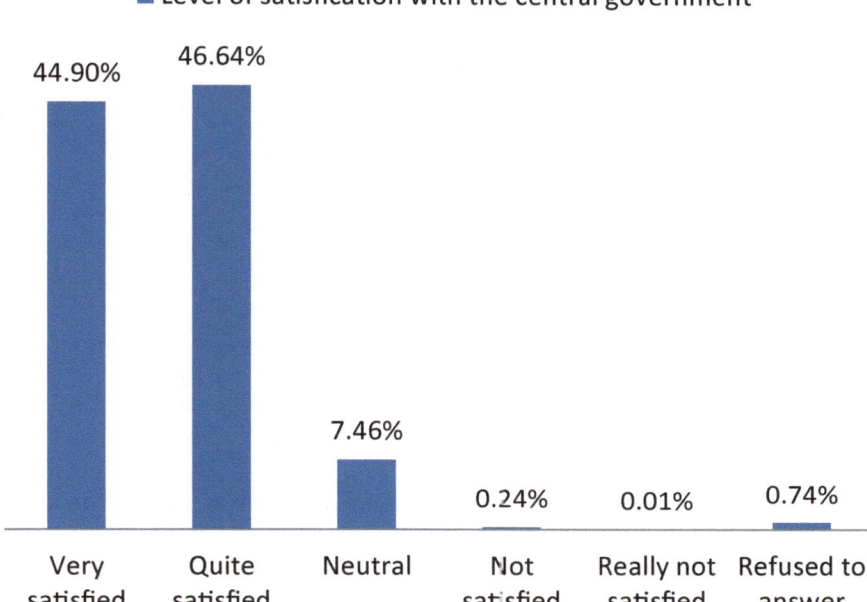

Fig. 7.1 Public's satisfaction in the central government's response to Influenza A (H1N1)

with the government's response efforts, 46.64% expressed they were quite satisfied, and 0.25% stated they were dissatisfied with the efforts (Fig. 7.1).

As can be seen in the data, individual characteristics within the public didn't significantly impact their assessment of the central government's response efforts, and it is evident that satisfaction with the state's efforts was prevalent among the masses. In regards to overall satisfaction, we investigated the impact demographics and other characteristics may have on the public's assessment. Using one-way analysis of variance, we found that factors such as gender, age, educational background, income, residence, experience with infectious disease, and having children had no significant impact on the level of satisfaction in regards to the central government's responses. After dividing the respondents according to age, income, and gender respectively, we found that more than 90% of the respondents felt satisfied with the government, which was accordance with the overall situation.

There were some significant differences in the level of satisfaction among different occupations and industries. The results of the study showed that middle to upper level management in enterprises expressed higher satisfaction than their peers in government bodies and public institutions. Over 90% of enterprise management expressed their satisfaction with the central government, while over 80% in government bodies and public institutions answered as being satisfied. After separating the groups by industry, we found that the education sector and the hotel and restaurant sector had lower levels of satisfaction than the average value (Fig. 7.2).

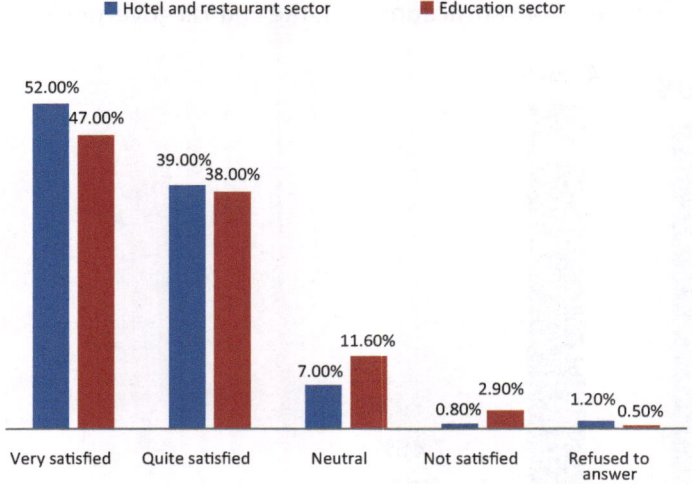

Fig. 7.2 Hotel and restaurant sector's and education sector's satisfaction with the central government's response efforts (Unit: %)

7.1.1.2 Ninety-Three Percent of the Public Aware of the Prevention and Control Mechanism Found It to Be Effective

In our assessment, we paid special attention to the public's level of satisfaction with the Prevention and Control Mechanism, as it played a pivotal role in the central government's response efforts. Among the respondents, 36.13% knew that the State Council had established such a mechanism, out of those who were aware of it, 57.09% believed it to be successful and 35.79% found it to be very successful. As shown in Fig. 7.3, it is evident that most of the people who knew about the mechanism believed in its efficacy.

7.1.1.3 Eighty-Five Percent of the Public Were Satisfied with Prevention and Control Efforts from Their Local Governments

The public was also satisfied with their local governments, as 85% were satisfied with their local government's overall performance, but generally not as much as they were satisfied with the central government. As you can see in Fig. 7.4, which shows the public's satisfaction towards the central government, the proportion of people who answered very satisfied declined, and overall satisfaction dropped by 7%, while more people answered as being neutral to not being satisfied with their local government's performance.

In line with the satisfaction found with the central government, demographic factors such as gender, age, educational background, income, and family

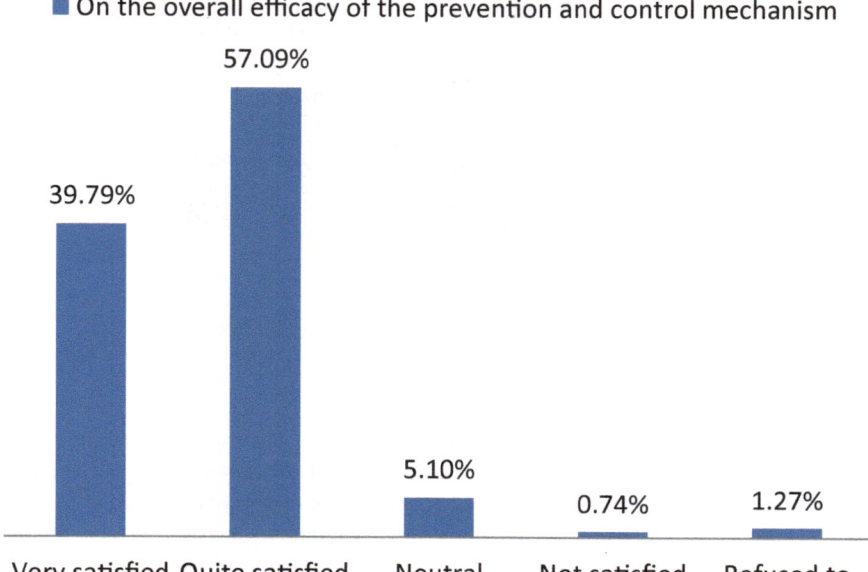

Fig. 7.3 Assessments by respondents aware of the prevention and control mechanism of its efficacy in Influenza A (H1N1) response efforts

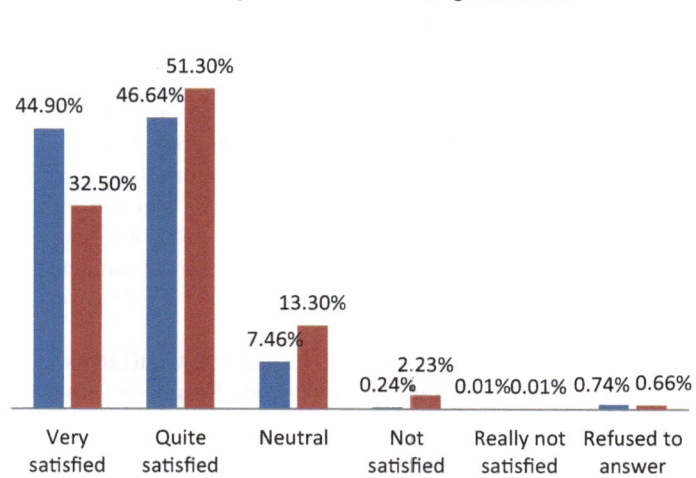

Fig. 7.4 The public's satisfaction in the local government's responses to Influenza A (H1N1) (Unit: %)

background had no significant impact on the level of satisfaction. Occupations, however, did have a relatively significant impact as 12.4% of service members as well as the same percentage of police officers were neutral or dissatisfied with the local government's overall performance. The participants working in education had the highest level of dissatisfaction among the groups, with 9.1% answering as dissatisfied.

In terms of a regional comparison, residents in the central region were slightly less satisfied with local government than residents in the eastern and western regions, while the proportion of eastern respondents expressing "not very satisfied" with the performance of local governments was higher than those of the central and western regions.

7.1.2   The Public's Assessment on the Credibility of the Government

Credibility in a government is a type of soft resource. It's the amount of trust the public has in their state institutions. It's an important guarantee of a government's usefulness and its improvement, and enhancing this credibility is mutually beneficial for both the government and the public. Enhancing credibility can happen through the government proactively improving its performance, or it can happen through communication with the public. Therefore, we took two factors into consideration when assessing the state's prevention and control efforts and their impact on government credibility. One was measuring the level of trust, or change in trust by the public in their government's emergency response capabilities after they experienced the Influenza A (H1N1) outbreak, which showed the impact of the state's emergency management response on the government's credibility. Second was measuring the level of public trust in the information provided by the government which showed the impact of communication on government credibility.

In order to assess credibility in the state's prevention and control efforts, this assessment team measured the change in trust by the public after they experienced the Influenza A (H1N1) in regards to the central and local government's capabilities in emergency management. We also compared the level of trust during the SARS period with this epidemic. The results of the survey showed that the public generally expressed confidence in the government's emergency response capacity, and the public became significantly more trusting of local governments and their capabilities.

7.1.2.1   Ninety-Six Percent of the Public Expressed Confidence in the Central Government's Emergency Response Capabilities

In regards to the central government's emergency response capabilities, the following results were found: 32.3% of the public polled felt "the same amount of trust as before;" 44.7% felt they "trusted in the past, and have a little more trust in them now;" 19.1% felt "no trust in the past, and now there is trust;" and only 2.1% felt that they did not trust in the central government (see Table 7.1).

Table 7.1 Public's assessment on the credibility of central and local government's prevention and control efforts

	After Influenza A (H1N1) (%)		Comparison with the time of SARS(%)	
	Central government	Local government	Central government	Local government
Trust even less than before	0.2	0.3	0.1	0.4
No change: still no trust	1.9	3.8	2.1	4.2
No change: same amount of trust as before	32.3	35.9	29.3	34.0
Change: no trust before, now there is trust	19.1	30.7	22.3	29.1
Change: trust before, but even more trust now	44.7	27.4	43.8	29.6
Refused to answer/don't know	1.8	1.9	2.4	2.7

7.1.2.2   Ninety-Four Percent of the Public Expressed Confidence in Their Local Government's Emergency Response Capabilities

As shown in Table 7.1, in regards to local government's emergency response capabilities, the following results were found: 35.9% felt "the same amount of trust as before;" 30.6% felt they "trusted in the past, and have a little more trust in them now;" 27.4% "felt no trust in the past, and now there is trust;" and only 4.1% expressed no trust in their local governments, which is two percentage points higher than those who expressed the same for the central government.

7.1.2.3   There Was a Relatively High Level of Credibility of the Central Government Along with a Significant Increase in the Credibility of Local Governments

The central government's credibility has been relatively high in regards to emergency response, with 77% of respondents expressing they had confidence or even more confidence than before in the government's capabilities. After experiencing the outbreak of Influenza A (H1N1), the ratio of respondents that felt "no trust before, but now there is trust" was much higher for local governments (30.6% of respondents) than for the central government (19.1%). Although the credibility of local governments overall was relatively lower, after the outbreak there was a significant increase in the trust in local governments' response capabilities.

7.1.2.4   Government-Released Information Became the Public's Most Trusted News Source

In the surveys, we asked respondents about the reliability of news from different sources including the central government, local government, experts, grassroots communities, village groups, working units, and news by word of mouth. The results clearly showed that during this epidemic, the public's most trusted news source was still the government, and the trust in the central government was higher than in local governments (as seen in Fig. 7.5).

Similar to the assessment on the public's satisfaction towards their government, demographic factors such as gender, age, educational background, income, family background, and residence had no significant impact on their perception of the government's credibility. What did make a significant impact on the perception of the credibility of the central government was whether the respondent or any of the respondent's family members had been infected in the past by a contagious virus. However, this one factor did not seem to have any significant impact on the respondents' confidence in their local governments.

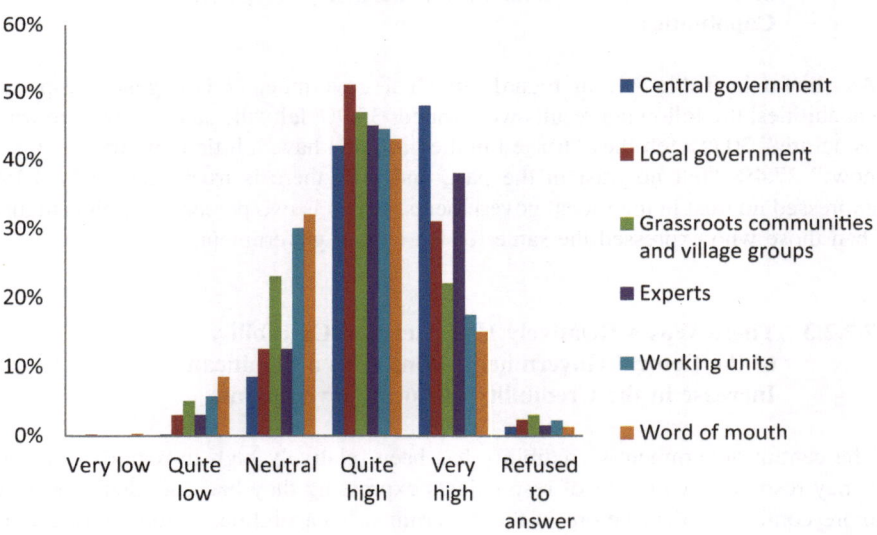

Fig. 7.5 The level of trust the public showed in different news sources (Unit: %)

7.1.3 The Public's Specific Evaluation on the Government's Prevention and Control Measures

7.1.3.1 Over 90% of the Public Recognized the Necessity for the Prevention and Control Measures

The government adopted relevant measures in each of the four distinct epidemic phases, and these measures included the following: customs health inspection, patient isolation, close contact isolation, class suspension where the virus was prevalent, the promotion of wearing masks and frequent hand washing, inoculations, more exercise, and the use of traditional Chinese medicine. The majority of the respondents recognized the need for these measures, especially the customs health inspection, patient isolation, close contact isolation, class suspension, and the promotion of exercise. Over half of the respondents felt that these measures were necessary as can be seen in Fig. 7.6. It is clear that there was a wide acceptance by the public of these prevention and control measures and that the implementation personified humanistic care. However, Fig. 7.7 shows that one third of the respondents felt that these measures were inconvenient to a certain extent for their daily routines.

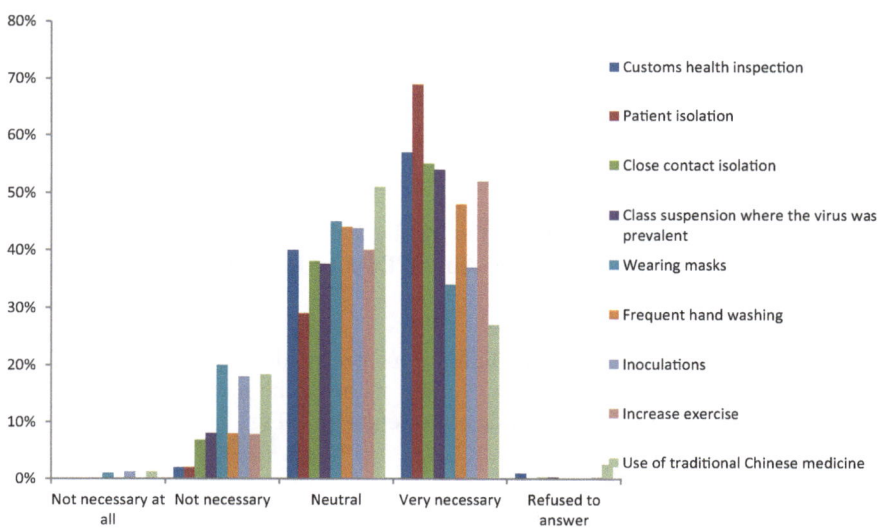

Fig. 7.6 Analysis on the necessity of state-led prevention and control efforts during the four phases of the epidemic

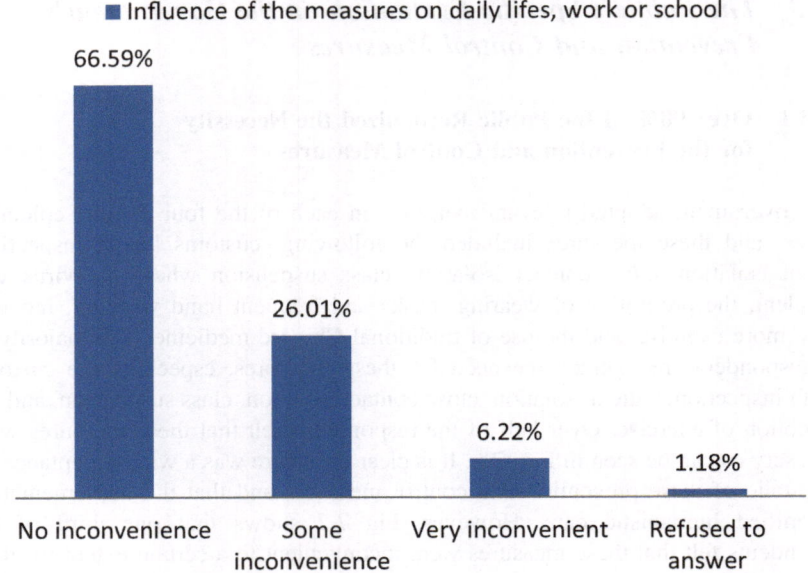

Fig. 7.7 Study on the effects of Influenza A (H1N1) prevention and control measures on daily lives, work, or school

7.1.3.2 Nearly Seventy Percent of the Public Recognized the Effective Results of the Prevention and Control Measures

Close to 70% of respondents felt that the state-led prevention and control strategies and measures in each of the four phases produced good to very good results, and this sentiment remained consistent throughout all four phases (Fig. 7.8).

7.1.3.3 Roughly Fifty Percent of the Public Felt that the Measures Were Appropriate, While About Twenty Percent Felt Them to Be Relatively Strict

About 50% of the respondents felt that the measures adopted were appropriate in terms of their intensity, but the ratio of those who felt the measures partially strict did rise in the peak and slow periods of the epidemic (Fig. 7.9).

7.1.3.4 Roughly Seventy Percent of the Public Felt that There Were Timely Adjustments to Prevention and Control Strategies

As seen in Fig. 7.10, 67.9% of the public felt that the government strategies and measures in place before the first imported case on May 5th were timely; 76.3% of

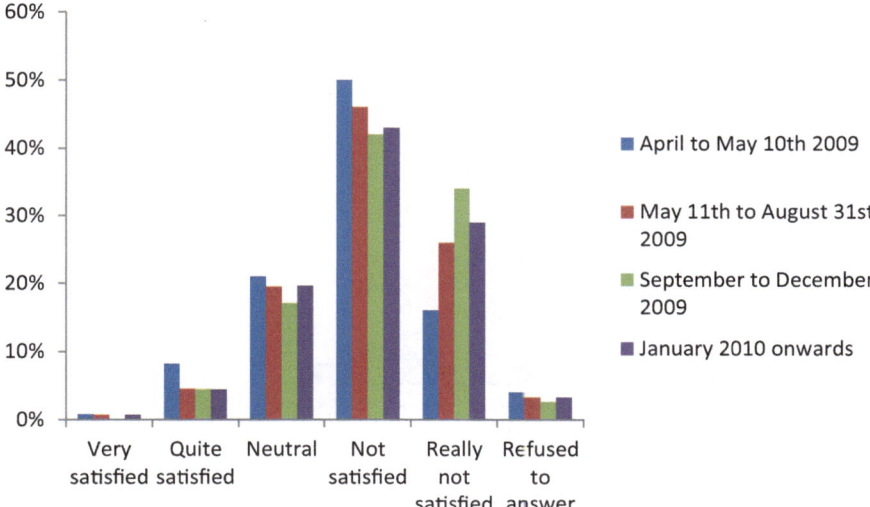

Fig. 7.8 The public's assessment on the results of the state's prevention and control strategies and measures in the four epidemic phases

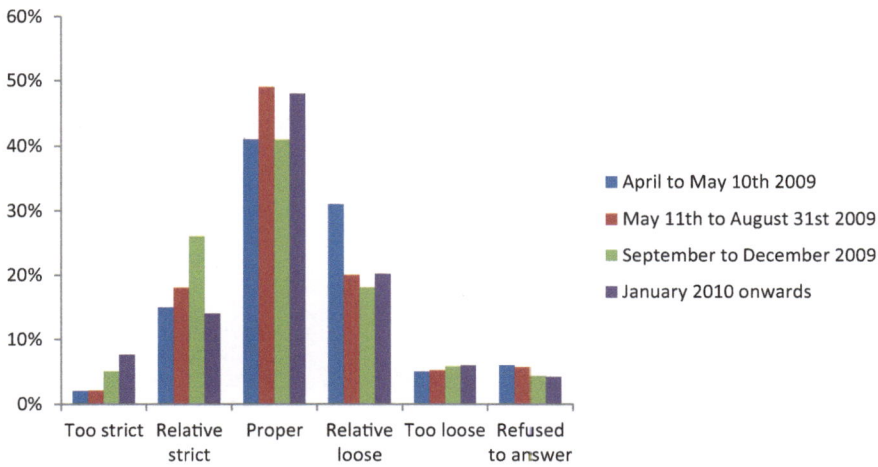

Fig. 7.9 The public's assessment on the overall intensity of prevention and control measures during the four epidemic phases

the public felt that timely adjustments were made to prevention and control measures between May 11th and August 31st; 80.1% of the public felt that timely adjustments were also made during the epidemic's peak period from September to December 2009; and 75.1% of the public felt the same after January 2010.

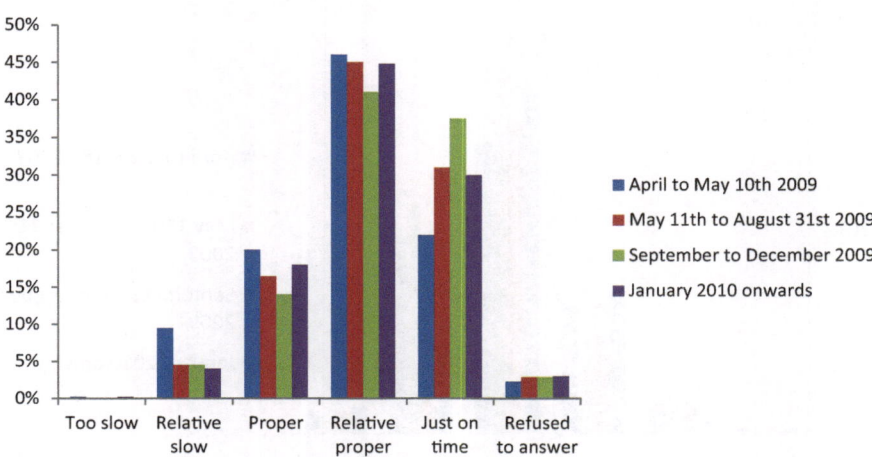

Fig. 7.10 Public's analysis on the timeliness of the prevention and control measures within the four epidemic phases

7.1.3.5   Roughly Thirty Percent of the Public Felt that the Government Invested a Lot in Prevention and Control of Influenza A (H1N1)

As seen in Fig. 7.11, 25.2% of the public felt that the government invested a lot before the first imported case on May 5th; 29.4% felt the same for the time period between May 11th and August 31st; 34.9% for September to December; and 30.5% for after January 2010.

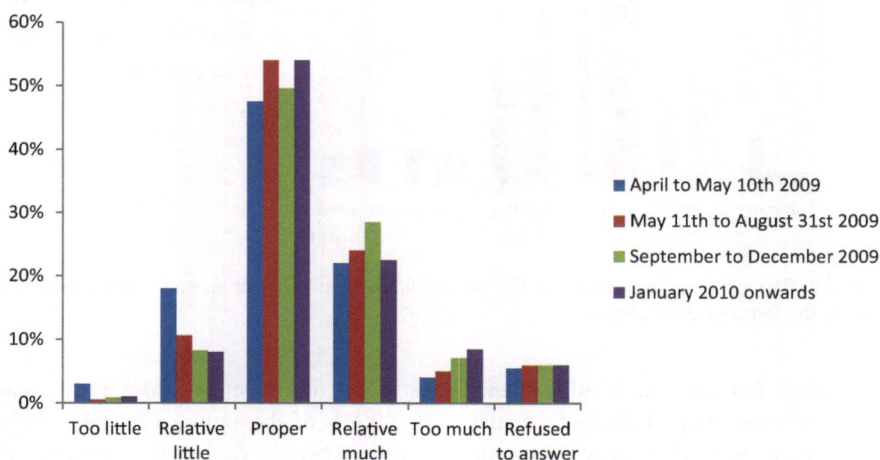

Fig. 7.11 Public's analysis on the government's investment during the four epidemic phases

7.1.3.6   The Public Approved of the Government Disclosing Information Regarding the Epidemic

Information disclosure to the public had a direct impact on their level of awareness and behaviors surrounding the epidemic. The government disclosed information not only regarding trends in the domestic spread of the virus, and scientific information regarding prevention and control, they also disseminated information on the measures adopted as well as the provided information to relevant agencies.

As seen in Fig. 7.12, the public generally approved of the government's disclosure on epidemic information, and over 80% of respondents approved of the information regarding their local epidemic situation, the domestic and international trends updates, and the use of self-protection in preventing the spread of the virus. All of those who had been infected with SARS, the Avian Flu, or Influenza A (H1N1) felt that the government did very well in disclosing the right information to the public.

From a regional perspective, people in the eastern regions showed the smallest amount of satisfaction in the local information disclosure regarding the epidemic; the highest level of satisfaction was found in the western regions; and satisfaction in the northern regions was slightly higher than in the southern regions as seen in Figs. 7.13 and 7.14.

7.1.3.7   Evaluation of Implementation of Prevention and Control Measures in Key Areas

Prevention and control in public places was the focal point of post-epidemic measures, which included disinfecting, temperature testing, isolation, prevention and control information dissemination, and the retention of personal data. As

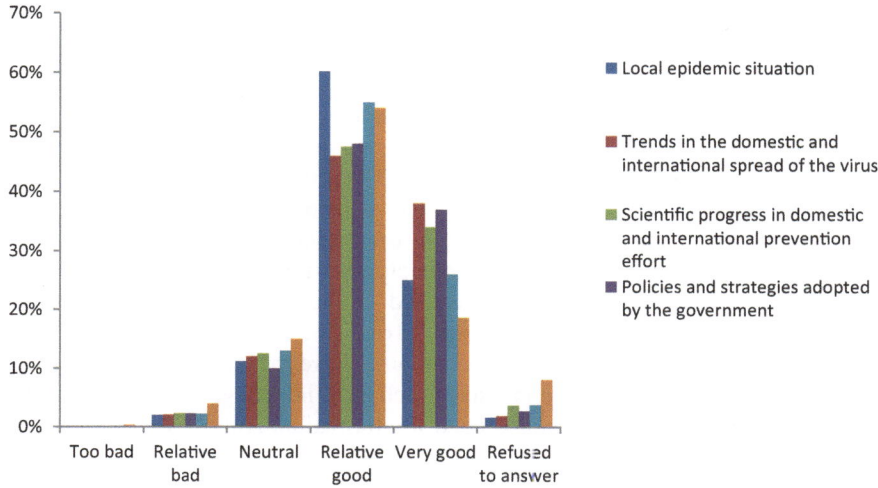

Fig. 7.12 The public's assessment on the government's information disclosure

Fig. 7.13 Satisfaction in information disclosure in the eastern, middle, and western regions

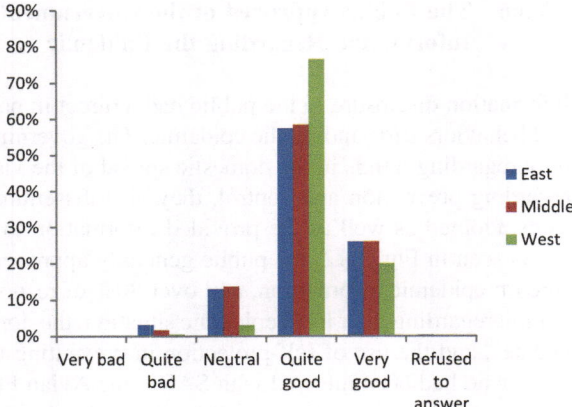

Fig. 7.14 Satisfaction in information disclosure in the northern and southern regions

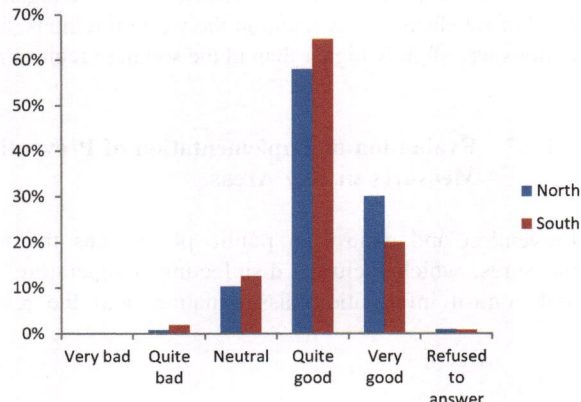

Fig. 7.15 shows, over half of the respondents' communities adopted measures such as disinfecting areas and disseminating prevention and control information, which were the focus of the prevention and control efforts during this phase.

Schools are also focus of the middle- to late-stage prevention and control efforts, and the implementation of these measures was fairly comprehensive. Most schools took measures including disinfecting, temperature testing, as well as prevention and control information dissemination. One third of the schools employed isolation measures and retained personal data (Fig. 7.16).

Hospital-led prevention and control measures were the most comprehensive in scope, as most hospitals adopted measures such as disinfecting, temperature testing, and dissemination of prevention and control information. Almost 40% of hospitals adopted isolation measures as well (Fig. 7.17).

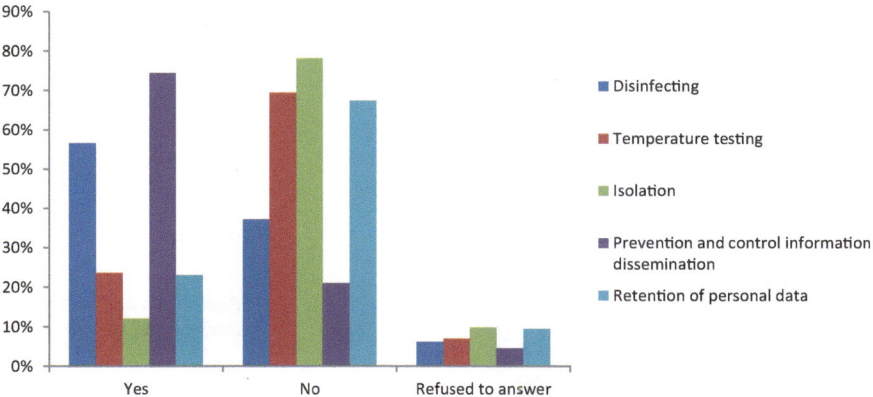

Fig. 7.15 Implementation of community prevention and control measures

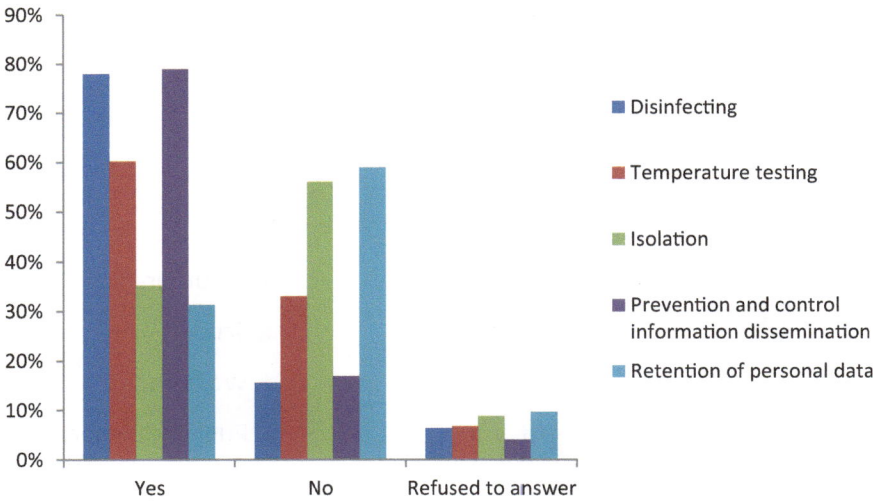

Fig. 7.16 Implementation of school prevention and control measures

A horizontal comparison was done on the same data for different prevention and control measures, and it was found that implementation of disinfecting and temperature testing in schools and hospitals was more comprehensive (Fig. 7.18). As a portion of the respondents lacked any interaction or understanding of hotels, it is understandable that there was a high rate of "refused to answer/don't know" responses.

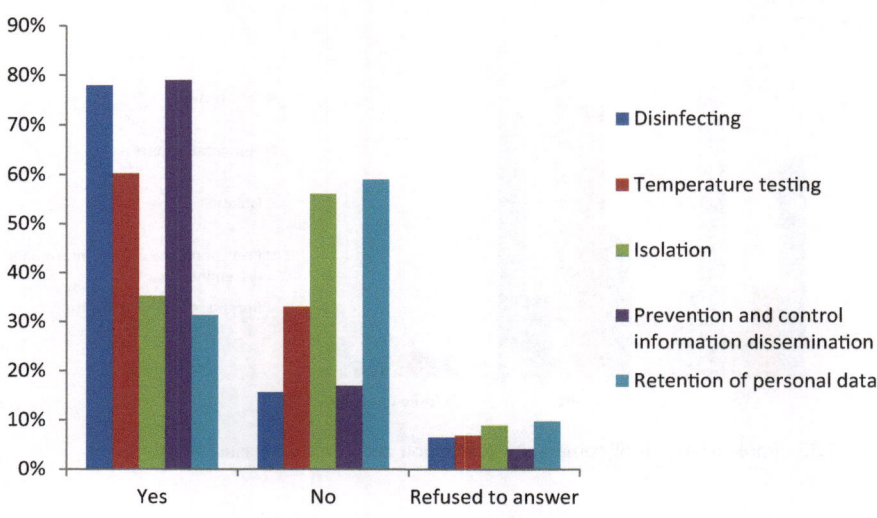

Fig. 7.17 Implementation of hospital prevention and control measures

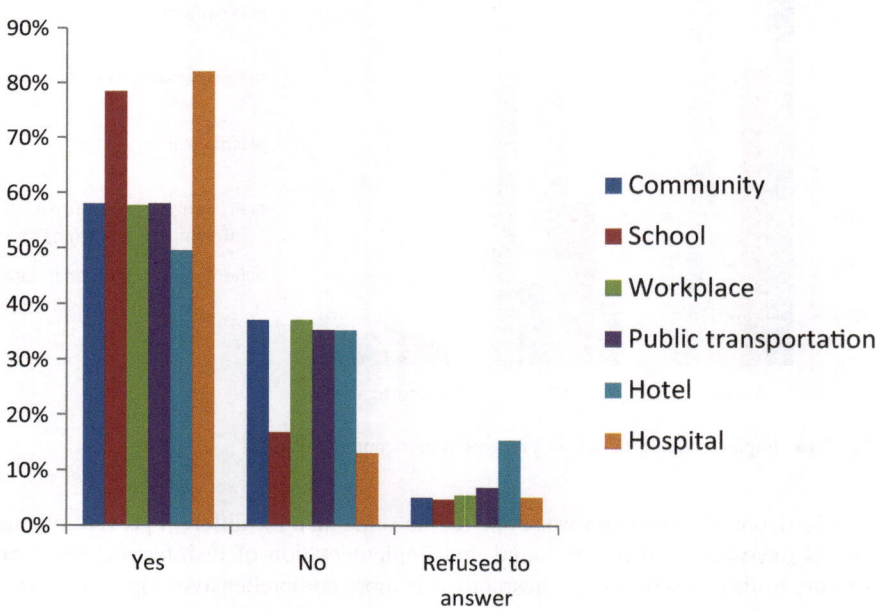

Fig. 7.18 Comparison chart of implemented disinfection measures

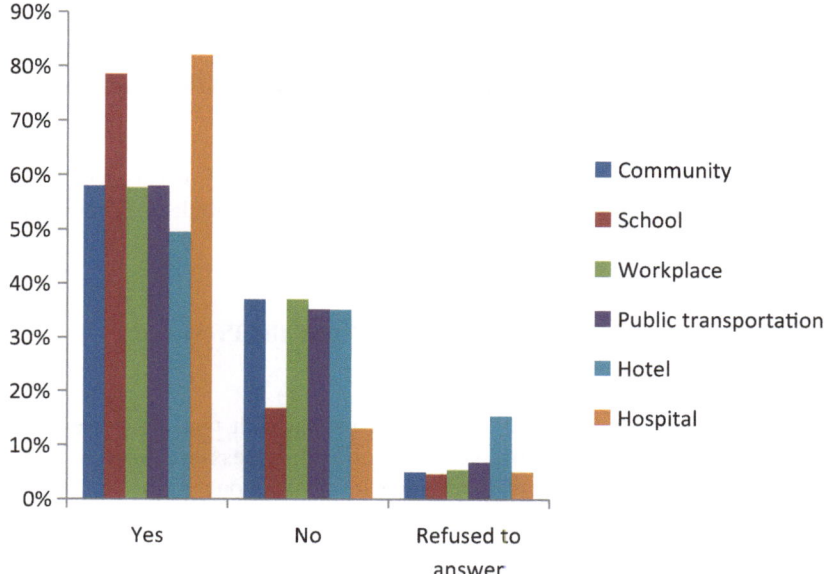

Fig. 7.19 Comparison chart of implemented temperature testing measures

7.2   Assessments from Influenza A (H1N1) Patients and Close Contacts

Patients and close contacts of Influenza A (H1N1) were the direct beneficiaries of the state's prevention and control strategies and measures, and their attitudes, feelings, and levels of satisfaction with these policies directly reflect the outcome of the government's response efforts. Understanding the implementation of these prevention and control strategies for patients and close contacts, and understanding the attitudes, feelings, and levels of satisfaction from these affected people towards national strategies, will provide useful references for future emergency response policies. Based on the four different epidemic phases, we employed a stratified sampling method and conducted phone interviews with 893 patients and 646 close contacts from the three areas in the national disease monitoring information report management system: Beijing, Fujian, and Henan. The interview included topics covering implementation of quarantine and treatment policies during different epidemic phases, the implementation of discharge standard policies, the implementation of humanistic care policies, and medical treatment costs. We also investigated the attitudes of the close contacts in regards to medical observation management and humanistic care policy implementation.

7.2.1 Assessments from Patients with Influenza A (H1N1)

7.2.1.1 Sixty-Five Percent of Patients Were Satisfied with Prevention and Control Efforts

The study showed that 65% of patients were either satisfied or very satisfied with the national prevention and control efforts; 26% were neutral; and 9% were dissatisfied or very dissatisfied (Table 7.2).

7.2.1.2 Ninety-Three Percent of Patients Found the Prevention and Control Measures Necessary

As seen in Tables 7.3, 7.4, and 7.5, 93% of patients felt that the prevention and control measures adopted by the government were necessary; however, 25% of them felt that these measures caused some level of inconvenience to their daily lives, and among them 79% felt that they could tolerate this inconvenience. Among those patients who believed the measures were inconvenient, most (75%) found the isolation measures to be the most inconvenient, followed by triage, diagnosis, and treatment measures. Lastly, measures such as control of public opinion, information disclosures, and class suspensions did have a certain impact on people's daily lives.

Table 7.2 Influenza A (H1N1) patients' satisfaction assessments with prevention and control efforts

Province	N	Very dissatisfied	Dissatisfied	Neutral	Satisfied	Very satisfied
Beijing	306	15(5%)	5(2%)	77(25%)	140(46%)	69(22%)
Fujian	288	9(3%)	20(7%)	82(28%)	95(34%)	82(28%)
Henan	299	10(3%)	24(8%)	75(25%)	122(41%)	68(23%)
Total	893	34(4%)	49(5%)	234(26%)	357(40%)	219(25%)

Table 7.3 Influenza A (H1N1) patients' assessment on the necessity of prevention and control measures

Province	N	The necessity in adopting prevention and control measures against Influenza A (H1N1)	
		Yes	No
Beijing	306	278(91%)	28(9%)
Fujian	287	272(95%)	15(5%)
Henan	293	272(93%)	21(7%)
Total	886	822(93%)	64(7%)

Table 7.4 Influenza A (H1N1) patients' assessment on convenience of prevention and control measures

Province	N	Did the national prevention and control measures cause any inconvenience?		
		Yes	No	Hard to say
Beijing	303	76(25%)	185(61%)	42(14%)
Fujian	288	65(23%)	206(72%)	17(6%)
Henan	298	79(27%)	212(71%)	7(2%)
Total	889	220(25%)	603(68%)	66(7%)

Table 7.5 Evaluation of the tolerance for inconvenience of Influenza A (H1N1) patients

Province	N	Toleration for inconvenience	
		Can	Cannot
Beijing	76	57(75%)	19(25%)
Fujian	65	50(77%)	15(23%)
Henan	79	66(84%)	13(16%)
Total	220	173(79%)	47(21%)

7.2.1.3 Fifty-Seven Percent of Patients Felt that the Prevention and Control Measures Were Appropriate

Table 7.6 shows that 17% of patients felt that state-led prevention and control measures were a little strict during the onset of the epidemic. During our investigations into assessments of early prevention and control, we discovered that respondents in in the central province of Henan felt that these measures were a little strict and it also was evident that there was a certain rationality and necessity to adjusting regional policies according to regional differences.

Table 7.7 shows that 42% of patients felt that the prevention and control measures taken against the Influenza A (H1N1) epidemic were fair or very fair; 37% were neutral; 13% felt it was hard to say; and 7% felt that they were unfair or very unfair. Among those, respondents' overall evaluations in Henan were lower than those found in Beijing and Fujian, and thus it is clear that distinct differences existed in the implementation and adjustments of regional policies.

Table 7.6 Influenza A (H1N1) patient's evaluation on the adequacy of early prevention and control measures

Province	N	The adequacy of early prevention and control measures			
		Relatively strict	Relatively relaxed	Appropriate	Hard to say
Beijing	306	50(16%)	29(9%)	159(52%)	68(22%)
Fujian	287	50(17%)	26(9%)	173(60%)	38(13%)
Henan	298	50(7%)	29(10%)	176(59%)	43(14%)
Total	891	150(17%)	84(9%)	508(57%)	149(17%)

Table 7.7 Influenza A (H1N1) patients' assessment on the fairness of the prevention and control measures

Province	N	Fairness in Influenza A (H1N1) prevention and control measures					
		Very unfair	Somewhat unfair	Neutral	Somewhat fair	Very fair	Hard to say
Beijing	306	4(1%)	4(1%)	92(30%)	77(25%)	89(29%)	40(13%)
Fujian	286	5(2%)	15(5%)	75(26%)	107(37%)	36(13%)	48(17%)
Henan	297	5(2%)	31(10%)	163(55%)	49(16%)	17(6%)	32(11%)
Total	889	14(2%)	50(5%)	330(37%)	233(26%)	142 (16%)	120 (13%)

7.2.1.4   Eighty-Four Percent of Patients Felt that the State's Investment into Influenza A (H1N1) Prevention and Control Was Worth It

In regards to investment into prevention and control efforts, Table 7.8 shows that 84% of patients felt that the cost of these measures was worth it. It is clear that state investments into the prevention and control measure were widely supported and accepted by patients.

7.2.1.5   Eighty-Two Percent of Patients Felt that Progress Was Made in the State's Public Emergency Response Capabilities

In addition to SARS, the Influenza A (H1N1) pandemic was another test in global public health emergency management. In comparison with SARS, 82% of Influenza A (H1N1) patients felt that the government had made improvements in its public health emergency response capabilities. Among those, Beijing had the highest number of respondents (87%) who felt that progress had been made (Table 7.9).

Table 7.10 shows that after experiencing the prevention and control, 79% of patients felt they could trust in the government's response capabilities; 15% stated it was hard to say; and 6% expressed distrust in the government's capabilities.

Table 7.8 Influenza A (H1N1) patients' assessment on the necessity of state investment in prevention and control measures

Province	N	Necessity of state investment into prevention and control measures			
		Worth it	Not worth it	Neutral	Hard to say
Beijing	307	250(81%)	11(4%)	18(6%)	28(9%)
Fujian	289	250(86%)	3(1%)	10(3%)	26(9%)
Henan	297	253(85%)	10(3%)	12(4%)	22(7%)
Total	893	753(84%)	24(3%)	40(4%)	76(9%)

Table 7.9 Influenza A (H1N1) patient's assessment in public health emergency response capabilities

Province	N	Progress in response capabilities since SARS				
		A lot of progress	Some progress	No progress	Some regression	A lot of regression
Beijing	305	71(23%)	195(64%)	31(10%)	6(2%)	2(1%)
Fujian	287	38(13%)	194(68%)	24(8%)	28(10%)	3(1%)
Henan	299	36(12%)	197(66%)	56(19%)	8(3%)	2(1%)
Total	891	145(16%)	586(66%)	111(12%)	42(5%)	7(1%)

Table 7.10 Assessment of trust in emergency response after the outbreak of Influenza A (H1N1)

Province	N	Trust in state emergency response capabilities after Influenza A (H1N1) outbreak		
		Yes	No	Hard to say
Beijing	306	236(77%)	16(5%)	54(18%)
Fujian	288	227(79%)	16(6%)	45(16%)
Henan	285	230(81%)	25(9%)	30(11%)
Total	879	693(79%)	57(6%)	129(15%)

Table 7.11 Close contacts' satisfaction assessments with prevention and control efforts

Province	N	Very dissatisfied	Dissatisfied	Neutral	Satisfied	Very satisfied
Beijing	247	2(1%)	1(0%)	27(11%)	125(51%)	92(37%)
Fujian	198	5(3%)	0(0%)	38(19%)	97(49%)	58(29%)
Henan	199	2(1%)	2(1%)	26(13%)	77(39%)	92(46%)
Total	644	9(1%)	3(0%)	91(14%)	299(46%)	242(38%)

7.2.2   Assessments from Close Contacts of Influenza A (H1N1)

7.2.2.1   Eighty-Four Percent of Close Contacts Expressed Satisfaction in Prevention and Control Efforts

Our research discovered that 84% of close contacts felt satisfied or very satisfied with the state's prevention and control efforts against Influenza A (H1N1); 14% were neutral; and 2% felt dissatisfied or very dissatisfied.

7.2.2.2 Ninety-Three Percent of Close Contacts Felt
that the Prevention and Control Efforts Were Necessary

As seen in Tables 7.12, 7.13, and 7.14, 93% of close contacts polled felt that the prevention and control measures directed towards them were necessary, but 23% of them also felt that these efforts caused to some extent inconvenience to their daily lives. Among those that felt inconvenienced, 92% of them felt they could tolerate it.

7.2.2.3 Seventy-One Percent of Close Contacts Felt that the Prevention
and Control Measures Were Appropriate

Regarding the prevention and control measures adopted by the government at the start of the epidemic, 11% of close contacts felt that they were a little strict; 71% felt them to be appropriate; only 3% found them to be too relaxed; and 15% stated it

Table 7.12 Close contacts' assessment on the necessity of prevention and control measures

Province	N	The necessity of prevention and control measures directed towards close contacts	
		Yes	No
Beijing	248	224(90%)	24(10%)
Fujian	199	188(94%)	11(6%)
Henan	199	191(96%)	8(4%)
Total	646	603(93%)	43(7%)

Table 7.13 Close contacts' assessment on convenience of prevention and control measures

Province	N	Did the national prevention and control measures directed towards close contacts cause any inconvenience?		
		Yes	No	Hard to say
Beijing	248	70(28%)	147(59%)	31(13%)
Fujian	199	38(19%)	156(78%)	5(3%)
Henan	198	40(20%)	158(80%)	0(0%)
Total	645	148(23%)	461(71%)	36(6%)

Table 7.14 Evaluation of the tolerance for inconvenience of close contacts

Province	N	Is the inconvenience tolerable?	
		Yes	No
Beijing	69	60(87%)	9(13%)
Fujian	28	27(27%)	1(4%)
Henan	35	34(97%)	1(3%)
Total	132	121(92%)	11(8%)

Table 7.15 Close contacts' evaluation on the adequacy of early prevention and control measures

Province	N	The adequacy of prevention and control measures adopted at the start of the epidemic			
		Relatively strict	Relatively relaxed	Appropriate	Hard to say
Beijing	248	40(16%)	9(4%)	166(67%)	33(13%)
Fujian	199	8(4%)	10(5%)	130(65%)	51(26%)
Henan	197	21(11%)	3(2%)	161(82%)	12(6%)
Total	644	69(11%)	22(3%)	457(71%)	96(15%)

Table 7.16 Close contacts' evaluation on the fairness of prevention and control measures

Province	N	Fairness in prevention and control measures					
		Very unfair	Unfair	Neutral	Fair	Very fair	Hard to say
Beijing	247	3(1%)	4(2%)	38(15%)	92(37%)	85(34%)	25(10%)
Fujian	199	0(0%)	6(3%)	49(25%)	88(44%)	13(7%)	43(22%)
Henan	198	1(1%)	5(3%)	101(51%)	79(40%)	4(2%)	8(4%)
Total	644	4(1%)	15(2%)	188(29%)	259(40%)	102(16%)	76(12%)

was hard to say. Also, 56% of close contacts felt that the prevention and control measures adopted were fair or very fair, and only 3% felt that they were unfair (Tables 7.15 and 7.16).

7.2.2.4   Eighty-Two Percent of Close Contacts Felt that the State Investment into Influenza A (H1N1) Prevention and Control Was Worth It

Among the close contacts, 82% felt that the state investment into Influenza A (H1N1) prevention and control was worth it, while only 3% felt it was not (Table 7.17).

Table 7.17 Close contacts' approval assessment on the state investment in prevention and control measures

Province	N	The worthiness of the cost of state prevention and control efforts			
		Worth it	Not worth it	Neutral	Hard to say
Beijing	248	180(73%)	15(6%)	23(9%)	30(12%)
Fujian	199	170(85%)	4(2%)	6(3%)	19(10%)
Henan	199	177(89%)	3(2%)	9(5%)	10(5%)
Total	646	527(82%)	22(3%)	38(6%)	59(9%)

7.2.2.5 Ninety-Five Percent of Close Contacts Felt that the State Had Made Progress in Their Public Health Emergency Response Capabilities

In comparison with the response to SARS, 95% of close contacts felt that the state had made progress in its public health emergency response capabilities (as seen in Table 7.18).

After experiencing the prevention and control measures against the Influenza A (H1N1) epidemic, 84% of close contacts felt they could trust the state's health emergency response capabilities; 15% stated it was hard to say; and 6% expressed distrust as seen in Table 7.19.

7.3 Assessments from Medical Personnel and Agencies

Medical agencies and disease prevention and control mechanisms were the core organizations in the response efforts against Influenza A (H1N1), as they were responsible for policy advice and implementation during the epidemic. Thus, medical personnel working for these agencies were directly involved in the process and should be able to make judgments concerning these policies. Their assessments on the timeliness, necessity, rationality, feasibility, sustainability, and comprehensiveness of these policies will better reflect the implementation and effects of these policies and measures. In order to gain an understanding of assessments from

Table 7.18 Close contacts' approval assessment of progress made in response measures since SARS

Province	N	Progress in response capabilities since SARS				
		A lot of progress	Some progress	No progress	Some regression	A lot of regression
Beijing	246	105(43%)	131(53%)	7(3%)	0(0%)	3(1%)
Fujian	197	25(13%)	162(82%)	6(3%)	0(0%)	4(2%)
Henan	199	42(21%)	141(71%)	16(8%)	0(0%)	0(0%)
Total	642	172(27%)	434(67%)	29(5%)	0(0%)	7(1%)

Table 7.19 Close contacts' evaluation of health emergency response capabilities after Influenza A (H1N1)

Province	N	Trust in state's emergency response capabilities after Influenza A (H1N1)		
		Trust	Don't trust	Hard to say
Beijing	248	212(85%)	4(2%)	32(13%)
Fujian	199	141(71%)	6(3%)	52(26%)
Henan	197	191(97%)	1(1%)	5(3%)
Total	644	544(84%)	11(2%)	89(14%)

medical personnel on national prevention and control policies, we provided a questionnaire to the following entities: the heads of the comprehensive team, the medical treatment team, and the safeguarding team from the Prevention and Control Mechanism; managers and leaders from 29 designated hospitals for Influenza A (H1N1) cases and hospitals that received and treated severe cases of Influenza A (H1N1); and relevant personnel from 31 disease prevention and control agencies all within Beijing, Fujian, Guangdong, Sichuan, and Henan. The questionnaire covered the evaluation and analysis for medical agencies and disease prevention and control departments on the distribution, adjustments, implementation, and enforceability of national medical treatment policies.

7.3.1 Assessments from Medical Agency Personnel

Tables 7.20, 7.21, and 7.22 display the scores given to prevention and control policies and medical policy implementation by medical personnel in the 29 designated hospitals that treated Influenza A (H1N1). These personnel assessed the policies' timeliness, necessity, rationality, feasibility, sustainability, and comprehensiveness.

Table 7.20 Assessments by medical personnel in key hospitals on early prevention and control policies and plans for the phase with mostly imported cases (n = 243)

Score	Timeliness	Necessity	Rationality	Feasibility	Sustainability	Comprehensiveness
1	0	0	0	0	2	0
2	0	0	1	2	6	5
3	17	11	37	45	65	68
4	61	53	109	104	103	101
5	165	179	96	92	67	69
Average score	4.6	4.7	4.2	4.2	3.9	4.0

Table 7.21 Assessments by medical personnel in designated hospitals on prevention and control policies and plans for the phase with mild domestic cases (n = 189)

Score	Timeliness	Necessity	Rationality	Feasibility	Sustainability	Comprehensiveness
1	0	0	0	0	0	0
2	0	0	0	1	1	1
3	17	15	25	33	38	44
4	52	49	89	84	88	77
5	120	125	75	71	62	67
Average Score	4.5	4.6	4.3	4.2	4.1	4.1

Table 7.22 Assessments by medical personnel in designated hospitals on prevention and control policies and plans during peak periods of the epidemic with severe cases (n = 54)

Score	Timeliness	Necessity	Rationality	Feasibility	Sustainability	Comprehensiveness
1	0	0	0	0	0	0
2	2	0	0	0	0	0
3	6	4	5	8	8	9
4	13	15	22	20	21	22
5	33	35	27	26	25	23
Average Score	4.4	4.6	4.4	4.3	4.3	4.3

7.3.1.1 Roughly Ninety Percent of Medical Personnel in Designated Hospitals Approved of the Timeliness of the Medical Treatment Measures

The results of this study showed that 93% of the medical personnel polled felt that the medical treatment policies and measures during the imported case phase of the epidemic were timely or very timely, and no respondent felt that the measures were untimely or very untimely; 91% of the respondents felt that the measures were timely or very timely during the light domestic cases phase of the epidemic, again with no one finding them untimely or very untimely; and during the peak phase of the epidemic, 85% of those personnel felt that the measures were timely or very timely, with 4% feeling that the measures were untimely. There was a trend of declining approval of the timeliness of the measures shown in the responses.

7.3.1.2 Over Ninety-Two Percent of Medical Personnel in Designated Hospitals Felt the Medical Treatment Measures Were Necessary

The results of this study produced the following: 95% of medical personnel polled felt that the prevention and control along with medical treatment measures implemented during the imported case phase were necessary or very necessary, and no one felt them to be unnecessary; 92% of the respondents felt that the measures were necessary or very necessary during the light domestic case phase of the epidemic, again with no one feeling that they were unnecessary; and 93% felt the measures to be necessary or very necessary during the peak phase of the epidemic, with no one finding them unnecessary. The assessments regarding the necessity of these policies and measures remain relatively high.

7.3.1.3 Over Eighty-Four Percent of Medical Personnel in Designated Hospitals Approved of the Rationality of the Medical Treatment Measures

The results of this study showed that 84% of medical personnel polled felt that the prevention and control as well as the medical treatment measures implemented during the imported case phase of the epidemic were either rational or very rational, with 0.4% who felt the measures were not rational; 87% of respondents felt that the measures implemented during the light domestic case phase were rational or very rational, with no one finding them to be not rational; and 91% of respondents felt the measures implemented during the peak phase of the epidemic to be rational or very rational, with no one finding them not rational. There was an upwards trend of more people believing in the rationality of the measures implemented.

7.3.1.4 Over Eighty Percent of Medical Personnel in Designated Hospitals Approved of the Feasibility of the Medical Treatment Measures

The results of this study showed that 80% of medical personnel polled felt that the prevention and control as well as the medical treatment measures implemented during the imported case phase of the epidemic were feasible or very feasible, with 0.8% finding the measures infeasible; 82% of the respondents felt the measures implemented during the light domestic case phase were feasible or very feasible, with a few individuals finding them infeasible; and 85% of the respondents felt the measures implemented during the peak phase of the epidemic were feasible or very feasible, with no one finding them infeasible. There was also an upwards trend in the perceived feasibility for these measures.

7.3.1.5 Over Seventy Percent of Medical Personnel in Designated Hospitals Felt that the Medical Treatment Measures Were Sustainable

The results of this study showed that 70% of the medical personnel polled felt that the prevention and control as well as the medical treatment measures implemented during the imported case phase of the epidemic were sustainable or very sustainable, with 3% finding the measures to be unsustainable; 79% of the respondents felt the measures implemented during the light domestic case phase were sustainable or very sustainable, with a few individuals finding the measures to be unsustainable; and 85% of respondents felt the measures implemented during the peak phases of the epidemic were sustainable or very sustainable, with no one finding them unsustainable. There was an upwards trend of perceived sustainability for these measures.

7.3.1.6   Over Seventy Percent of Medical Personnel in Designated Hospitals Felt that the Medical Treatment Measures Were Comprehensive

The results of this study showed that 70% of medical personnel polled felt that the prevention and control as well as the medical treatment measures implemented during the imported case phase of the epidemic were comprehensive or very comprehensive, with 2% finding them uncomprehensive or very uncomprehensive; 76% of respondents felt the measures implemented during the light domestic case phase were comprehensive or very comprehensive, with only a few individuals finding them uncomprehensive; and 83% of respondents felt the measures implemented during the peak phase of the epidemic were comprehensive or very comprehensive, with no one finding them to be uncomprehensive. There was an upwards trend in the perceived comprehensiveness of these measures.

7.3.1.7   A Comparison of Policy Assessments for Different Epidemic Phases

Figure 7.20 outlines policy assessments for the first three phases of the epidemic, and from this comparison we can see that there is a downwards trend in perceived timeliness and necessity of the policies, and so the timing of policy adjustments may need further consideration. There is an upwards trend in believing in the rationality of the policies as well as their feasibility, sustainability and comprehensiveness. This shows that the entire process of Influenza A (H1N1) prevention and control was rational, and as we gained a deeper understanding of the virus and epidemic information, the medical policies gradually improved and became more sustainable.

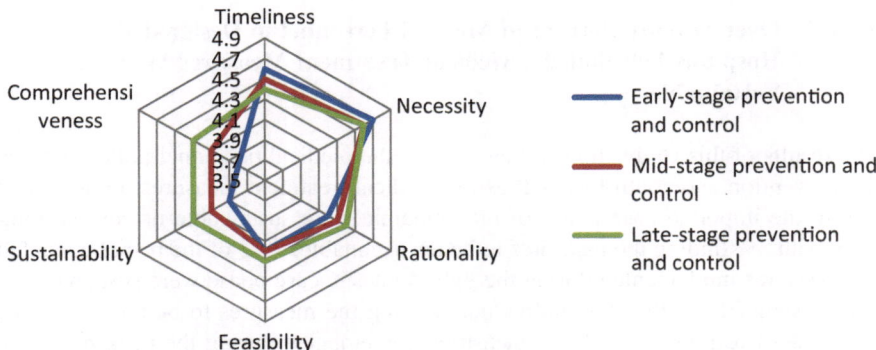

Fig. 7.20 Diagram of policy assessment for Influenza A (H1N1) prevention and control during the first three epidemic phases

7.3.2   *Assessments from Personnel in the Disease Prevention and Control Agencies*

This study conducted surveys on 519 disease control personnel from Fujian, Guangdong, Sichuan, Henan, and Beijing to find out their understanding and assessment of prevention and control policies and measures. The results are as follows:

7.3.2.1   Ninety-Five Percent of the Disease Control Personnel Felt that the Prevention and Control Efforts Against Influenza A (H1N1) Were Successful

The results show that 95% of disease control personnel felt overall that the prevention and control of Influenza A (H1N1) was successful, and 67% felt that the overall input/output ratio for these efforts was proper. In comparison with the prevention and control of SARS, 75% felt the measures were timelier; 72% felt they were more open; 69% felt they were more transparent; 59% felt they were more rational; and 57% felt they were more effective (Table 7.23).

Among the disease control personnel, 95% felt that the national strategies for the different phases were "fully consistent" or "mostly consistent" with the epidemic situation; 95% felt that the strategies were consistent with objectives; 94% felt that the measures were consistent with the strategies; and 90% felt that the measures were in line with the epidemic situation as seen in Table 7.24.

7.3.2.2   Forty-Four Percent of Disease Control Personnel Felt It Was Necessary to Take Class a Infectious Diseases Management Measures

Among the respondents, 90% felt it was necessary to make Influenza A (H1N1) a statutory epidemic under the country's legislation. Among those, 70% thought Influenza A (H1N1) should be dealt with as a Class B infectious disease, and only 44% felt it was necessary to respond to it with Class A infectious disease management measures; 85% felt that the timing was appropriate in dropping it from Class A to Class B infectious disease and 83% felt that in the future it should be dropped from Class A to Class C (see Table 7.25).

Table 7.23 Assessments from disease control personnel on overall results of prevention and control efforts

Assessment item		Province		City		County		Total	
		Number of respondents	%	Number of respondents	%	Number of respondents	%	Number of respondents	%
Overall assessment	Proper input/output ratio	102		126	64	113	68	341	67
	Prevention and control success	150		175	94	158	95	483	95
In comparison with SARS prevention and control	Timelier	117		145	71	123	78	385	75
	More open	121		135	74	115	73	371	72
	More transparent	118		129	72	111	70	358	69
	More rational	76		118	46	113	64	307	68
	More effective	85		100	52	107	54	292	64

Table 7.24 Assessment by the disease control personnel on overall strategies and measures

Assessment item		Province		City		County		Total	
		Number of respondents	%	Number of respondents	%	Number of respondents	%	Number of respondents	%
Were national strategies for different phases consistent with the epidemic situation	Fully consistent	13	8	42	23	20	12	75	15
	Mostly consistent	136	86	133	72	137	83	406	80
	A little consistent	5	3	9	5	8	5	22	4
	Completely inconsistent	4	3	2	1	0		6	1
	Total	158	100	186	100	165	100	509	100
Strategies consistent with objectives		153	94	180	96	159	95	492	95
Measures consistent with strategies		151	93	180	96	155	93	486	94
Measures consistent with epidemic situation		150	93	162	88	149	90	461	90

Table 7.25 Assessment by disease control personnel on incorporating legal management

Assessment item	Province		City		County		Total	
	Number of respondents	%	Number of respondents	%	Number of respondents	%	Number of respondents	%
Necessary to make Influenza A (H1N1) a statutory epidemic under the country's legislation	142	89	170	94	143	87	455	90
Necessary to incorporate it into class B infectious diseases	111	77	138	82	88	62	337	74
Necessary to manage it as a class A infectious disease	67	49	87	54	34	26	188	44
It's time to reclassify it to class B	106	87	131	91	86	76	323	85
Necessary to incorporate it into class C in future	131	82	144	81	139	87	414	83
Necessary to list it into entry/exit quarantined diseases	35	22	75	41	53	33	163	32
Necessary to list it into entry/exit monitored diseases	64	41	100	56	100	61	264	53
It's time to reclassify it from quarantined diseases to monitored diseases	99	80	119	88	104	78	322	82

7.3.2.3 Ninety-One Percent of Disease Control Personnel Felt Adjustments in Close Contact Policies Suited the Epidemic Situation

Table 7.26 shows that 81% of respondents thought that the management of close contacts was only necessary in the early days of the epidemic; 91% felt that adjustments in close contact measures suited the epidemic situation at that time; 84% felt the adjustment suited local conditions; and 85% felt that the timing was appropriate in adjusting close contact policies during the different epidemic phases.

7.3.2.4 Eighty-Four Percent of the Disease Control Personnel Felt It Was Necessary to Expand the Epidemic Monitoring Network

As show in Table 7.27, 84% of respondents felt that the epidemic monitoring network needed to be expanded; 76% felt that the proper amount of expansion was conducted; and 78% felt that the expansion was realistic. What cannot be ignored is that 20% of respondents did not approve of this expansion, stating in the interviews that a large-scale expansion simply wasn't necessary and that choosing a few representative areas would suffice. These respondents felt that it was a waste of resources and that it would be unsustainable after the epidemic. In regards to the number of sentinel hospitals and laboratories along with the coverage of the monitoring network, how to distribute resources to properly meet the demands of prevention and control, and at the same time reduce inputs to ensure sustainability is an issue that requires further study.

7.3.2.5 Comparison of Assessment on Several Major Prevention and Control Measures

As Fig. 7.21 shows, concrete measures received fairly high approval rates of four and above. Building on this, in comparison we see that close contact management measures and adjustments received the lowest ratings, followed by case diagnostic processing and expansion measures for the epidemic monitoring network. Law-based management scored the highest among the assessments. Necessity and importance of these measures also received high ratings, however sustainability, comprehensiveness, and fairness scored relatively low which need to be strengthened in future policy formulation.

7.3.2.6 Comparison of Assessment on Prevention and Control in Different Epidemic Phases

In scoring the different epidemic phases, necessity, importance, and timeliness all received   high   ratings,   but   the   rationality,   feasibility,   sustainability,

Table 7.26 Assessment on close contact management and policy implementation

Assessment item		Province		City		County		Total	
		Number of respondents	%	Number of respondents	%	Number of respondents	%	Number of respondents	%
Close contact isolation	Necessary in early days	128	88	137	79	117	76	382	81
	Necessary in later days	5	3	0		1	1	6	1
	Always necessary	13	9	36	21	36	23	85	18
	Total	146	100	173	100	154	100	473	100
Close contact policy adjustments suited current epidemic situations		140	89	164	92	149	92	453	91
Close contact policy adjustments suited local conditions		134	85	148	83	135	83	417	84
Close contact measures adjustments in different phases were timed appropriately		126	80	150	84	150	84	426	85

Table 7.27 Assessment on the expansion of the epidemic monitoring network

Assessment item	Province		City		County		Total	
	Number of respondents	%	Number of respondents	%	Number of respondents	%	Number of respondents	%
Necessary to expand epidemic monitoring network	134	85	159	87	128	78	421	84
Scale of expansion was appropriate	105	67	151	83	126	77	382	76
Expansion policies were realistic	111	71	154	85	127	77	392	78

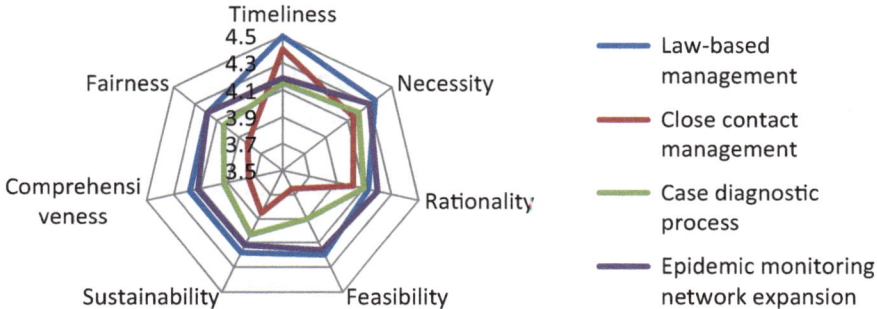

Fig. 7.21 Comparison diagram of Influenza A (H1N1) prevention and control policies

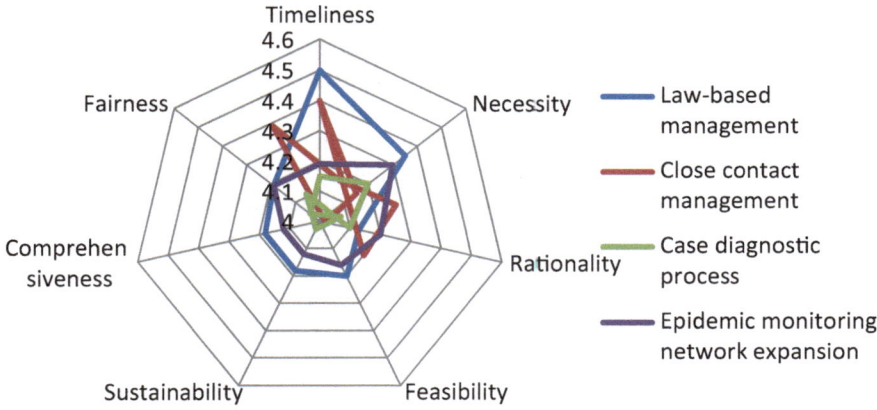

Fig. 7.22 Comparison diagram of assessment on prevention and control polices in the different epidemic phases

comprehensiveness, and fairness of the policies and measures scored relatively low. Among those, besides the high score of "timeliness" in the imported case phase, all other items scored relatively low in this phase (as seen in Fig. 7.22).

7.4   Assessments from the International Community

One key characteristic of the prevention and control efforts against the Influenza A (H1N1) pandemic was widespread and strategic international cooperation. Understanding international assessments on the national prevention and control efforts will provide us with a more comprehensive and objective view into our own successes and setbacks. Therefore, we conducted in depth interviews with WHO officials stationed in Beijing and we conducted a literature review on the international media surrounding the pandemic.

7.4.1   WHO's Assessment on Our National Influenza A (H1N1) Prevention and Control Efforts

7.4.1.1   China's Overall Prevention and Control Strategies Were Consistent with Their Domestic Realities

Looking at the overall picture of their prevention and control strategies, from the very beginning China adopted a containment strategy and also adopted other control measures like close contact isolation, and held these measures in place over a long period of time. The transition to the mitigation phase did take a little longer than in other countries as this decision took into consideration China's domestic realities. China's medical treatment capabilities are weaker than developed countries like the U.S., and thus the country needs to strengthen its first line of defense. However, this type of containment strategy expends a large amount of resources and manpower, and as soon as the epidemic spreads, containment is no longer efficient. In regards to vaccinations, China was the first developing country to successfully research and implement inoculations. The WHO offered guidance to many countries as well as information to help with decision-making, and China's prevention and control measures in many areas were quite stringent.

7.4.1.2   China's Influenza A (H1N1) Monitoring Capabilities Garnered Worldwide Recognition

In comparison with other developing countries, China possesses strong monitoring capabilities. China's disease surveillance is part of the WHO system, and both the

WHO and the China CDC have enjoyed a long period of close collaboration. Both kept close contact through phone conferences during this pandemic. The collaboration between the China CDC and the WHO is already in its second Five-Year Plan (2005–2010); the WHO helped China build their disease monitoring system, including the construction of monitoring sites in 23 provinces and sites in some cities. In November 2010, Chinese National Influenza Center (CNIC) of National Institute for Viral Disease Control and Prevention under the Chinese Center for Disease Control and Prevention, through the WHO Evaluation, became the fifth WHO Collaborating Centre for Reference and Research on Influenza and also the first developing country to enter the "core circle" for the international disease monitoring network. Because of this, China's disease monitoring capabilities have garnered worldwide recognition.

7.4.1.3   It Would Be Difficult to Respond to a Severe Epidemic with China's Current Medical Treatment Capabilities

During the Influenza A (H1N1) epidemic, China's medical treatment capabilities did improve on a national scale; however, overall, the requirements for these capabilities were relatively low since this epidemic was mild with few severe cases. If a severe epidemic did occur, there would be risks with China's current treatment capabilities. Additionally, in comparison with other countries, China has a smaller stockpile of the drug Tamiflu.

7.4.1.4   There Was Significant Progress in the Chinese Government's Risk Communication Capabilities

Each country has its own contextual history, and for China, there has been a significant improvement in its crisis communication capacity since the SARS outbreak. At the very start of the Influenza A (H1N1) epidemic, the Ministry of Health and the China CDC were in close communication with the WHO, as China and the WHO had already begun risk communication collaboration as outlined in the Five-Year Plan. Risk communication must start at the beginning of an outbreak, and public understanding of decision-making is only achieved on the basis of strong communication with the public. The U.S., which was still able to provide leadership and guidance for the public and medical agencies at the onset of the epidemic even though there were still many uncertainties as to the nature and danger of the virus. China's government, on the other hand, did not effectively assume this role at the beginning of the epidemic.

7.4.2 The International Media's Assessment on China's Influenza A (H1N1) Prevention and Control

Generally speaking, mainstream media worldwide and some experts evaluated China's Influenza A (H1N1) prevention and control positively, but they have expressed reservations about the effects of the measures.

7.4.2.1 Mainstream Media "Mostly Positive"

The mainstream media did not provide a lot of judgments on the actions of the Chinese government for this epidemic, nor were there any clear criticisms. The majority of news reports were objective and rational, and simply covered the facts; there were few that provided any evaluations. In other words, most of the reports focused on a few key countries, including China, and provided introductions to the outbreaks, developments, and prevention and control efforts; there were very few that provided any assessments of these developments. In a sense, this phenomenon could mean that China's emergency management was suited to the task this time around which left little for the media to criticize. Taking into account mainstream media leans more towards "criticism and not praise" and the influx of criticism from foreign media for the SARS outbreak, we could interpret this phenomenon as a more positive international response to China's Influenza A (H1N1) prevention and control efforts.

7.4.2.2 Most Expressed Understanding and Approval of the Prevention and Control Measures

Both public and expert opinion overall showed that, although there were criticisms, most understood and approved of the strict prevention and control measures China adopted in response to the Influenza A (H1N1) epidemic.

During the onset of the outbreak, the Chinese government's decision to segregate and isolate all of the passengers on the plane was criticized. Of course, the most intense criticism came from the Mexican government, especially the Minister of Foreign Affairs, Patricia Espinosa. She stated that the treatment of Mexican citizens in China was "discriminatory" and that some of the quarantined people were in "unacceptable conditions."[1] U.S. Congress also criticized the isolation procedures by issuing tactful travel warnings. The isolation and medical detention adopted by China was called an "offensive" prevention and control measure in *The New York Times,* and China was also criticized for being inflexible, as the author

---

[1]Austin Ramzy, China and Swine Flu: Are Mexicans Being Singled Out? http://www.time.com/time/world/article/0,8599,1895659,00.html#ixzz13bdWvTmF, May 4, 2009.

felt these type of measures "are easy to implement in authoritarian countries."[2] Other foreign professionals who experienced isolation measures also expressed their dissatisfaction. Psychiatry professor Jonathan M. Metzl from the University of Michigan felt that the isolation he experienced was "against public health regulations and xenophobic in nature;" he also felt that the isolation measures adopted were "completely inappropriate."[3] Other public opinions felt that the measures were "redundant." *The Wall Street Journal* also had criticisms on the state's actions: "The government's attempts to quarantine all arriving passengers suspected of carrying H1N1—and those seated around them on aircraft—has been overzealous."[4] On the other hand, CNN stated in a report on September 16th that "China has had perhaps the most extreme and active response to the virus than any other country in the world."[5]

However, a considerable amount of public opinion also reflected an understanding of these measures. On November 11th, 2009, *The New York Times* quoted a U.S. school teacher who had been isolated in this passage: "At the time, it seemed extreme, and it seemed restrictive, because I had never experienced an infectious disease outbreak. Now, looking back and seeing some of the measures that are being taken now in the U.S., the Chinese measures don't seem so extreme."[6] MSNBC also pointed out that, "China was hit hard before by SARS, it's understandable as to why they are so worried about another outbreak of an infectious disease." BBC News also stated that "This time the government has acted quickly and decisively."[7]

In November 2009, the head of the WHO Office in Beijing officially approved of China's response measures to Influenza A (H1N1) stating, "I think there were a variety of measures put in place by different countries, and it's difficult to say what worked best and what didn't, but China's has worked very well."[8]

---

[2]Edward Wong, *China's Tough Flu Measures Appear to Be Effective*, http://www.time.com/time/world/article/0,8599,1895659,00.html, November 11, 2009.

[3]Jonathan M. Metzl, *China's Ill-Considered Response to the H1N1 Virus,* http://articles.latimes.com/2009/jul/12/opinion/oe-metzl12, July 12, 2009.

[4]*Jeremy Chan, China Tries to Head Off Rural Flu Outbreak,* http://online.wsj.com/article/SB124656091632187681.html?KEYWORDS=China+H1N1, July 2009.

[5]Emily Chang, Inside China's H1N1 Vaccine Laboratories, http://articles.cnn.com/2009-09-16/world/china.swine.flu.vaccine_1_sars-vaccine-sinovac-biotech-h1n1?_s=PM:WORLD,September 16th, 2009.

[6]Edward Wong, *China's Tough Flu Measures Appear to Be Effective*, http://www.time.com/time/world/article/0,8599,1895659,00.html, November 11, 2009.

[7]Swine flu found on China mainland, http://news.bbc.co.uk/2/hi/asia-pacific/8043189.stm.

[8]Edward Wong, *China's Tough Flu Measures Appear to Be Effective*, http://www.time.com/time/world/article/0,8599,1895659,00.html, November 11, 2009.

Some media reported on foreign visitors who received top notch treatment from the Chinese government during isolation. On May 28th, 2009, *The New York Times* quoted a tourist who explained that the Chinese officials worked very hard to make the isolated tourists feel at home, that the Minister of Culture actually sent fruit and flowers and a band to play for the foreign students during isolation. Although the students naturally were bored and frustrated, they still felt that "the Chinese were very friendly."[9] *The Washington Post* also cited a tourist who stated, "I was definitely happy I was treated nicely."[10]

What received the most approval was the "unusual openness" of China's information disclosure both to the public and other countries. According to *The New York Times*, some researchers felt that the biggest difference between the SARS outbreak and the Influenza A (H1N1) pandemic was the amount of information disclosed by the government.

"Aggressive," "strict," "tough," and "all-court press" were the adjectives used by the international media to describe the actions by the Chinese government. The U. K.'s *The Times* described China's Influenza A (H1N1) prevention and control methods as "the world's most stringent."[11]

7.4.2.3   There Was Significant Progress in Prevention and Control Since SARS

All the praise garnered for China's Influenza A (H1N1) prevention and control efforts to a certain extent came from the comparison of their efforts in 2003 against SARS. When the international media assesses the Influenza A (H1N1) response, they always cite the measures adopted during SARS. A large portion of reports that talk about China's Influenza A (H1N1) epidemic draw comparisons to the 2003 SARS outbreak. One representative piece from the *Wall Street Journal* (July 2009) cited, "With fresh memories of its failed coverup of the SARS outbreak in 2002, China this time has been notably more open and aggressive in its response to H1N1."[12]

---

[9]Doug Donovan, Worried About Flu, China Confines U.S. Students, May 28, 2009.

[10]Ariana Eunjung Cha, Caught in China's Aggressive Swine Flu Net, *The Washington Post*, May 29, 2009.

[11]Jane Macartney, China Adopts Stringent Measures to Contain Spread of Swine Flu, http://www.timesonline.co.uk/tol/news/uk/health/article6719469.ece, July 20, 2009.

[12]Jeremy Chan, China Tries to Head Off Rural Flu Outbreak, http://online.wsj.com/article/SB124656091632187681.html?KEYWORDS=China+H1N1, July 2009.

7.4.2.4 Questions Arose Around the Isolation Measures and Vaccination Effectiveness

The international opinion around China's isolation measures were doubtful of its effectiveness and high cost. For example, the *Los Angeles Times* made their opinion clear: "So is China's aggressive approach, which has quarantined thousands of Americans and others, the proper way to protect its population from the new flu? No."[13] There was positive feedback regarding China's Influenza A (H1N1) vaccination, but there were also suspicions regarding its effectiveness. For example, Australia's *The Age* expressed the concern that although the vaccination is at the international forefront of development, it still poses a safety issue.[14]

7.4.2.5 Recommendations from International Public Opinion

The CSIS Commission on Smart Global Health Policy stated that when responding to an infectious disease outbreak, the public's trust in their government comes from "having no secrets." In view of the fact that the lack of trust in the government during the SARS period led to the rapid spread of the disease, this time around the Chinese government and media must learn from the past and promote public cooperation and trust through whatever effective measures are available.[15]

The Los Angeles Times also purported that, "Many countries—the U.S. included —have tended to see viral illness as coming from 'outside,' only to learn that pandemics show little respect for national borders in a globalized world. Chinese health authorities need to wake up to this lesson and develop China's ongoing H1N1 response in concert with, rather than in rejection of, international norms."[16]

7.5 Overall Evaluations from Different Parties

In combination with the survey results of satisfaction with state prevention and control efforts from patients, close contacts, and medical institutions, along with the survey findings on the impact of Influenza A (H1N1) on the credibility of the government and international assessments, the following conclusions can be made.

---

[13]Jonathan M. Metzl, China's Ill—Considered Response to the H1N1 Virus, http://articles.latimes.com/2009/jul/12/opinion/oe-metzl12, July 12, 2009.

[14]China Approves One—dose Homegrown Swine Flu Vaccine, http://news.theage.com.au/breaking-news-world/china-approves-onedose-homegrown-swine-flu-vaccine-20090903-f9qj.html.

[15]China's H1N1 Response and Public Opinion: Promise and Potential Challenges, http://www.smartglobalhealth.org/blog/entry/china.

[16]Jonathan M. Metzl, China's Ill—Considered Response to the H1N1 Virus, http://articles.latimes.com/2009/jul/12/opinion/oe-metzl12, July 12, 2009.

7.5.1   There Was High Praise for the State's Influenza A (H1N1) Response Measures

The results from this study showed that almost 92% of the public polled were satisfied with the central government's prevention and control efforts, among which 44.9% were very satisfied and only 0.25% expressed clear dissatisfaction; 85% of respondents also were satisfied with their local governments. Additionally, 95% of disease control professionals felt that the measures were an overall success, and 84% of close contacts along with 65% of patients expressed satisfaction towards the treatment they were given (The overall satisfaction of patients and close contacts was lower than the public's, which is understandable as they were the targets of these measures. They were constrained in the isolation and treatment process, their level of satisfaction naturally decreased).

7.5.2   There Was a General Consensus that There Was Significant Improvement in the State's Health Emergency Management Capabilities

The Chinese government's work in information disclosure and openness during the prevention and control of Influenza A (H1N1) garnered widespread approval as the information supplied by the government became the public's most trusted news source. The public also approved of the government's emergency response capabilities, especially in regards to their local governments, as there was a clear improvement in capabilities since SARS. After they experienced Influenza A (H1N1), 96.1% of the public polled expressed trust in the central government's emergency response capabilities, and 94% of the public expressed trust in their local governments' emergency response capabilities. Compared with the time of SARS, 63.8% of the public trusted the central government's emergency response capabilities more and 58.1% expressed more trust in their local governments' emergency response capabilities, which shows significant improvement. In addition, 95% of close contacts and 82% of patients felt that the government made improvements in their public health emergency management. The distinct transition of 30.7% of the respondents from distrust to trust of the local government's capabilities is a clear indication of the significant progress the state has made in emergency management and public communication.

7.5.3   There Was an Overall Recognition of the Necessity of the State's Prevention and Control Measures

Out of the population that was directly affected by the prevention and control measures, 93% of patients, 93% of close contacts, and 92% of medical personnel in designated hospitals all agreed to the necessity of these measures. Over 90% of the general public polled also saw the necessity of certain prevention and control measures. Over 84% of the medical personnel in designated hospitals approved of the rationality of the treatment measures adopted, and 91% of disease control personnel felt that the close contact measures adopted were consistent with the current epidemic situation. The WHO also felt that the overall strategy matched China's epidemic realities, and the disease monitoring system garnered worldwide recognition for its success.

7.5.4   Generally Speaking All Parties Approved of the Timeliness and Appropriateness of the Prevention and Control Measures, but Some Controversy Still Exists

Roughly 90% of medical personnel in designated hospitals felt that the prevention and control strategies and measures were adjusted in a timely manner; however, this proportion was lower in the general public, with only 70% feeling that the adjustments were timely. The WHO office in Beijing felt that the transition from "containment" to "mitigation" was a little slower than other countries, and that the cost for containment was rather high.

In regards to the measures adopted, only 50% of the public felt them to be appropriate, with roughly 20% stating the measures were relatively strict. Additionally, 17% of patients and 11% of close contacts felt that the measures adopted at the onset of the epidemic were relatively strict. Some industries and professionals felt the measures to be excessive, and the level of satisfaction was relatively low. For example, the overall satisfaction expressed from military members in regards to prevention and control efforts by the central and local government was relatively low. There was higher proportion of neutrality or dissatisfaction among people working in the hotel and restaurant sectors as well as education sector in regards to the central and local governments efforts against Influenza A (H1N1). This could be because the measures adopted placed more pressure on the military and education sectors, and also had a negative impact on the hotel/restaurant businesses.

Roughly 30% of the public polled felt that the government invested a lot into its prevention and control efforts. However, the proportion of patients and close contacts that felt the investment by the government was worth it is relatively higher than that of the public, with 84% of patients and 82% of close contacts seeing the worth of state investment. It's clear from these numbers that state investment in the prevention and control efforts was widely approved of and supported by the affected population.

7.5.5 There Were Some Differences in Assessments Regarding Other Specific Prevention and Control Measures

Taking management of Class A infectious diseases as an example, less than half of the disease control personnel felt that Influenza A (H1N1) needed to be classified for Class A management, most just felt that in the future this virus should be downgraded to a Class C infectious disease. At the same time, there were similar issues in diagnosis procedures. Almost 40% of respondents felt it was not necessary to ask the higher authorities to confirm the diagnosis; most respondents in fact felt this procedure wasted a large amount of manpower and resources, and that it was completely unnecessary. Thus, the formulation of certain prevention and control measures will need improving in the future.

Chapter 8
Evaluation Findings and Policy Suggestions

The foregoing Chaps. 3–7 have dealt with the five aspects of China's Influenza A (H1N1) prevention and control efforts respectively, namely, strategies, systems and mechanisms, emergency response measures, costs and benefits, and social comments. This chapter will summarize the evaluation team's findings in three respects of Influenza A (H1N1) prevention and control—main effects, basic experience, and inadequacies, and go on to raise issues worth further discussion and provide relevant policy suggestions.

8.1 Main Effects of Influenza A (H1N1) Prevention and Control

Compared with developed countries, China, as a big developing country with a population of more than 1.3 billion, confronted a wide variety of national conditions during the epidemic prevention and control, including, among others, a high population density, a high rate of population mobility, a considerable imbalance of economic development between urban and rural areas and between the east and west parts of the country, relative weak health care and public health infrastructure, and inadequacy of emergency materials and resources—especially in rural and remote areas, where capabilities of infectious disease prevention and control are lower. And what's more, Influenza A (H1N1) broke out against a series of complex international and domestic backgrounds such as the global financial crisis and the reconstruction in the aftermath of the 2008 Sichuan earthquake. The epidemic, once it spread widely in a short time, would cause serious consequences to the people's physical health and life safety as well as the country's economic and social order.

Despite the complex international and domestic situations and the huge pressure from the highly uncertain new influenza, the evaluation team thinks, the Chinese government actively took measures and obtained important results. So far as public

© Social Sciences Academic Press and Springer Nature Singapore Pte Ltd. 2019
L. Xue and G. Zeng, *A Comprehensive Evaluation on Emergency Response in China*, Research Series on the Chinese Dream and China's Development Path, https://doi.org/10.1007/978-981-13-0644-0_8

health effects are concerned, the prevention and control work delayed the spread of the epidemic in the country, reduced its harm to public health and improved the country's capabilities of health emergency management; as for economic and social effects, the prevention and control work mitigated the impact of the epidemic on the country's social and economic development, ensured the normal order of production and life and maintained social stability. These outcomes were not only satisfactory on the whole, but they also improved public trust in the government and the country's international image as well.

8.1.1 The Spread of the Epidemic Remained at a Relatively Low Level and Public Health Protected Maximally

Following the Influenza A (H1N1) outbreak, China quickly established the joint prevention and control mechanism, and in the early stages of the epidemic, adopted the strict "virus containment" strategy, the measures aimed to detect, isolate, diagnose, report and treat cases at the earliest possible time, and a combination of measures that gave equal importance to disease prevention and treatment. These efforts proved to be quite effective. As shown by the epidemiological curve of reported cases in China, cases didn't rise rapidly until well over 3 months after the emergency of the first case, the pandemic peak remained at a relatively low level, and the pandemic curve of this stage was relatively flat. That fully demonstrates that the country's early containment strategy reached the goal of "delaying the spread of the epidemic and winning more time". The evaluation team thinks of this as an effective practice in human history in which the means of human intervention was first ever adopted to alter the natural peak of an influenza pandemic.

Based on epidemic situations, the country actively adopted effective prevention and control strategies and adjusted prevention and control measures as appropriate, which greatly delayed the epidemic spread in the country and lowered the pandemic intensity, buying precious time for the country to get prepared for the development, production and storage of antivirals and vaccines needed to cope with possibly worse epidemic situations. The national effort on Influenza A (H1N1) treatment was quite fruitful, with a high cure rate and a lower case fatality rate than in many other countries. China became the world's first country to produce vaccines and vaccinate priority groups so that susceptible groups could all be well protected in time, a move that was highly thought of by the WHO and other countries and regions.

8.1.2   Input into Epidemic Prevention and Control Was Cost-Effective and Safeguarded Economic and Social Stability

The impact of Influenza A (H1N1) on economic and social development was determined a wide variety of factors such as epidemic severity, case fatality rates, and effects of comprehensive prevention and control. A rapid increase of cases and deaths in case of widespread outbreaks in a short time would not only threaten the health and life safety of the public, leading to a mass panic and social turmoil, but affect the economic operation of tourism and other industries and subsequently the normal order of the entire economy and society and produce obvious adverse effects on the realization of the country's economic and social development goals.[1] The adoption by the country of effective prevention and control measures minimized the ill effects of Influenza A (H1N1) on the economy and society.

Firstly, China saw relative fast economic growth in the aftermath of the global financial crisis. GDP growth remained at 7.1% in April–June 2009, and reached 9.1% for the year. According to the evaluation team's cost-benefit analysis, Influenza A (H1N1) prevention and control measures were estimated at 1 RMB cost in exchange for minimally 7.99 RMB benefit and maximally 11.55 RMB benefit, a remarkable outcome of input in epidemic prevention and control.

Secondly, the normal social order was maintained maximally. The epidemic in 2009–2010 didn't take a heavy toll on the society, and the social order was normal and stable. Survey findings showed that nearly 70% of the people interviewed thought that Influenza A (H1N1) didn't cause inconvenience to their work and life and only 6.22% of the respondents thought they were greatly affected by the epidemic.

8.1.3   Effective Prevention and Control Measures Ensured Success in Major Events

Influenza A (H1N1) broke out when China was preparing for such major events as the 60th anniversary of the founding of the People's Republic of China (October 1, 2009), the 11th National Games of China (October 16–28, 2009), and the Expo 2010 in Shanghai (May 1–October 31, 2010). The joint prevention and control mechanism and all sides involved in these important events took strict measures for

---

[1]According to the World Bank (WB), Influenza A (H1N1) may have caused a global GDP loss ranging from 0.7 to 4.8%, depending on the severity of epidemic situations. Based on 2003 SARS data and predictions by WB, UK and U.S. experts, Chinese experts estimated that Influenza A (H1N1) was likely to have serious effects on the country's economic and social development and, if not controlled by effective measures, to cause a GDP loss at 0.5–1%.

Influenza A (H1N1) prevention and control, with emergency materials such as Tamiflu and vaccines given first to meet the needs for these events.

Governments of Beijing, Shandong, Shanghai among other places watched closely epidemic situations, made detailed Influenza A (H1N1) prevention and control plans and contingency plans, carried out vaccination against Influenza A (H1N1), stockpiled emergency materials, and properly dealt with epidemic situations related to important events. The experience in and related measures for epidemic prevention and control in the run-up to the National Day celebrations and the 11th National Games of China in particular, laid a firm foundation for epidemic prevention and control measures intended for school opening, New Year's Day and Spring Festival holidays, the Expo 2010, etc. These efforts ensured that all major events proceeded safely and smoothly.

8.1.4 People-Centered Epidemic Response Strategy Was Widely Recognized, and Government Credibility and Global Image Significantly Increased

The Chinese government's efforts made to deal with Influenza A (H1N1), especially the specific practices which were people-centered and gave top priority to the health and life safety of the public, gained widespread understanding and support and greatly improved public trust in the government. In the entire process of epidemic prevention and control, the state of public opinion was calm and stable, there was no panic, and the public was largely satisfied with the effects of epidemic prevention and control efforts. According to survey findings, 92% of the respondents said they were satisfied or very satisfied with the overall performance of the central government in Influenza A (H1N1) prevention and control, and only 0.25% were not much satisfied or were very unsatisfied; 85% of the respondents expressed satisfaction with the overall performance of local governments in Influenza A (H1N1) prevention and control; the central government always enjoyed a high level of credibility, and local governments saw a remarkable uplift in credibility.

In addition to high satisfaction from the public at home, the country's work of handling Influenza A (H1N1) in a science-based and orderly manner also greatly heightened the image of the Chinese government and was widely recognized in the world. Margaret Chan Fung Fu-chun, WHO Director-General, noted that following the outbreak of the epidemic the Chinese government had played a strong role of leadership with active and effective measures of prevention and control. Western society in the beginning accused China of over-response but later opined that "The Chinese people did a smart thing" and "China is the sole country that is able to have adopted so strict measures". Besides, China also played an active role in international collaboration and assistance regarding epidemic prevention and control, establishing an image as a responsible big country.

8.1.5   Capabilities of Public Health Emergency Management Was Greatly Strengthened

Crisis is the best classroom for learning. In dealing with all kinds of crisis, both the government and the society could learn more intensively and efficiently than at usual times. The experience learned from the combat against the 2003 SARS crisis suggests that investment in disease prevention and medical treatment during an epidemic is in the long run of great benefit. The work of Influenza A (H1N1) prevention and control, into which the central government and local governments at all levels stepped up financial investment, improved the country's capacity for Influenza A (H1N1) surveillance, field epidemic management and medical treatment, built up professional teams in various fields, and will have a far-reaching effect on the country's capacity building for infectious disease prevention and control and public health emergency management.

Firstly, the work of Influenza A (H1N1) prevention and control boosted the country's capacity building for influenza surveillance. In the wake of the epidemic outbreak, China invested nearly 400 million RMB to expand the influenza monitoring network to include 411 influenza monitoring network laboratories and 556 sentinel hospitals—a network which covered all prefectural-level cities and some priority districts and counties, and initially established "a border port inspection and quarantine system targeted at major respiratory infectious diseases". In December 2009, the WHO agreed to make the Chinese National Influenza Center (CNIC) a WHO Collaborating Centre for Reference and Research on Influenza (WHOCC), the first of its kind in a developing country. In September 2010, the Ministry of Health (MOH) announced a new influenza surveillance program according to which by 2015 over 90% of the provincial centers for disease control and prevention will build a provincial-level center for reference and research on Influenza And over 90% of the network laboratories will be able to perform virus separation dependently, which will greatly improve the country's capacity for influenza surveillance.

Secondly, the work of Influenza A (H1N1) prevention improved national capacity for medical treatment, disease detection, and vaccine research and development. The effort in negative pressure rooms research and development and in purchasing medical apparatuses will play an important role in future prevention and control of avian influenza, Influenza A (H1N1) and other infectious diseases. Moreover, world-leading achievements were made in several fields including vaccine research and development. The country's effort towards vaccine development and clinical research was quite fruitful. It was one of the first countries to develop an Influenza A vaccine, and on August 21 declared to the world that a single injection of Influenza A (H1N1) vaccine had proved to be effective; its fast influenza testing technology also reached the world-leading level. Commenting on a study by Chinese scholars, *The New England Journal of Medicine* wrote that China's effort on Influenza A (H1N1) prevention and control and research is very fruitful, and that China had built a robust surveillance and response system in a relatively short period and its ability for early detection and handling new infectious diseases had been significantly improved.

8.2 Basic Experience in Influenza Prevention and Control

During the Influenza A (H1N1) prevention and control, governments at all levels and social organizations made active explorations and efforts from which a wealth of experience has been accumulated. Among other things, the joint prevention and control mechanism in which "the government takes the lead with the participation of the whole society", the prevention and control idea of "emphasizing people and relying on science and technology", and the communication strategy of "openness, transparency, and active collaboration" played a crucial role and also will be of great reference value to coping with similar emergencies in the future.

8.2.1 Strengthening Emergency System Building, Laying a Solid Foundation for Influenza A (H1N1) Prevention and Control

Since the SARS epidemic that broke out in 2003, remarkable progress has been made in the country's emergency management effort structured around preparedness plans, systems, mechanisms and legislation. The CPC Central Committee and the State Council made clear the principle of giving equal importance to prevention and management and combining the routine measures and exceptional measures, under which principle the following was done: establishing a comprehensive contingency plans system and a preliminary emergency management system; strengthening operations in various respects—surveillance and early warning, information reporting and announcement, emergency management, and medical treatment; promulgating and implementing related laws and regulations, such as the Emergency Response Law; strengthening the building of emergency workforce, emergency materials storage; stepping up the dissemination of emergency management knowledge; and initially creating a situation where the whole society participated in disease prevention and control. After years of effort, the country had seen a considerable uplift in its capacity for emergency management as well as remarkable effects of emergency management.

Public health input had been ramped up at central and local levels, especially since the country's success in handling the 2003 SARS crisis, giving a boost to the development of disease prevention and control institutions and hospitals. The establishment of public health emergency response mechanisms, the improvement of public health emergency legislation and preparedness system building, the strengthening of health emergency monitoring and warning capabilities, and the broadening of international and regional communication and cooperation, laid a good foundation for the country's success in Influenza A (H1N1) prevention and control.

8.2.2 Taping System Strengths, Creating a Disease Prevention and Control Climate in Which the Government Took the Lead with the Participation of the Whole Society

Following the Influenza A (H1N1) outbreak, the country gave full play to its system strength of "bringing together forces to do big things" and tapped fully into national health resources. Concerted efforts from governments, health care institutions and the rest of the society created a disease prevention and control climate where the government took the lead with the participation of the whole society and epidemic prevention and control measures were carried out in an efficient, orderly and effective manner.

On the one hand, the central government played a decisively leading role in the national work of epidemic prevention and control. The CPC Central Committee and the State Council took Influenza A (H1N1) prevention and control very seriously. General Secretary Hu Jintao made important instructions specifically on epidemic prevention, while Premier Wen Jiabao presided over State Council executive meetings to study and arrange the national epidemic control work. The joint prevention and control mechanism adopted effective measures in actively dealing with the epidemic. Local governments made explorations and innovations based on local actual situations, sparing no effort to combat the disease. On the whole, the Chinese government performed outstandingly worldwide, especially among developing countries, for its strict prevention and control measures, rapid implementation of measures, and huge investment in the combat against the disease.

On the other hand, communities, NPOs, the general public, drug storage enterprises, reagent manufacturers, places used for quarantine purposes, and infrastructure enterprises all participated in epidemic prevention and control in various forms. With the country's response effort entering its second stage, the 13th meeting of the national joint prevention and control mechanism, held on June 10, 2009, proposed establishing responsibility systems and prevention and control mechanisms with the participation of urban communities, schools, enterprises and villages, disseminating knowledge about and measures for family and personal protection against Influenza A (H1N1), and improving measures intended to maintain the normal operation of infrastructure, the society and the economy. Enterprises, communities, volunteers among other groups all played a crucial role. For instance, Beijing's and Henan's practices, which stressed the disease prevention and control responsibility of every unit and individual, offered valuable experience in social involvement in epidemic prevention and control.

8.2.3   Establishing the Joint Prevention and Control Mechanism to Strengthen Inter-departmental Coordination and Collaboration

To cope with Influenza A (H1N1) which in the beginning was of tremendous uncertainty, under the leadership of the CPC Central Committee and the State Council, the country established the joint prevention and control mechanism to strengthen coordination and information communication between all departments involved, so that response efforts could be carried out in a coordinated, orderly manner. As a multi-departmental emergency coordination model that lay between a national public health emergency operations center at national level and a MOH emergency operations center at departmental level, the joint prevention and control mechanism convened 33 meetings altogether, through which the following work was done: elevating the degree of importance that related departments and governments at all levels placed on Influenza A (H1N1) prevention and control; giving full play the important roles of specialized departments and making governmental and departmental duties clear; strengthening communication and collaboration between departments; introducing a series of prevention and control policies which were issued and implemented at local levels after being jointly signed; addressing issues concerning funding, manpower and emergency materials; and increasing the efficiency of introducing and implementing all kinds of prevention and control measures.

Based on local epidemic situations and economic and social development levels, local governments established their own joint prevention and control mechanisms, emergency operations centers or leading groups, specified governmental and departmental duties and stepped up coordination and communication between participants. Such institutional innovation not only helped to ensure the authority, unity and stability of the country's epidemic prevention and control work on the whole and push for the effective implementation of prevention and control strategies and measures countrywide, but it also helped to motivate local governments to take measures as appropriate for local situations.

8.2.4   Striving to Safeguard the Life and Health of the Public and the Interests of Special Groups of People

In the process of Influenza A (H1N1) prevention and control, governments at all levels and related departments and agencies acted prudently and responsibly and adopted a wide range of prevention and control measures, starting by lowering the risks and potential harm that the epidemic might cause to public health—and using it as the basis on which decisions and measures were made. The implementation of these measures gave full consideration to the interests and needs of various special groups:

The first was the policy of giving priority to the disadvantaged in terms of medical treatment and vaccination. When antiviral drugs and vaccines were limited in amount, the measure was taken of first giving treatment and vaccination to special groups like the elderly. Moreover, policies were also made locally based on actual circumstances on the medical treatment and vaccination of special groups. For instance, Beijing got migrant workers vaccinated, while Shanxi distributed for free TCM preparations against Influenza A (H1N1) among people aged 60 and older, people with disabilities, laid-off workers, etc. These policies were welcomed by local people. The evaluation team found in surveys that 96.7% of the respondents thought that the government's different disease prevention and control measures adopted in the four stages of Influenza A (H1N1) prevention and control fully embodied an attitude of high responsibility and the spirit of humanity.

The second was ensuring that some ethnic and religious events were carried out normally. For instance, from October 30 through December 23, 2009, about 12,000 Chinese people went on a pilgrimage to Mecca. It was when Influenza A (H1N1) was raging globally. The Chinese government formulated the Influenza A (H1N1) Prevention and Control Plan for Chinese Pilgrims in 2009, conducted health publicity among the pilgrims about Influenza A (H1N1) prevention and control, and gave them priority to receive vaccination and epidemic prevention materials, giving considerate support to ethnic religious activities.

The third was stressing support measures for the quarantine policy. People placed under quarantine were provided with good living conditions and considerate services, as well as psychological counseling, and their employers were not permitted to stop paying them while kept in quarantine. This was also a full display of human values. Foreigners were also provided with good diagnosis, treatment and living conditions as well as necessary amenities.

8.2.5   Employing Science and Technology to Make Disease Prevention and Control More Rational and Effective

As an emerging strain of uncertainty, Influenza A (H1N1) was little understood. The country made full use of science and technology in epidemic prevention and control to make prevention and control measures as rational and effective as possible.

The first was strengthening epidemic surveillance and early warning by which to provide scientific basis for decision-making about prevention and control. On the early epidemic monitoring and warning, China CDC and other specialized agencies displayed good professionalism; in the later stages of monitoring, the country upgraded the epidemic monitoring and reporting networks, increased the number of influenza monitoring sentinel hospitals and expanded the influenza monitoring system in time; added the monitoring of outpatient and emergency service trends at Grade-2 and higher medical institutions countrywide; launched national quick serological surveys on infection with the Influenza A (H1N1) virus; and predicted epidemic developments and trends. Multi-side epidemic monitoring provided first-hand scientific basis for decision-making about Influenza A (H1N1) prevention and control, and all prevention and control measures were actively arranged in advance.

The second was quickly launching emergency research projects. Following the Influenza A (H1N1) outbreak, the country soon launched emergency research projects, tackling key issues in respect of etiology, epidemiology, clinical diagnosis and treatment, laboratory testing, new drug development, etc. concerning Influenza A (H1N1). Research results were applied to the prevention and control work in time and provided scientific basis for effectively controlling the epidemic and improving relate prevention and control measures.

The third was relying full on the expertise of experts in making and improving epidemic prevention and control plans. In the entire process of Influenza A (H1N1) prevention and control, governments at all levels took seriously the roles of experts so that policies could be more rational and feasible. The national joint prevention and control mechanism specifically set up the Expert Advisory Committee which was tasked with proposing suggestions on Influenza A (H1N1) emergency preparedness, trend analysis and control measures, participating in making plans for epidemic prevention and control and medical treatment, and providing technical guidance on epidemic management and medical treatment; and introduced a series of diagnosis rules, treatment criteria and technical guidance, so that medical techniques and guiding policies could be updated and adjusted dynamically. According to surveys by the evaluation team, over 84% of the medical workers interviewed in designated hospitals thought of medical treatment measures as scientific, and 91% disease control personnel deemed the adjustments to close contacts measures appropriate to epidemic situations.

8.2.6 Sticking to Openness and Transparency, Improving Risk Communication and Health Education

As information on the work of Influenza A (H1N1) prevention and control was sensitive information to which the society paid great attention, epidemic information releasing and risk communication became a strongly strategic job. Ineffective communication probably would intensify the public fear of the epidemic and lead to a social panic.[2] In dealing with the Influenza A (H1N1) epidemic, the country stuck to the principle of "timeliness and accuracy, openness and transparency, positive

---

[2]For instance, media in Japan, France and some other countries exaggerated pandemic situations in their news reports to embellish "the widespread transmission" of the pandemic influenza virus in home countries through imported cases, making people panic-stricken and the whole society nervous. After announcing a state of health emergency, Mexico failed to conduct risk communication in time and effectively, leaving its capital Mexico City almost paralyzed.

guidance, moderateness in amount" when it comes to epidemic publicity and risk communication, publishing information on epidemic situations and prevention and control efforts in time and accurately, explaining questions and doubts, and pushing prevention and control efforts efficiently and in an orderly manner. The risk communication efforts strengthened epidemic monitoring and guided public participation in epidemic prevention and control while maintaining the stability of the society as a whole.

First, ideas and methods of risk communication were first applied systematically and successfully in the country. When the pandemic influenza was raging abroad and spreading to China, related departments made meticulous arrangements and put risk communication ideas into use through scientific organization—including publishing updates on domestic and foreign epidemic situations, making work arrangements and developments known to the public and explaining topics about which the public were concerned, making the work of risk communication over Influenza A (H1N1) proceed smoothly and in an orderly manner. The risk communication work allowed the public to have quite a good understanding of the epidemic, removed some unnecessary worries and fears, and strengthened public confidence and resolve to defeat the epidemic.

Secondly, epidemic information was published in time and opinion guidance done actively. The government's work on information disclosure was widely recognized, and information the government published became the most trustworthy source of information to the public. Related departments actively carried out opinion monitoring and adjusted their publicity strategies in time through timely analysis. According to survey findings, there was widespread public approval of governments' emergency management capabilities; after having experienced the Influenza A (H1N1) epidemic, 96% of the respondents expressed trust in the central government's emergency management capabilities, and 94% showed trust in local governments' emergency management capabilities—of them, 30.6% previously had not trusted in local governments, indicating that governments had made remarkable progress in emergency management and communication with the public.

Thirdly, health education was strengthened. During the Influenza A (H1N1) prevention and control, a wide variety of publicity and communication measures were taken to increase public understanding of the disease and awareness of protection against it, including giving related lectures in hospitals, communities and schools, compiling and distributing leaflets, broadcasting publicity advertisements and televised lecturers, setting up Influenza A (H1N1) prevention and control columns, sending mobile messages about influenza knowledge, etc.

8.2.7 Stepping up International and Regional Collaboration

Influenza A (H1N1) prevention and control was a global combat, and the disease' characteristic of cross-border, cross-continent transmission required global collaboration on fighting against it. In light of this, the MOH actively participated in international exchanges and collaboration and acted upon the International Health Regulations 2005 (IHR 2005). The joint prevention and control mechanism set up the International Collaboration Group in the early days of the epidemic, which was tasked with collaborating with other countries as well as Hong Kong, Macao and Taiwan in epidemic prevention and control and collecting related information. On behalf of China, the MOH actively collaborated and communicated with the WHO, reported to the WHO and related countries about the home epidemic situation, and provided Mexico with support and assistance at the earliest possible time following the epidemic outbreak there. China also received timely technical guidance from the WHO as well as great support from the United States, Canada and Mexico. During the epidemic prevention and control, the country properly handled such affairs as suspending Mexican flights, placing under quarantine foreigners entering China, arranging for visiting delegations from abroad, and communicating over foreign-related prevention and control measures, and removed in time the misunderstanding and displeasure that relative countries and people had about the country's related prevention and control measures.

In the meantime, China participated in the World Health Assembly and in the high-level meeting on global Influenza A (H1N1) prevention and control held in Mexico; it also actively supported and attended the "ASEAN Plus Three" (the three being China, Japan, and South Korea) health ministers' special meeting on Influenza A (H1N1), provided technical training and donated test kits to laboratories of ASEAN countries, and discussed with these countries about collaboration on prevention and control measures, in an effort to push for implementation of strategies and the fast and extensive information communication. These efforts helped boost capacity building for emergency response teams and obtain international resources and support necessary for Influenza A (H1N1) prevention and control.

8.3   Inadequacies of Influenza A (H1N1) Prevention and Control

The country's Influenza A (H1N1) prevention and control efforts, though quite fruitful up to now, have revealed some problems and inadequacies that exist in the making of prevention and control policies, the running of the joint prevention and control mechanism, the availability of supporting policies, the application of laws and emergency response plans, scientific and technological input, etc.

8.3.1 The Switch Mechanism Is not Smooth and the Joint Prevention and Control Mechanism Is not Clearly Legally Defined

The prevention and control mechanism is successful on the whole and has played an important part in organizational support for effectively coping with Influenza A (H1N1) epidemic. But in practice there exist problems with it, such as inadequacy of authority, unsound switch into motion, lack of regulation for some prevention and control acts, policy measures not being rational enough, and inadequate flexibility and suitability.

Firstly, the legal status of the prevention and control mechanism is not definite. As a multi-departmental emergency coordination model that was between a national public health emergency operations center at national level and a MOH emergency operations center at departmental level, the joint prevention and control mechanism is not provided for in either the Emergency Response Law or the National General Contingency Plan for Public Emergencies, so that it doesn't enjoy a definite legal status. Because there was no official work seal specifically used for the joint prevention and control mechanism, policy documents could only be issued bearing the seal of a department (or departments) in the name of the joint prevention and control mechanism, or issued in the name of a department (departments). Because there were no corresponding normative documents that were available for its implementation at local level, there were no unified standards on the name, content, form of establishment, and system composition for local governments' prevention and control bodies.

Secondly, the joint prevention and control mechanism is apparently inadequate in terms of decision-making and command. The joint prevention and control mechanism that stresses consultation and communication had its limitations when it comes to departmental interest, division of duty, policy execution, etc. Within the prevention and control mechanism, the introduction of policies, strategies and measures would usually undergo a process of discussion by representatives of multiple departments, which to a certain degree delayed the introduction of and timely adjustment to some policies and measures and even led to phenomena that departments didn't synchronize with one another in timing and contents of plan adjustment. The evaluation team found that in the two most volatile months that lasted from April 28 to June, documents were issued frequently and in some cases were in conflict with one another, and prevention and control measures were lacking in continuity.

Thirdly, existing permanent emergency mechanisms were not fully tapped. After the 2003 SARS epidemic, all local governments established public health emergency response departments and corresponding work mechanisms as permanent bodies to deal with public health emergencies. The current Emergency Response Law, Public Health Emergency Response Regulation, National Overall Preparedness Plan for Public Emergency, National Preparedness Plan for Public Health Emergencies among others, though with provisions relating to such aspects as emergency warning and response, are still lacking in explicit provisions concerning—for instance—procedures from emergency warning to response and for how to switch between peacetime and wartime, making it rather difficult in practice to declare a state of emergency and launch corresponding command and decision-making systems. In the process of their coping with Influenza A (H1N1), most provinces didn't put into motion existing emergency command mechanisms but instead assembled prevention and control leading groups after the central government established the joint prevention and control mechanism, which didn't help carry out epidemic prevention and control efforts in an orderly manner and at the same time caused a waste of human, financial and material resources.

Fourthly, the multidisciplinary decision-making mechanism still need be further improved. No multidisciplinary expert decision-making and participation mechanism has been fully established when it comes to coping with public health emergencies. Most of the members of the expert committee under the prevention and control mechanism are experts in the health care fields, and though there were occasions that experts in other fields like economics, politics, law, public administration, press, ethics and international relations were requested to participate in decision-making, their roles could hardly be truly tapped since they were not always involved.

8.3.2 Legal and Planning Systems Need to Be Further Improved and Some Prevention and Control Actions Further Regulated

During the Influenza A (H1N1) prevention and control, though laws and emergency contingency plans were given greater importance than in the past so that response measures could be carried out according to law, there were still problems such as the inadequacy of the legal system, inadequate attention paid to laws and contingency plans, and inadequate regulation of some prevention and control actions.

Firstly, contingency plans are less forward-looking and operable. There are still many issues which urgently need to be clarified or addressed in the preparation, update and rehearsal of contingency plans: The nature, status and functions of these plans are not clear, making it difficult to demand their execution; emergency contingency plans are less operable and relevant, containing more principles and requirements but less specific operations and measures; and especially, criteria for launching these plans are vague, and there are no clear provisions concerning management authority. In dealing with the Influenza A (H1N1) epidemic, the former influenza pandemic preparedness plan and emergency response plan were both made based on related guidance documents of the WHO, and as the plans were mainly targeted at the highly pathogenic avian Influenza A (H5N1) virus, they were not very suitable for the Influenza A (H1N1) pandemic and less operable. Also, former contingency plans were departmental plans, not national ones, and the problem widely existed, from the central to local governments, that their influenza emergency response plans didn't work as they were expected.

Secondly, some prevention and control measures were not well grounded, whether legally or from the angle of response plans. Because the country has no explicit standards and systems concerning the classification of alert and response for emergencies, on many occasions policy measures were lacking in inadequate basis, legally and in terms of response plans. During the Influenza A (H1N1) prevention and control, there had been no national announcement about epidemic alert and response levels. The downgrading of Influenza A (H1N1) from Category A to Category 6 B infectious diseases management was only notified via telephone, which was procedurally not up to standard and caused difficulties in policy execution by local governments. On the other hand, since the Influenza A (H1N1) pandemic is over now, there is no longer need to manage the disease as a Category B infectious disease, and it should be listed as a Category C infectious disease like other types of influenza—which, though scientifically justifiable, has not yet been done due to restrictions by the unreasonable change clause of the infectious disease prevention and control law.

Thirdly, the use of discretion by governments was not adequately regulated, and procedures for emergency requisition and compensation were not much clear and definite. In the process of Influenza A (H1N1) prevention and control, governments predominantly used administrative powers, which were largely of a compulsory nature and hence posted a risk of abusing civil rights. As citizens have a growing law and rights awareness with constant economic and social development, the excessive use of discretion by governments would risk causing controversy. It is therefore necessary to improve laws in a way that enables a balance between administrative powers and civil rights.

8.3.3 Decision-Making Mechanisms Were Flawed, Making Some Prevention and Control Measures Lacking in Flexibility, Timeliness and Suitability

During the Influenza A (H1N1) prevention and control, though the country made clear the principle of "taking seriously, responding actively to, and coping with the epidemic in a scientific manner and according to law through joint prevention and control efforts" and the making and implementation of most policy measures was rational and effective, there exists the problem of inadequate flexibility, suitability and timeliness for some policy measures.

Firstly, some policy-making mechanisms were not scientific enough, so that policies from multiple sources made it necessary to be executed flexibly. When national policies were adjusted, departments sometimes failed to sync with one another to this end. Discrepancies existed also in the implementation by local governments of specific measures. When national policies were not consistent with local epidemic situations, nearly a half of the local disease control authorities stuck strictly to national policies, 35% made their own strategies and measures, and 23% didn't make written rules but took measures flexibly to suit local situations. Furthermore, the phenomenon that policies came from multiple sources also led to confusion to disease prevention and control efforts at the grass-roots level.

Secondly, some national prevention and control measures were not suitable for local situations for being lacking in pertinence and operability. On the making of policies and measures in various stages, the country formulated and issued a lot of policy documents providing detailed specifications of prevention and control strategies, measures, etc., and made adjustments in time. Nevertheless, it was widely claimed that the nationally unified policies, strategies and measures couldn't fit into local epidemic situations and prevention and control capabilities so that local disease control authorities were unable to adapt well to those policies and measures; national policies were often formulated and adjusted either ahead of or behind local actual situations and prevention and control needs. On medical treatment, though the country issued related guidance documents in time, according to survey findings, those guidance documents could have been further improved in terms of guidance, feasibility, sustainability and comprehensiveness. Some experts deemed that whether related WHO recommendations were appropriate in China was worth discussion.

Thirdly, the adjustment of prevention and control measures was not timely enough. Because of lacking understanding of Influenza A (H1N1) as well as a full picture of epidemic situations in the course of its introduction to and spread in the country, strategic adjustments were not timely enough. Survey findings showed that nearly 30% of the respondents thought of policy adjustments as not timely enough. The WHO Beijing Office held that China took a longer time than other countries to enter the "epidemic mitigation" stage from the "containment" stage and had higher containment costs.

8.3.4 Public Health Input Are Lacking in Pertinence, and the Foundation Is Still Weak in Terms of Epidemic Prevention and Control

After the country's success in fighting against SARS in 2003, the public health system saw rapid development. But, due to inadequate input into the system for quite a long time, the public health foundation was still rather weak. The imbalance of regional development, of economic and social development, and especially of urban-rural development, heavily hindered public health development in some remote and poor regions whose capabilities of dealing with public health emergencies—which had long been weak—were not fundamentally changed.

Firstly, there were inadequate emergency reserves and preparedness in terms of human, financial and material resources, and grass-roots disease prevention and control workers were especially in shortage. Before the Influenza A (H1N1) outbreak, there were only 0.5 million doses of Tamiflu in the national stockpile, local stockpiles of Tamiflu combined were only 37,900 doses, and the amount of N95 masks was also very limited. According to survey findings, Influenza A (H1N1) prevention and control brought a considerable pressure in human resources to grass-roots disease control institutions: 90% of the institutions suffered shortages of manpower; 45% experienced financial shortages, and 26% were faced with shortages of materials such as test kits, protective equipment and laboratory consumables after the epidemic broke out. Also, human, financial and material input into health service for the national education system, for grass-roots schools in particular, had long been inadequate; township health care centers and hospitals had weak capabilities of medical treatment.

Secondly, capabilities of medical treatment against pandemic diseases were still apparently inadequate. Currently, the country's capabilities of pre-hospital emergency aid for pandemic diseases are rather weak, and hospitals' medical treatment capabilities are inadequate. General hospitals are not strong enough in terms of detecting and diagnosing clinical cases. In some regions, especially less-developed ones, medical resources are limited, there are severe shortages of medical equipment and facilities, anti-virus drugs, and protective appliances, and intensive care unit (ICU) facilities and equipment can hardly meet medical needs to deal with pandemic diseases; grass-roots medical treatment capabilities are weak. WHO Beijing Office officials think that China's "capabilities of medical treatment can hardly deal with more severe epidemics".

Thirdly, monitoring and warning systems still need to be strengthened. There still is an imbalance among provinces in terms of influenza monitoring network development. Influenza monitoring has not yet been started in Tibet, and some influenza network laboratories are of poor monitoring qualities. An integrated monitoring system that enables full coverage, high quality, and epidemiology and laboratory monitoring has not truly been established in the country. Capabilities of comprehensive and in-depth monitoring data analysis as well as of detecting public health emergencies are not adequate. China has not yet established a global health monitoring system; considerable work is to be done to build a global health monitoring system like the U.S. CDC.

Fourthly, the country's scientific and technological input for epidemic prevention and control purposes is inadequate. Data have showed that research into life sciences and the frontiers of medicine is very costly. Though the country increased expenditure on science and technology, it was far not enough on the whole, especially when it comes to research concerning life sciences, medical frontiers, public health, disease prevention and control, emergency management, etc.

8.3.5   Support Systems Are Inadequate and Emergency Support Capacity Is Weak

During the Influenza A (H1N1) prevention and control, though the country's timely and powerful funding and material reserve measures bolstered up confidence in epidemic prevention and control and ensured that Influenza A (H1N1) prevention and control efforts were carried out in an orderly, efficient and effective manner, problems also existed, such as inadequate resource reserves and flawed policies on local government procurement payment and prevention and control compensation.

Firstly, there was a lack of policies on compensation for medical services delivered against pandemic diseases. Consequently, there was no definite policy as to the financial channel, responsibility, procedure, and time limits of compensation to the designated hospitals for expenses they paid for transportation, treatment, living, etc. when shouldering the task of curing a pandemic disease. Of the 26 designated hospitals surveyed by the evaluation team, only 55% received government subsidies, and nearly 84% paid medical expenses on behalf of the patients; the 26 hospitals paid 14,235,500 RMB in medical expenses altogether, about 550,000 RMB per hospital on average. Up to now, some provinces still have not yet addressed the issue of payments that designated hospitals made on behalf of patients, and some places have not paid vaccine manufacturers for the Influenza A (H1N1) vaccine purchased.

Secondly, there are still considerable gaps in appropriations for medical treatment of pandemic diseases. During the Influenza A (H1N1) prevention and control, the country's mechanisms for financial compensation to enterprises and local governments remained unsound, and problems in this respect which had existed during the time of SARS remained. For instance, local governments together still have arrears of 700 million RMB on payments for Influenza A (H1N1) vaccines. In October 2010, the MOH proposed to the State Council that "local governments continue to execute and complete the vaccine supply plans issued under the joint prevention and control mechanism", with the intention of urging local governments to solve arrears issues. Though the proposal was issued in the form of document to provinces, except a few provinces such as Guangdong which have solved part of their arrears, all others have so far made little progress in this respect.

Thirdly, drug stockpile mechanisms for pandemic diseases still need to be improved. National drug stockpiling at central and local levels was not fully implemented. National funding for emergency materials stockpiling still could not completely meet the needs of health emergency materials stockpiling, and in states of emergency, related ministries could not have a full picture of both the national and the local stockpiles. More work needs to be done in terms of health emergency materials reserving standards, forms and types, and there is a lack of reserve reporting and management mechanisms as well as principles governing the use of funds. Problems exist also about grass-roots stockpiles of such materials as antiviral drugs, e.g. few varieties and inadequate amounts. Moreover, the relationship between capacity buildup and material stockpiling still need to be improved, alongside drug bidding and rotation systems.

8.4   Issues to Be Discussed Further

Dealing with a global pandemic like Influenza A (H1N1), especially improving the capability of understanding, studying and making judgment and decision in highly uncertain situations, is a common challenge for all countries in the world. The evaluation team believed that further discussions are necessary on many aspects of China's efforts of Influenza A (H1N1) prevention and control, including further clarifying the emergency management system and mechanism, balancing administrative pressure with scientific countermeasure, making appropriate reactions to emergencies, and matching rigid policies with flexibility. More comprehensive and in-depth discussions about those matters will help us better understand and improve our work.

8.4.1   How to Improve the Health Emergency System and Mechanism

Since China won the battle against SARS in 2003, it has established a public health emergency commanding system characterized by "government leadership, centralized command, local management, layered responsibility, inter-departmental coordination and categorized treatment", and special groups responsible for health emergency management, handling and consulting are formed on local level. The joint Influenza A (H1N1) prevention and control mechanism established this time has played an important role. But actual work indicates that China's system and mechanism of dealing with public health emergencies has some problems that need further study and addressing, and the joint prevention and control mechanism to deal with major emergencies has to be improved.

First of all, how to properly position comprehensive emergency organizations and special departments to make their emergency management work complementary? To deal with the Influenza A (H1N1) epidemic this time, the MOH took the lead in setting up the joint prevention and control mechanism that involved 38 departments and commissions. It was a comprehensive coordination mechanism formed in accordance with the social hazards caused by the epidemic, and was positioned between the State Council's emergency command center (as in the SARS epidemic in 2003) and the MOH's special emergency command center. As the initiator of the joint prevention and control mechanism, special emergency organizations such as the MOH or local health authorities have to do more to straighten out their relation with comprehensive emergency organizations such as the emergency office under the State Council or provincial government. This relation isn't a problem on the State Council level, but it causes prominent problems on local execution level. As comprehensive and special emergency organizations report to different leaders, they inevitably have overlapping, segmentation and even conflict during execution (e.g. vice governor in charge of health care and executive vice governor in charge of emergency management of a province have to coordinate with each other). The emergency office in some local governments only serves as a duty room and cannot effectively lead and command emergency work owing to its low administrative level and understaffing. Therefore, the relation, including division of duty and cooperation, between comprehensive and special emergency organizations has to be clarified further and adjusted and improved timely during emergency response.

Second, how to quickly shift between emergency state and routine working state in government departments? The joint prevention and control mechanism against Influenza A (H1N1) is a temporary comprehensive emergency model that takes up a lot of administrative resources in relevant government departments, so it's only applicable in special periods when an epidemic breaks out on a large scale and not suitable for sustained implementation. But there isn't a clear and definite mechanism as to when to enter and exit the emergency state, such as dealing with Influenza A (H1N1), and no scientific and standard definition or explanations in this regard can be found in any law, rule or emergency plan. If the emergency state for Influenza A (H1N1) isn't called off, the emergency work at departments involved will continue, which will be a waste of precious government resources when the epidemic isn't that serious. Therefore, we have to study how to scientifically shift between the joint prevention and control mechanism and everyday work, put in place a sound mechanism that accommodates both emergency and normal states, and minimize the interference in and impact on normal work imposed by emergencies.

8.4.2 How to Make More Scientific and Effective Decisions

For emergency management, government decision makers on all levels, when faced with highly uncertain situations, must strike a balance between administrative pressure and scientific countermeasure. Government decision on prevention and control must be based on science, but "non-technical" factors such as administrative pressure from above and public opinions must be taken into account too. Many decisions made during the Influenza A (H1N1) prevention and control this time had to strike a balance like this, and reality showed that administrative pressure usually outweighed other factors in local government's decision making.

First of all, how to establish a scientific emergency management assessment and evaluation system? Due to the high level of uncertainty of emergencies, emergency efforts are usually disproportional to the final results, so higher-level government should avoid setting rigid targets for lower-level ones in emergency management because instead of inspiring and motivating them, the targets would put unnecessary pressure on lower-level governments and consequently distort their emergency actions and cause unnecessary losses. During the prevention and control of Influenza A (H1N1) this time, some local governments imposed too much pressure on lower-level governments and led to distorted implementation of some policies. For example, disease control authority included indicators on the prevention and control of infectious disease in the performance assessment for medical department, which burdened local disease control departments. Some local governments blindly pursued the goal of "zero death", which was irrational and put excessive administrative pressure on lower-level governments and medical staff, and seriously affected scientific policy making and implementation. Higher-level government also put pressure on lower-level ones in vaccine promotion, setting specific indicators and deadlines and even publishing a ranking list. The result was that some policies were issued and carried out completely based on administrative decisions instead of professional analysis, judgment and technical decision.

Second, how to combine technical and administrative factors? This Influenza A (H1N1) epidemic is a widespread global public health emergency. When the Chinese government made decisions, which may have an impact on the relation with international organizations like WHO and with other countries and regions and the domestic economic and social development, it had to keep in mind the possible political and international consequences when issuing policies. Moreover, when an epidemic first broke out, the media would report on it intensively, which formed public opinion pressure in uncertain conditions and in a way affected decision making, but governments on all levels still had to take immediate measures to keep the epidemic from escalation and diffusion. Under such circumstances, technical considerations usually gave way to administrative ones when decisions were made, which led to the phenomenon that countermeasures were often more rigorous than necessary and resources were wasted to some extent. This shows that how to balance technical and administrative factors in emergency management and fully respect science while making overall considerations is a topic worth careful and deep study.

8.4.3   How to Evaluate the Appropriateness of Emergency Response Amid High Uncertainties

How to react appropriately to highly risky and uncertain emergencies, in other words, how to keep the situation from worsening due to insufficient reaction and avoid waste of resources because of excessive reaction, is a difficult question faced by emergency managers and decision makers. The Influenza A (H1N1) epidemic is the first influenza epidemic in the world for 40 years. It wasn't as serious as originally imagined, and some people questioned the countermeasures adopted by the WHO. Meanwhile, some developed countries attached more importance to "treatment" than "control" and didn't take more rigorous measures in border entry quarantine and medical observation of suspected cases, which caused arguments about the appropriateness of China's prevention and control measures.

The evaluation team discovered through survey that people had different opinions and comments regarding whether China overreacted to the Influenza A (H1N1) epidemic and whether its prevention and control measures were appropriate. In terms of government input in Influenza A (H1N1) prevention and control, about 30% of the public thought it excessive, but a larger proportion of Influenza A (H1N1) patients (84%) and close contacts (82%) believed government input was worthwhile. In terms of the appropriateness of prevention and control measures, only 50% of the public thought them appropriate and about 20% thought them too rigorous. In terms of local governments' reaction to Influenza A (H1N1), overreaction was common due to administrative pressure and the great importance attached by leaders, and they tended to adopt more rigorous measures than the national government. For example, the central government demanded that large-scale events should be avoided unless absolutely necessary, but local governments prohibited large-scale events of all kind.

On the other hand, decision makers had to make tough choices when in face with unknown epidemics like SARS and Influenza A (H1N1). If the countermeasures were loose but the virus was highly hazardous, that would lead to immense losses of life and properties, which would be hard to accept. If the countermeasures were rigorous and costly but the virus wasn't very hazardous, that would be a more acceptable scenario. Since public health emergencies concern people's life and health, governments of all countries tend to adopt rigorous measures when it is unclear how harmful the virus or bacteria is, so as to avoid massive losses because of insufficient reaction. If the reaction was costly and turned out excessive afterwards, the high cost could be understood as the premium needed to prevent the worst scenario and was therefore worthwhile.[3] As WHO Director-General Margaret Chan Fung Fu-chun said, "we are not exaggerating the epidemic, but if we are underprepared because of my mistake, that would be unacceptable. I'd rather be over-prepared than under-prepared."

8.4.4   How to View the Influenza A (H1N1) Prevention and Control This Time

This Influenza A (H1N1) epidemic marked the first global cooperation on coping with public health emergency. It achieved important results, but also displayed various defects and deficiencies. On the whole, the Influenza A (H1N1) prevention and control this time provided valuable experience. The whole country worked in

---

[3]A case in point is the strategies adopted by the U.S. government during the 1976 swine flu outbreak.

unison, we shortened the vaccine's time to market, and China became the first country in the world that completed the clinical test of Influenza A (H1N1) vaccine and vaccinated its people on a large scale, but we couldn't neglect the fact that chance may have played a part in our success. For example, it was by accident that China participated in the global defensive battle against Influenza A (H1N1) at an early stage and its participation had preconditions. We obtained the latest epidemic information from Mexico, and got the virus strain from the United States to develop diagnostic reagent and vaccine, which gave us sufficient time to make preparation. The next influenza epidemic won't necessarily have the same conditions, and our experience today won't necessarily be useful tomorrow. Meanwhile, China's capability of vaccine production is quite limited compared with developed countries, so we cannot take our vaccine success this time as a normal phenomenon. We cannot just focus on the medical interventions against influenza epidemic and vaccine development and production, but neglect social interventions. An effective and reliable strategy is to put equal stress on them both. Furthermore, short-term measures or those temporarily adopted this time should not be taken as regular measures to deal with similar public health emergencies in the future.

We should look at both the positive and negative sides of this prevention and control campaign against Influenza A (H1N1) scientifically, and use the experience and lessons learnt to better guide the prevention and control of infectious diseases and health emergency responses in the future. We should scientifically evaluate the achievements, experience and problems of this campaign from such angles as coping strategy, operating features of the joint prevention and control mechanism, cost effectiveness of prevention and control, and overall social effects. We should establish a sound emergency response evaluation and learning mechanism and improve our learning ability during each emergency response, so as to turn risks into opportunities and turn current experience into valuable lessons that enhance our ability to deal with public health emergencies.

8.5 Policy Suggestions for the Future

Based on the findings stated above, the evaluation team proposed the following policy suggestions for the reference of relevant parties.

8.5.1 Laws on Epidemic Prevention and Control and Public Health Emergency Response Should Be Revised and Improved

The terms on rating new infectious disease in the Infectious Disease Prevention and Treatment Law should be revised, and the health departments should be given more decision-making and adjusting power so that they can timely adjust the prevention and control strategy when a new infectious disease breaks out. Meanwhile, to deal with sustained public health emergencies like Influenza A (H1N1) in a more standard way, the criteria on pre-warning and emergency response classification and the corresponding management systems should be further clarified in the Emergency Response Law, National Preparedness Plan for Public Health Emergencies and other emergency plans, and the criteria and management system should be properly differentiated and aligned. We should further clarify the authority of relevant government departments in emergency state, especially serious emergency state, and standardize the procedures on formulating and adjusting emergency response policies.

To enable local governments to deal with public health emergencies in a more timely, active and effective way, we suggest delegating the power of releasing news about epidemic or event in an appropriate scope. For example, prefecture-level and municipal government, with the approval of provincial government, will be allowed to release news on suspected epidemic or emergency state. Moreover, while intensifying the unified leadership and coordination on the central level or at higher-level government, local governments should be allowed room for independent decision-making, so that they can determine the pre-warning and response level based on actual situations. Other contents that should be revised include the improvement of prevention and control commanding and decision-making system and of the joint emergency response mechanism among various departments, betterment of pre-warning and response classification mechanism, local government's power of determining the criteria for pre-warning, and human resource, financial, material and technical guarantee for prevention and control. Regulations on communicating the risks of the epidemic, guiding public opinions and mass publicity and education will also be revised.

8.5.2 Plans for Epidemic Prevention and Control and Against Pandemic Influenza Should Be Revised and Updated

The Infectious Disease Prevention and Treatment Law and its implementing rules should be revised and improved in order to conduct flexible and standard management of Influenza A (H1N1) and other epidemics. The existing preparation and response plans for the prevention and control of pandemic Influenza And other infectious diseases should be revised comprehensively at an early date, and the emergency plan for pandemic influenza should be elevated from the Ministry of Health's level to state level, so that it can better guide the prevention and control actions taken by relevant departments. Meanwhile, government departments on all levels, government bodies, public institutions, enterprises, social units, grass-roots-level communities and other relevant organizations should all work out their own prevention and control plans against pandemic Influenza And other infectious diseases based on local situations, so as to form an all-round, connected and coordinated epidemic prevention and control system. Moreover, given the uncertainty and complexity of emerging infectious diseases for which the existing single-disease emergency response plans are not suitable, it is suggested that the country make emergency response plans dedicated to emerging infectious diseases, regulate universal measures, procedures, and rights and responsibilities of participating agencies in prevention and control of emerging infectious diseases, and establish as fast as possible mechanisms that allow flexible adjustment in strategies against unknown diseases. On that basis, more efforts should be made to disseminate relevant laws and plans and, depending on the necessity, organize drills within or among relevant departments.

8.5.3 The National Commanding System and Working Codes for Major Public Health Emergencies Should Be Improved

To improve the commanding system for major public health emergencies, there are three key aspects: state-level emergency response system, relation and alignment between state-level and local emergency response systems, and relation of joint prevention and control among the government, enterprises and the public. While drawing on the experience of the joint prevention and control mechanism against Influenza A (H1N1) this time, we can also learn from China's mature experience in other emergency management areas including flood control and drought relief and earthquake relief.

8.5.3.1 Cross-Departmental National Command Center for Public Health Emergencies Should Be Set up as a Standing Organization

A cross-departmental national command center for public health emergencies should be set up as a standing organization, and the current innovative joint prevention and control mechanism should be made its special decision-making and coordinating mechanism and be combined with the existing emergency management system. This center has its office at the Ministry of Health (MOH) which also works as its convener, providing related service guidance and specialized coordination services and accepting work guidance from the Emergency Management Office of the State Council. Meanwhile, rules concerning the initiation of the cross-departmental national command center for public health emergencies should be revised, and the level of response should be determined not only based on possible hazards, but also on the scope involved, and the response level should be adjusted as the emergency evolves.

8.5.3.2 Corresponding Public Health Emergency Commanding Organization Should Be Set up on Local Level

Based on their specific conditions and the state-level system, local governments can set up standing emergency organizations accordingly. To more effectively integrate regional resources and prevent and control the cross-regional impact of public health emergencies, the state should encourage and push local governments to form a cross-regional health emergency coordination and joint prevention and control mechanism according to actual needs. Besides, local emergency organizations should participate in the decision-making at state emergency command center, so that the prevention and control policies made by the center will be suitable for local conditions and truly workable. Flexibility in local prevention and control measures should also be maintained.

8.5.3.3 Abide by the Principle of Responsibility by Level and Jurisdiction, Further Clarify the Scope of Authority and Operational Rules Concerning Emergency Management for Governments at Central, Local or Other Levels, Delegate, as Necessary, the Power to Release Information on an Epidemic and Other Events, and Further Strengthen Timeliness, Pertinence and Flexibility of Epidemic Response

In the process of the Influenza A (H1N1) prevention and control this time, the WHO provided China with prevention and control measures in good time based on global epidemic developments, and China made clear the principle of "taking threats to public health seriously, responding actively, and coping with the epidemic in a scientific manner according to law through joint prevention and control efforts", organized experts to conduct surveys in time according to epidemic developments, and came up with measures for timely adjustment in prevention and control strategies. However, due to China's vast territory and the varied situations in different places, some local governments and departments couldn't take local or their own conditions into full consideration when understanding and implementing the policies and measures, and their responses and disposals were not flexible, timely and adaptive enough. Therefore, the general epidemic prevention and control policies adopted by the state should be more targeted and operable on local and departmental level. The survey conducted by the evaluation team showed that 70% of the public thought the prevention and control measures were adjusted timely, indicating room for improvement.

The evaluation team gave the following suggestions. On one hand, when decisions were made on the central level, local disparity in epidemic development and response capability should be taken into account to leave room for local adjustment. On the other hand, targeted efforts should be made to improve local government's capability of making scientific decisions based on local conditions and keep them from being irrational.

8.5.3.4 The Mechanism and System of Effective Coordination and Interaction Among the Government, Enterprises and the Society Should Be Standardized

Given the complicated composition of enterprises and the society, we need to focus on three aspects when trying to realize effective coordination and joint prevention and control among the government, enterprises and the society. First, the rights and obligations of enterprises and social entities in handling public health emergencies should be clarified on the legal level. Second, when formulating and exercising emergency plans, approaches should be explored for enterprises and social entities to take part in the prevention and control effectively, and relevant working mechanisms should be put in place. Third, in the working mechanism of national and local public health emergency commanding organizations, an emergency meeting mechanism involving the government, enterprises and the society should be considered, which can provide consultation and suggestions on how to coordinate their actions in the prevention and control.

8.5.4 Emergency Management Mechanism Should Be Improved and Enhanced

When dealing with public health emergencies such as SARS, bird flu and Influenza A (H1N1), the central and local governments established a string of effective emergency management mechanisms, which played an important role in the Influenza A (H1N1) prevention and control this time. In light of the work this time, we believe special attention should be paid to the following aspects in the future.

8.5.4.1 Internal Information Reporting Mechanism Should Be Improved

The Influenza A (H1N1) response this time revealed a serious problem in the health system, or the entire government system, namely epidemic information was reported by multiple departments. IT application should be strengthened in the national emergency commanding and decision-making system, and in medical health organizations on the basis of resource integration. Information sharing should be reinforced among higher-level and lower-level authorities, departments on all levels, professional organizations and monitoring outlets to make health care more IT-based. We should fully utilize the current direct reporting system for public health events, unify the standards, channels and approaches of epidemic and event information reporting, and ensure information sharing among all relevant departments.

8.5.4.2 The Mechanism of Making Scientific Decisions for Health Emergency Involving Experts on Multiple Disciplines Should Be Emphasized

China formed the expert consulting committee for national public health emergency management in 2006, and the expert committee in the joint prevention and control mechanism against Influenza A (H1N1) this time played an important role. However, members of this expert committee were mostly medical experts, and not enough experts specializing in other disciplines were brought onboard, which should be changed in future. Meanwhile, the working mechanism and approach for experts to participate in decision-making should be improved, and more attention should be paid to the opinions of middle-aged and young experts as well as local ones.

8.5.4.3 Opinions and Suggestions from All Walks of Life Should Be Collected Through Various Channels

When dealing with public health emergencies in the future, we should pay more attention to the opinions, papers and interviews of experts on different disciplines, and collect their professional opinions on specific health emergency issues through the internal information system.

8.5.4.4 International and Inter-regional Communication, Exchange and Cooperation Should Continue to Be Intensified

To deal with Influenza A (H1N1) this time, relevant departments in China stepped up the communication, exchange and cooperation with the WHO, the U.S. Centers for Disease Control and Prevention and relevant organizations in Hong Kong, Macao and Taiwan, and benefited a lot from that. Going forward, we should continue to strengthen international and inter-regional coordination, learn from the "going global" strategy for health prevention and control adopted by the U.S., and proactively weave a network of epidemic monitoring, prevention and control with other countries and regions concerned. This way we can grasp the global epidemic developments more comprehensively, make our prevention and control work more active and better deal with public health emergencies of all kinds. While doing that, we should keep our head clear and maintain independent thinking instead of blindly believing and following other countries' moves. We should prevent and control epidemics independently based on our own situations and under the guidance of the WHO and other international organizations.

8.5.4.5 The Awareness of Public Health Crisis Should Be Enhanced and Regular Health Risk Evaluation Should Be Carried Out

In the age of economic globalization today, we should stay highly alert to all kinds of old and new infectious diseases that may cause major public health threats. Regular or irregular public health risk evaluation should be promoted in the health system of all levels, and concrete steps should be taken to enhance people's health risk and crisis awareness. We must take precautions and prepare for the worst.

8.5.5 In Light of the New Round of Medical System Reform, the Mix of Public Health Input Should Be Improved and a Fiscal Fund Appropriation and Compensation Mechanism Should Be Established

China's input in public health has increased significantly since 2003. While continuing to invest more in public health, we should also improve the input mix, attach more importance to health emergency response and pay special attention to the following matters.

8.5.5.1 Fiscal Input and Compensation Mechanism for Public Health Emergency Should Be Established as Soon as Possible

The central government made resolute decisions and earmarked fiscal fund timely to fight Influenza A (H1N1) this time, and governments on all levels, enterprises, public institutions and individuals all contributed immensely to the prevention and control by investing a huge amount of manpower, materials and capital. However, government purchase fund and relevant compensation policies for epidemic prevention, control and treatment were not completely in place. The compensation for government bodies, enterprises, social groups and individuals was far from enough, and the fund used to purchase Influenza A (H1N1) vaccine was still not paid to the providers. If such situation continues, it will seriously dampen the enthusiasm of governments at all levels, enterprises and public institutions for joining the public health emergency response and leave a major hazard for that work. This problem has existed and never been completely solved since SARS.

The basic medical insurance should be expanded to cover more people, and commercial medical insurance system should be improved to provide more coverage of pandemics. A public health emergency fund and compensation mechanism should be established on provincial and municipal level as soon as possible to make sure that there will always be enough capital for emergency handling, and the investment by local governments, enterprises, public institutions and individuals in public health emergency response will be reasonably compensated for. We should establish stable and effective mechanisms for multi-channel compensation to medical institutions at grass-roots level, and establish funding and compensation tracking and supervision mechanisms. Furthermore, local government's fiscal input in fighting Influenza A (H1N1) and financial compensation for concerned hospitals and vaccine suppliers should be inspected to enhance government credibility. Only when we mobilize the whole society to participate in health emergency response can we promote the sustainability of this work and raise public trust in the government.

8.5.5.2 Ability of Health Emergency Response in the Health Industry and Key Areas of Non-health Industry Should Be Strengthened

While investing more in public health, we should first and foremost strengthen comprehensive hospitals' capability of detecting, diagnosing and treating clinical cases, and the diagnostic and treating capability of special hospitals such as children's hospital. We should pay special attention to strengthening the capability of health emergency response in key areas of non-health industry, such as education system, large construction site and important traffic hub. For example, 70% of public health emergencies in China happened in the education system, mainly schools, but the evaluation team discovered in the survey that the education system's human resources, financial and physical input in health care, especially at schoolsat the grass-roots level, has always been deficient, and it is extremely weak in handling public health emergencies. It is therefore suggested that the Ministry of Education and Ministry of Health should work out policies that request more health care input in the education system and more input in public health publicity and health education in schools of all types, so as to straighten out the public health management mechanism in the education system.

8.5.6 More Should Be Done to Improve the Communication on Public Health Risks and Health Education

8.5.6.1 Public Health Education Strategy Should Be Strongly Promoted

During the Influenza A (H1N1) prevention and control, some expert said "health education is the best vaccine against Influenza A (H1N1)". It is indeed a key step to raise the whole society's health level. Therefore, we suggest continuing to increase the input in public health education and taking effective measures to enhance people's awareness, knowledge and capability of prevention and control.

8.5.6.2 Full-Process Risk Communication During Emergency Management Should Be Carried Out

Risk communication during the Influenza A (H1N1) prevention and control this time displayed considerable progress, but revealed some problems as well. For instance, risk communication in the later stage wasn't as well conducted as in the early stage, risks related to vaccine safety were understated while vaccine safety was excessively pledged, and epidemic information from overseas was over-emphasized when the severity of the influenza was explained to the public.

We suggest that the health and other related authorities should attach due importance to full-process risk communication, especially pre-event risk communication, to help people perceive and deal with risks rationally. When communicating about highly uncertain risks, the government should not intentionally understate the risks for fear of public panic and excessively vouch that the epidemic is "preventable, controllable and curable", but should objectively tell the truth (including uncertainties) and the measures already and to be adopted by the government. The government had better avoid such words as "preventable, controllable and curable", and leave it to the experts to guide the public and all sectors of society to make their own judgment.

8.5.6.3 Emerging Media Should Be Brought into Full Play

Online media plays an increasingly important role today. During the fight against Influenza A (H1N1), the health authority opened a special web page on the epidemic, which was upgraded frequently at first but not so much later, and the information was very limited compared with special web pages on commercial websites in China. As a result, the web page didn't play its due role as the main channel of communicating and disseminating the epidemic prevention and control. Therefore, it is suggested that national health authority develop special websites or web pages for serious health emergencies at an early date either by itself or in cooperation with mainstream websites. It should enrich the page contents and update them timely throughout the emergency to facilitate people's search for authoritative information and prevention and control knowledge and fully play the role as the main channel of epidemic or event communication.